T0281537

Uncommon Psychiatric Syndromes

This book explores the historical background to, and present-day under-standing of, a number of unusual psychiatric disorders. This fully revised new edition contains a new chapter on a range of recently emerging conditions as well as updated literature and a collection of new and updated cases.

Since the publication of the fourth edition, there have been many developments in the field of psychiatry, including changes in the *Diagnostic and Statistical Manual of Mental Disorders* (*DSM-5*) and the advancement of neuroimaging and related research, which have been incorporated into the fifth edition. In this now classic text, each chapter covers an individual disorder in detail, using several case studies gathered by the authors them-selves to illustrate and exemplify the disorders discussed. The clear and easy-to-understand writing style ensures that this text is accessible for the wide range of studies and professions who will find it useful.

Uncommon Psychiatric Syndromes, Fifth Edition, is essential reading for psychiatrists, clinical psychologists, psychiatric nurses, psychiatric social workers, social workers and other mental health professionals. It will also be of interest to graduate students in the fields of psychiatry and psychology as well as those enrolled in psychiatry resident courses.

Dr David Enoch, formerly senior consultant psychiatrist at the Royal Liverpool Hospital, is an internationally acknowledged authority and pioneer of uncommon psychiatric syndromes, the title of his best-selling book. A broadcaster and author, his other titles include *Healing the Hurt Mind* (seventh edition), *Schizophrenia: Voices in the Dark*, *Psychiatric Disorders in Dental Practice* and *I Want a Christian Psychiatrist*.

Prof. Basant K. Puri currently works in academic research and practises clinically.

Dr Hadrian Ball is a consultant forensic psychiatrist having worked in Norwich, UK, and Hobart, Tasmania. He is considered an international authority on sexual offending against older victims. He has retired from clinical practice.

Uncommon Psychiatric Syndromes

Fifth Edition

David Enoch, Basant K. Puri and Hadrian Ball

Routledge
Taylor & Francis Group

LONDON AND NEW YORK

Fifth edition published 2021
by Routledge
2 Park Square, Milton Park, Abingdon, Oxon, OX14 4RN

and by Routledge
52 Vanderbilt Avenue, New York, NY 10017

Routledge is an imprint of the Taylor & Francis Group, an informa business

First edition published by John Wright & Sons 1967
Fourth edition published by CRC Press 2001

British Library Cataloguing-in-Publication Data
A catalogue record for this book is available from the British Library

Library of Congress Cataloging-in-Publication Data
A catalog record has been requested for this book

ISBN: 978-1-138-06288-7 (hbk)
ISBN: 978-1-4987-8795-6 (pbk)
ISBN: 978-1-315-38114-5 (ebk)

Typeset in Garamond
by MPS Limited, Dehradun

Contents

Preface to the Fifth Edition

Although it is over half a century since the first edition was published, the demand for this book continues unabated.

It is still widely considered a classic text for psychiatrists, psychologists, psychiatric nurses, social workers and all those practitioners in the field of mental health. It continues to be increasingly valued as a definitive source of information regarding these fascinating and important uncommon syndromes (although accepting that some of the syndromes are no longer uncommon) as demonstrated by the increasing references made to the book by authors of published works. In 2013 the translation into Turkish appeared.

The London correspondent of *The New Yorker*, in its spring 2019 issue, refers to the book as a 'minor classic, the case studies ... having a fable like poetic quality'. This reiterated John Pollit's remarks in his review of the first edition that 'it deserves to become a classic'. It was included in Hodder's list of modern medical classics.

The content of the book has been shown to be increasingly important legally and socially. The chapter on de Clérambault's syndrome which deals with stalkers has been used as an authoritative source of information in the preparation of the Harassment Bill in 2011, and the information within the Ekbom's syndrome and body dysmorphia disorder sections has been used in the preparation of guidelines of cosmetic procedures. The first case of the victim taking part in the murder of the perpetrator, in the case of Munchausen's by proxy, is described, the victim being imprisoned for a number of years while her male partner was given a life sentence.

The form of the chapters has been preserved for each syndrome for historical background, and the present-day understanding and worldwide literature are reviewed. Each account gives the main features of the condition, its causation, epidemiology, psychopathology and treatment and management.

For this fifth edition, all the chapters have been extensively rewritten, fully updated to include the latest research findings in genetics, neuroimaging, functional anatomy and other research developments. One new chapter describing four new syndromes of importance are included. All the syndromes have been under the personal overview of the authors.

During the last decade, the book has also continued to capture a wider readership, although it was never meant to be a popular publication, satisfying an appetite for sensationalism. As with previous editions, it has continued to be mentioned in radio and TV programmes and other works. In 2019, the case of Munchausen's by proxy where the victim had 'escaped' and arranged for the murder of the perpetrator was the first case of its kind, and an eight-part documentary/drama based on this case on USA TV has drawn an enthusiastic audience. The writer and director Charlie Kaufman has used Cotard's syndrome and Capgras' syndrome as the basis of his films *Synechdoche, New York* and *Anomalisa*.

A further change has occurred in authorship. Hadrian Ball has continued to co-author the book, and Professor Basant Puri has joined us for this version, this fact being registered on the title face. We wish to thank Robert Jagger for his help in researching recent developments. We are grateful to the editors of Taylor & Francis, Nina Guttapalle, Olivia Powers, Grace McDonald and Charlotte Mapp for encouraging the writing of this fifth edition and their continued enthusiastic and patient support.

M David Enoch

Preface to the First Edition

The reader may wonder what are the reasons underlying the choice of syndromes described in this book. The first is that although accounts of them can be found in various journals they are, on the whole, not particularly well dealt with in standard psychiatric textbooks and in several are hardly mentioned at all. In some cases this is due to the rarity of their occurrence. The Capgras' syndrome, for example, is extremely rare; the Ganser's and Gilles de la Tourette's syndromes very uncommon. In contrast, the Couvade syndrome is, in its minor manifestations, of very frequent occurrence, though possibly almost as frequently missed owing to the relatively slight and transient nature of the symptoms. Grosser cases with severe and disabling symptoms are much less common. The Othello syndrome than it is usually considered to be. de Clérambault's syndrome ("pure" erotomania), although possibly quite common, has received relatively little attention in current works, although it is of interest to observe that erotomania in its various forms was quite extensively dealt with by nineteenth-century psychiatric authors. All the seven syndromes, including the Munchausen's syndrome, can, however, be regarded as "uncommon" in the sense of being remarkable or in some way unusual, though not necessarily rare.

There are, of course, a number of other conditions which could have been chosen as well those considered here. The number has been limited by the need to produce a volume of limited size. The most important reason governing the choice of contents is that one or more of the authors has made a particular study and has had considerable first-hand experience of each of the disorders described. Most of the case histories presented as illustrative examples are entirely new; a few only have been described before in papers published at one time or another by the authors themselves.

Three of the seven syndromes described (the Capgras' syndrome, the Othello syndrome, and de Clérambault's syndrome) are similar in the respect that they are all variants of paranoid states, the relationship between psychotic jealousy and the paranoid form of erotomania being particularly close. The others form a more heterogeneous group which can be classified under the heading of "neurotic or personality disorders". The Ganser's syndrome, though sometimes wrongly regarded as a psychotic state, is a hysterical pseudo-psychosis. Gilles de la Tourette's syndrome is an obscure manifestation of an obsessive-compulsive disorder which may in some cases have an organic background. The Couvade syndrome differs somewhat in that it is essentially a psychosomatic reaction which may occur in those who at other times are regarded as "normal". It is, however, rather more prone to affect those who are neurotic and also occasionally gives a pathoplastic colouring to a schizophrenic or other psychotic illness. The Munchausen's syndrome is a striking example of a type of "acting-out" found in certain hysterical psychopaths.

An attempt has been made to lay out the presentation of each syndrome in a consistent pattern. Where appropriate, historical data are dealt with including reference in some instances to relevant literary or dramatic works. This is followed by as comprehensive a review as space has permitted of the scientific literature, delving back as far as practicable and including, whenever possible, reference to original sources. Illustrative case histories are then given, followed by a clinical description of the main features of each syndrome together, where necessary, with a discussion of the differential diagnosis. A section on psychopathology in which an attempt has been made to maintain an eclectic approach considering both phenomenological and psychodynamic theories of causation and content. In most instances a short note on treatment and prognosis is given.

It is hoped that this small collection of unusual psychiatric syndromes will not merely be regarded as some kind of esoteric exercise but will provide some food for thought on the matter of the present chaotic state of psychiatric nosology. As Sir Harold Himsworth (1949, Lancet, 1, 465) once stated:

> We are now witnessing a liberation of medical thought by the substitution of syndromes for various "disease entities" as the units of illness. Disease entity implies that any particular illness has a specific cause, a sort of invariable prerequisite for illness. The syndrome has, as its philosophical basis, not specific disease factors but a chain of physiological processes, interference with which at any point introduces the same impairment of bodily function. The same syndrome may thus arise from many different causes. The revision of medical thought entailed by this application has hardly begun.

If to the above passage we add the words "and psychological" after "physiological" and later in the same sentence substitute "mental" in lieu of "bodily" function Himsworth's words then apply equally well to psychiatric as to physical disorders, for it is becoming ever more apparent that to continue to regard psychiatric illnesses as "disease entities" means squeezing square pegs into round holes and leads to inflexibility and retardation in the progress of our thinking.

Capgras' syndrome

You're like him, very like him, perhaps you are a relation – only mine is a bright falcon and a prince, and you're an owl and a shopman.

F. Dostoevsky, The Possessed (1871)

Capgras' syndrome is an uncommon, colourful syndrome in which the patient believes that a person, usually closely related to him, has been replaced by an exact double.

Historical

The condition was first described in 1923 by Capgras and Reboul-Lachaux, who used the term *l'illusion des sosies*, the illusion of doubles. The case they presented was that of a woman with a chronic paranoid psychosis who complained that "doubles" had replaced various persons in her environment.

The term "illusion of doubles" is a misnomer as the central pathology is a delusional belief and not a disorder of perception; a more accurate term is the "delusion of doubles." (*Sosie* is a French word meaning "double" and is derived from Plautus' play *Amphitryon* in which the god Mercury assumes the appearance of *Sosie*, the servant of Amphitryon, and thus becomes his double.)

In 1924, Capgras and Carette described a second case in a woman diagnosed as suffering from schizophrenia. She was a solitary woman of low intelligence who expressed ideas of reference and delusions of persecution. Since childhood she had exhibited a striking attachment to her father and hostility towards her mother. She always improved in hospital but quickly relapsed on returning home. Later she developed ideas of incest and the delusion of doubles. She accused her parents, who visited her in hospital, of being "doubles" and of taking her parents' place.

Capgras' syndrome is the best known and most frequently occurring example of the *delusional misidentification syndromes*, which can be classified as follows:

- *Capgras' syndrome* – described above.
- *Illusion of Frégoli* – described by Courbon and Fail in 1927; the patient identifies his supposed persecutors in several persons – in the doctor, the nurses, the attendants, a neighbour, and a postman, the persecutor being accused of changing faces, as did the famous European actor Frégoli on the stage.
- *Illusion of intermetamorphosis* – described by Courbon and Tusques (1932); the patient believes that persons in his environment change with one another, i.e. A becomes B, B becomes C, C becomes A, and so on.
- *Syndromes of subjective doubles* (doubles of the self) – described by Christodoulou (1978); the patient believes that other people have transformed into his own self. This particular condition is further subdivided into three subtypes: 1. *Capgras type,* in which unseen doubles are active in the patient's environment (this was included in the Capgras'-Lachaux original 1923 description but never emphasised). 2. *Autoscopic type,* where the patient sees doubles of himself "projected" onto other people or objects (Raschka, 1981). 3. *Reverse type,* where the patient believes himself to be an impostor or in the process of being replaced (Simopoulos and Goldsmith, 1975).
- *Reduplicative paramnesia* – patients believe that a physical location has been duplicated. This term was introduced by Pick (1903) in reference to a hospitalised 67-year-old woman who, following a neurological illness, fever, diarrhoea and vomiting, came to believe that the entire hospital had been replicated at a new, second location at the instigation of her doctor. There exist three subtypes, which may occur singly or together (Politis and Loane, 2012) – 1. *Place reduplication,* as in Pick's description, two identically appearing places coexist in geographically distinct locations. 2. *Chimeric assimilation,* whereby two places become assimilated into one. 3. *Extravagant spatial localisation,* in which the patient believes that his location is different from its actual location. Reduplicative paramnesia is often associated with neurological lesions, particularly affecting the right cerebral hemisphere (Förstl et al., 1991; Devinsky, 2009).

Jacques Vie (1930) termed Capgras' syndrome the "illusion of negative doubles" and the illusion of Frégoli as the "illusion of positive doubles." In the former there is a perception of non-existent differences resulting in a negation of identities, whereas in the latter there is an affirmation of imaginary resemblances. Similarly Christodoulou (1976; 1977) regarded the syndrome of Capgras as a *hypoidentification* and the other types, including Frégoli, as *hyperidentification.* Other variants of delusional misidentification syndromes have been described (Joseph, 1986).

In contradistinction to British psychiatrists, considerable attention was initially given to Capgras' syndrome by French and German practitioners.

However, since the 1970s the balance has been redressed, and increasing numbers of case reports have been appearing in the English-language literature.

Other case reports soon followed the Capgras-Lachaux original description. For example, Larrive and Jasiensky (1931) described a woman with an unsystematised persecutory psychosis. She developed a delusion that her poorly endowed lover had a rich, aristocratic, handsome and potent double. Other cases include those of Halberstadt (1923), Dupouy and Montassut (1924), Bouvier (1926), Brochado (1936), Lévy-Valensi (1939) and Vie (1944).

In 1933 and 1944, Coleman wrote extensively on the phenomenon of misidentification and non-recognition which included a comprehensive description of Capgras' syndrome. He admitted that the case he described was not an entirely satisfactory example, because it did not concern the double of a person but letters written by an individual. The woman, aged 50 years, who was diagnosed as suffering from involutional melancholia with feelings of guilt and hopelessness and expressed feelings of depersonalisation, then developed an illusion of doubles in the form that she refused to recognise the letters of her daughter. She insisted that they were facsimiles written by someone else.

Such fragmentary forms of the Capgras' phenomenon are rare. Another example occurred in an intelligent university student, aged 22 years, who, while suffering from an acute attack of schizophrenia, was subsequently able to give a striking account of her primary delusional state and wrote, "I walked on until I came to a steep bank aligned with trees and a small stream at the bottom. I sat down and had a cigarette. ... I threw the empty packet into the stream then I examined my watch. I did not think it was mine, but a clever copy that the police had made so I threw it into the stream as well."

It is significant that all reports up until 1936 concerned women only. Then Murray (1936) reported the first example of the syndrome in a man. He was young, single, apparently homosexual and was diagnosed as suffering from schizophrenia. When his parents visited him in hospital, he insisted that they were not his real parents but doubles. Stern and MacNaughton (1945) described two new cases with special reference to the Rorschach findings. Todd (1957) and then Todd and Dewhurst (1955) described seven further cases: five associated with schizophrenia and allied illnesses and two associated with affective psychosis. They emphasised the role of depersonalisation in the psychopathology (Dewhurst, 1954).

Wagner (1966) presented a diagnostic case study of a young girl with a delusional system which he regarded as a variant of Capgras' syndrome. The patient, a young unmarried woman who had recently been jilted by a medical student, experienced great annoyance with acquaintances who would relate that they had met a married couple whose descriptions matched that of the estranged couple in all essential details. Wagner acknowledged that the case differed from Capgras' syndrome in that the experience was indirect; but one of the doubles was of the patient herself and that there were two doubles. Disertori and Piazza (1967) presented a case occurring in a woman and related it to the "Alcmene complex" or the "complex of innocent adultery."

Since 1970, an increasing number of cases of the Capgras' delusion and the illusion of Frégoli have been reported, often with an emphasis on co-existing overt organic brain disease. The list of organic disorders is now very long and includes drug intoxication and withdrawal, infection and encephalitis, endocrine disorders, epilepsy, serious and minor head injury, brain tumours, delirium, Alzheimer's disease, vascular dementia, multiple myeloma, Lewy body disease, lithium toxicity and migraine. More recently many of the reported cases have included the results of electrophysiological, neuroimaging and neuropsychological studies, and great interest has been aroused concerning a possible neurobiological basis for all of the misidentification syndromes.

The Capgras' phenomenon has also been described in fictional literature. For example, Dostoevsky gives a striking description of the phenomenon in his novel *The Possessed*. The psychopathic Marya Timofyevna has been secretly married to Stavrogin, but at a social function in their hometown he fails to acknowledge her, drawing her aside saying, "Only think you are a girl, and that though I am your devoted friend, I am an outsider not your husband, nor your father, nor your betrothed." When Stavrogin visits her a few days later, Marya, refusing to recognise him, laughs in his face. She speaks the words quoted at the head of this chapter and then accuses him of murdering her prince, stating, "When I saw your mean face after I had fallen down … it was like a worm crawling into my heart. It is not he, I thought, not he! My falcon would never have been ashamed of me a fashionable lady … tell me, you impostor, have you much bite? Did you need to be bribed to consent?"

Also, in Lord David Cecil's biography of Cowper, *The Stricken Deer* (Cecil, 1943), there is an example of the Capgras' phenomenon. It is clear that Cowper suffered from an affective psychosis with paranoid features. The Reverend Newton had been a close friend and confidant for many years. About one of the later depressive phases, Cecil writes, "He still believed he was damned. So little hold he had on reality that years after this he could never be sure if the Newton he saw was the real Newton or some phantom masquerading in his shape."

Case reports

Case 1

A 50-year-old painter began to act strange, "listening" at the walls of his home and believing that the police were persecuting him. On admission to hospital, he was tense and perplexed, was hallucinating and had delusions of persecution. He believed that the doctors were conspiring with the police and that other patients were spies and that his wife was trying to get to him at night but that some harm had occurred to her. The most probable diagnosis was of paranoid psychosis with some depression. Although psychometry revealed a slight intellectual impairment, all physical investigations including an EEG and blood bromide levels were normal. The element of organic confusion present cleared within a month of his admission, and psychometry a year later confirmed this.

Now he began to exhibit Capgras' syndrome. He protested that his wife who visited him "is not my wife but a double." He believed that 'something had happened to her: she might have been replaced'. He added, "I love my wife very much but not the woman double." Later the delusion extended. Modified ECT resulted in the depression and agitation clearing, and his delusions were less prominent. The delusion of doubles persisted, but later this also remitted with haloperidol therapy.

The patient was a quiet introverted personality, while his wife was more forceful and domineering. It appeared that there had always been some conflict between them, although superficially the marriage seems to have been successful. A few months before his illness, however, he had become increasingly affectionate towards his wife, more demonstrative and more demanding sexually. He appeared to be continually seeking reassurance regarding her affections. This only tended to aggravate the situation, and the wife became colder towards him and repulsed by his behaviour. His attitude became even more pronounced later, and she exhibited active hostility towards his returning home even for short periods. The husband found it most difficult to accept this hostility and reacted by protesting his love for her. When this was further thwarted, feelings of aggression and hate were produced in him. Thus love and hate existed together, and he solved the problem of ambivalence by producing the phenomenon of Capgras.

Striking similarities can be seen in the second case, that of a 30-year-old German woman. Capgras' syndrome was the most dominating feature of her psychotic illness.

Case 2

On admission she was weepy, depressed and tense with a manneristic nervous smile that possibly revealed an incongruity of affect, but most marked was the shallowness of her feelings. In addition to the Capgras' delusion regarding her husband, she had other paranoid delusions and ideas of influence. There was no evidence whatsoever of clouding of consciousness. She was diagnosed as suffering from a paranoid schizophrenic reaction. Psychometry confirmed the presence of a paranoid state with a depressive component of a mild degree being secondary to the delusion and hospitalisation. She improved on chlorpromazine therapy, and a steady diminution of her projective thinking, including the Capgras' delusion, occurred. She was discharged after a month, still showing affective shallowness but no evidence of the Capgras' phenomenon. Two years later she needed further hospitalisation because of a reoccurrence of her psychosis, including the delusion of Capgras'.

In this case the Capgras' delusion dominates the symptomatology, for the patient's principal complaint was of the change in her husband's identity. He had always been a quiet, undemonstrative, brooding, morose man, rather rigid and always on the defensive, was shy and hypersensitive and intensely jealous. Immediately before her illness, she had become increasingly demonstrative and demanding sexually, craving for reassurance from her husband of his love for her at the same time she had already feared him. Here again the patient faced the problem of ambivalence which is basic to this condition.

The third case is different in that it occurs in a depressive illness, although there are secondary paranoid features.

Case 3

A woman aged 40, having had numerous admissions to hospital, was diagnosed as suffering from a recurrent endogenous depression. She was of low intelligence and on her sixth admission in 1963, with severe depression, and began to complain that her husband was not her real husband but someone who had taken his place. Her depression cleared following a course of ECT and imipramine, as did the Capgras' delusion. When her depression recurred about a year later, there was no evidence of the Capgras' delusion.

These cases show the main features of Capgras' syndrome, resembling the 10 cases described in detail by Enoch (1963).

Epidemiology

Historically, Capgras' syndrome has been considered to be a rare phenomenon. However, in recent years it was been increasingly and more frequently recognised and reported. Indeed, some studies have revealed that it may be present in up to 4% of psychotic patients (Cutting, 1987; 1994; Frazer and Roberts, 1994; Kirov et al., 1994), rising to 14% of first-episode psychotic-disorder patients (Salvatore et al., 2014). Furthermore, up to a third of all sufferers with Alzheimer's disease may display the phenomenon at some point during the course of their disease (Ballard, 1995; Ballard et al., 1995; Harciarek and Kertesz, 2008). The syndrome occurs in all age groups. There is an increased incidence in women, although this has not been reported in all studies (Oyebode and Sargeant, 1996). A Turkish university hospital psychiatric inpatient study reported that, out of 920 admissions over a five-year period, 12 were patients with Capgras' syndrome, giving a crude five-year prevalence of 1.3% (1.8% for females and 0.9% for males); schizophrenia was the principal diagnosis in 50% of these cases, while an organic aetiology underlying Capgras' syndrome was found in only 17% of the cases (Tamam et al., 2003).

Clinical features

* Capgras' syndrome rarely occurs in a *pure state*. It usually accompanies or occurs in the context of another recognised psychotic illness.
* Despite the intense interest in the possible organic aetiology, 70% of reported cases occur in association with a functional psychosis.
* In the majority of cases, the functional psychosis is of a paranoid schizophrenic type (Wallis, 1986; Signer, 1987). It can, however, also occur as a paranoid feature of an affective psychosis in both the manic and depressive phases.

The *onset* of Capgras' syndrome is not dependent on the length of illness which it accompanies. It can occur at any time during the course of such a psychosis. One man suffering from a schizophrenic illness for 20 years developed Capgras' syndrome only after discharge from hospital. Soon after leaving hospital his father died, and he demanded permission to exhume the body. His mother refused, and he began to believe that she opposed him because she was not his real mother but an impostor. In another instance, a man who had been in hospital for several years following the death of his wife began to believe that his brother who visited him was not his brother but a double. When Capgras' syndrome occurs, even in the presence of other psychotic symptoms, it tends to dominate the clinical picture. It is significant how often the patients themselves use the word 'double' and 'impostor' to describe the misidentified person. One patient categorically affirmed: "She is her double."

Another important feature of the clinical state is the considerable personal specificity of the (alleged) double. Often one person is implicated and persistently misidentified. In most married patients, the spouse is the main double. In widows, relatives other than spouses become the main double. In single persons it is usually the parent or sibling.

If there is any *spread* of the double phenomenon (which is more common than formerly thought) it is restricted to near relatives or persons closely involved with the patient, such as nurses and doctors. The double is obviously a key figure in the life of a patient at that time, and often there is an emotional element.

Rarely, misidentification syndromes have been reported for animals. Darby and Caplan (2016) reported the case of a 73-year-old man with right posterior frontal and bilateral anteromedial frontal damage resulting from trauma who believed that his pet cat had been replaced by an impostor. The authors jokingly referred to this manifestation of Capgras' syndrome as a "cat-gras" delusion.

Parallel symptoms for inanimate objects have also been reported, as noted earlier in this chapter, when Coleman described the delusion in the form of letters and also in the case referred to of the 22-year-old student believing that her watch was a "clever copy." Anderson (1988) has described the case of an elderly man, with a large pituitary tumour, who believed that his wife and nephew had replaced more than 300 of his possessions with similar but inferior doubles.

Although in the cases of those exhibiting functional psychosis organic type confusion is absent, a state of perplexity and bewilderment is often widespread and constant.

Aetiology and psychopathology

Traditionally Capgras' syndrome has been considered to have its origins in a psychodynamic conflict. However, since Gluckman (1968) described a case occurring in the setting of apparent organic disease with radiologically-proven cerebral atrophy, although implicating psychological factors as well, an advanced advocacy for an organic aetiology has grown. Now it is estimated that 25–40% of cases are associated with organic disorders, which include dementia, head trauma, epilepsy, and cerebrovascular disease. Neuroimaging evidence suggests a link between Capgras' syndrome and right hemisphere abnormalities, particularly in the frontal and temporal regions. Neuropsychological research has provided empirical support for these findings by consistently reporting the presence of impairments in facial recognition processes – an established right hemisphere function – although there is no universal agreement regarding the exact nature of this impairment.

We remain convinced that the study of the aetiology of Capgras' and other syndromes will lead to a greater understanding of the psychoses, especially the paranoid. This should include both the neuropsychological and the psychodynamic elements. Such study may reveal the link between mood and thought, affect and cognition and even explain the very nature of belief within normal as well as pathological populations.

In spite of the sharp increase in the number of published cases accompanied by various suggestions regarding an organic aetiology, no specific universal lesion has been described. To explain fully the delusion, it is still necessary to embrace the psychodynamic as well as the organic. Even if eventually a specific neuropsychological lesion is found, the psychodynamics of the individual will still be pertinent. Indeed, the relevance of the affect, especially in relation to cognitive function, will remain of vital importance and will complement constructs explaining the nature of the belief.

However, the present state of knowledge can be summarised under the following headings:

- Functional settings
- Organic settings: (a) cerebral dysfunction (b) neuropsychology
- Face misidentification impairments
- Psychodynamics
- Role of affect

Functional settings

Capgras' syndrome predominately occurs in the setting of schizophrenia, particularly of the paranoid type, and less frequently in association with schizoaffective and affective disorders. It is still a fact that a majority of cases present as a functional psychosis. Increasingly it has been noted that an organic condition may trigger the development of the phenomenon, but in such cases there will be some signs of cognitive impairment typical of a psycho-organic syndrome. However, often, when these signs clear, the Capgras' delusion will persist, thus emphasising the precipitant role of the organic element.

Lansky (1974) demonstrated the inadequacy of the organic explanation by emphasising that in any condition such as Capgras' syndrome where *belief* has become the central symptom, to understand the phenomenon we will first need to know more about belief itself and its role in normal and pathological states. Thus even in cases where the organic component is a prominent factor, the comprehensive description of the psychopathology is still relevant. As Berson (1983) emphasised, "the organic factors in themselves, however, seem neither necessary or sufficient to explain the particular and peculiar content of the delusion."

Organic settings

Since Gluckman (1968) first described a case of Capgras' syndrome occurring in the setting of organic disease, a sharp increase in the number of published cases with an organic aetiology has followed. It is estimated that they now account for 25–40% of all case reports (MacCallum, 1973; Todd et al., 1981; Berson, 1983; Bienenfield and Brott, 1989; Cutting, 1994; Forstl et al., 1994; Signer, 1994). A great number of neuropsychiatric conditions have been described as being associated with the syndrome, including Alzheimer's disease, Lewy body dementia, multi-infarct dementia, Parkinson's disease, Fahr syndrome (idiopathic basal ganglia calcification), head trauma, ischaemic stroke, epilepsy, cerebrovascular disease, pituitary tumour, multiple myeloma, multiple sclerosis, viral encephalitis, frontal lobe pathology, neurosyphilis and AIDS. Other medical associations include

hypothyroidism, pseudohypoparathyroidism, diabetes mellitus, hepatic encephalopathy, copper toxicity, homocystinuria, chloroquine-induced psychosis, therapeutic doses of lithium as well as lithium toxicity, therapeutic
doses of cardidopa-L-dopa, disulfiram, ketamine, pneumonia, Klinefelter
syndrome, reactive hypoglycaemia, vitamin B_{12} deficiency, ECT-induced
psychosis, postpartum depression, pre-eclampsia and pulmonary embolism.

Cerebral dysfunction

It has been long proposed that cerebral dysfunction can be the central
factor in the development of Capgras' syndrome (Christodoulou, 1977).
The evidence supporting a neuropathological basis for Capgras symptomatology and other misidentification syndromes has been comprehensively
reviewed by Edelstyn and Oyebode (1999).

It appears that unilateral right hemisphere lesions, particularly affecting
the temporo-limbic regions, may occur more frequently than the left
(Jackson et al., 1992; Förstl et al., 1994; Lebert et al., 1994; Feinberg and
Roane, 1997; Hillers Rodríguez et al., 2011). However, Peña-Salazar
et al. (2014) reported a case with exclusively left hemisphere neuropathology in a right-handed patient. The authors reported CT scan
findings in a 70-year-old woman who presented with Capgras features
(believing her husband and children had been replaced by impostors)
occurring against a background of affective symptomatology. Specifically,
scanning revealed a small lacunar image in the left thalamus along with
left frontal subcortical hypodensity. Nevertheless, in the majority of cases
there may be bilateral cerebral disease, particularly affecting the frontal
lobes (Signer, 1994; Silva et al., 1995; Hillers Rodríguez et al., 2011).

Thiel et al. (2014) carried out an fMRI study of a 70-year-old right-
handed female patient who believed that her husband was not her real
husband but another person who was completely similar to her husband
and who had helped her to recover from a right frontal intracerebral
haemorrhage which had occurred three years previously. Neural activity
to familiar and unfamiliar faces in this patient differed from that in
13 healthy volunteers (with a mean age of 65 years). Specifically, the
patient failed to show neural activation to her husband's face in a number
of cerebral areas (posterior cingulate cortex, posterior superior temporal
sulcus and the supra marginal gyrus). The authors concluded that "the
first factor in Capgras' delusion may be reduced neural activity in the
extended face processing system that deals with inference of mental states
while the second factor may be due to a lesion in the right middle frontal
gyrus" (Thiel et al., 2014).

A causal role for cerebral dysfunction is strengthened by the similarities
existing between Capgras' syndrome and reduplicative paramnesia, a
condition that has a well-established neurological basis. For example,

Joseph et al. (1999) carried out a neuroradiologically-blinded CT brain study comparing 10 consecutive psychiatric inpatients suffering from both reduplicative paramnesia and another principal psychiatric diagnosis with a control group of inpatients who did not suffer from reduplicative paramnesia but who were matched with the first group in terms of age, sex and principal psychiatric diagnosis; cortical atrophy, cortical fissure enlargement and deep brain atrophy in the first group significantly distinguished the two groups. Indeed, reduplicative paramnesia and Capgras' syndrome frequently co-exist in the same patient.

The cerebral disturbance need not be gross and in some cases may exist at the sub-structural level. In this regard there is a putative role for neuro-chemical disturbances. A number of studies have implicated dopamine or serotonin imbalance (Daniel et al., 1987; Potts, 1992; Shiotsuki et al., 2010).

However, no matter how much evidence of neuropathology is forth-coming, such cerebral pathology does not necessarily explain how the psychopathology arises. There still remains a need for an adequate theory of cognitive mechanisms, together with the role of affect. We are also still left with the psychodynamics of individual patients and the question of the nature of universal belief.

Neuropsychological factors

An association between Capgras' syndrome and depersonalisation has been considered to exist since the time when the disorder was first de-scribed (Capgras and Reboul-Lachaux, 1923). Christodoulou (1977) postulated that depersonalisation is the basis of the condition which *may* develop in some individuals depending on the presence of certain neu-ropsychological factors. Misidentification syndromes have also been ex-plained in terms of specific cognitive deficits such as impaired memory function, e.g. disconnection between stored memories and new percep-tions (Staton et al., 1982; Sno, 1994), and interhemispheric disconnec-tion (Joseph, 1986). These explanations, although providing good bases for experimental testing, do not as yet provide any comprehensive un-derstanding of the full range and depth of misidentification phenomena. Two main neuropsychological hypotheses relating to the manifestation mechanism of Capgras' syndrome are (i) one based on prosopagnosia (see below), and (ii) self-other confusion resulting from right hemisphere dysfunction (see above) (Ohigashi, 2006). On the basis of a pattern of bifrontal and right temporo-limbic dysfunction, Hillers Rodríguez et al. (2011) have recently proposed a neuropsychological battery for the assessment of Capgras' syndrome.

Koralus and Mascarenhas (2013) have put forward a novel theory of reasoning which connects formal semantics and the psychology of de-ductive inference. This *erotetic theory* of reasoning is based on the notion that central to our successes and to our failures of reasoning is the relationship between questions and answers, with our capacity for reasoning proceeding by treating successive premises as questions and maximally strong corresponding answers, while systematically asking a certain type of question as each new premise is interpreted allows reasoning to take place in a classically valid way. More recently, Parrott and Koralus (2015) have suggested that, in contrast to more conventional (Bayesian) models, the erotetic theory provides a much better explanation of the onset and persistence of the Capgras' delusion. A more cautious approach questioning this assertion has, in turn, been put forward by McKay (2015). Meanwhile, the important explanatory role for patient experience in understanding Capgras' syndrome has been emphasised by Young (2011), which therefore includes the psychological and psychopathological, an approach which we have taken in this chapter and indeed in the whole book.

Facial misidentification

Originally, it was suggested that the neuropsychological symptom *prosopagnosia* is the basis of the Capgras' delusion either alone or in combination with a psychotic state (Shraberg and Weitzel, 1979). However, the detailed studies of Bidault et al. (1986) have revealed that the misidentification syndromes are not associated with this symptom. Prosopagnosic patients do not become deluded over their disorder, and the clinical characteristics of the two conditions are very different. For example, patients with prosopagnosia search for resemblances, whereas Capgras' sufferers look for dis-similarities. Further, the provision to the sufferer of extra details aids identification in the former condition but hinders in the latter. Finally, the occurrence of the Capgras' delusion in a blind person should remove all further attempts to relate it to prosopagnosia.

Much work has been done by Ellis and others (Ellis and Young, 1990; Ellis and Sheperd, 1992; Ellis et al., 1992) in attempting to understand the ways in which some psychiatric and neurological patients perceive others. However, neither these models nor those concerned with normal face processing fully explain the development of any of the misidentification syndromes. It is essential to take cognisance of the very narrow specificity of the double in order to establish an adequate explanation for Capgras' syndrome's basic aetiology.

The neuropsychological approach to understanding the misidentification syndromes is currently in its infancy. If it is found to have a limited value explaining the misidentification syndromes, it must also be accepted that Capgras' syndrome and the other delusional misidentifications may well occur for different reasons. Clinical experience shows that patients often have quite different onset patterns and respond very differently to drug treatments. It is, therefore, possible that more than one explanation for the same symptom may be required.

Psychodynamics

In their review of aetiological models of Capgras' syndrome, Scholte-Stalenhoef and van den Bosch (2012) concluded that "a sensation of 'alienation' at a conscious or subconscious level, together with inadequate evaluation of beliefs, seems plausible. All models demonstrate some form of 'splitting' i.e. the separate processing of information in time, anatomy or mental representation." Capgras' syndrome can be interpreted as a disorder of ego function which permeates the whole personality. There is, in this, some resemblance to feelings of derealisation and depersonalisation. Christodoulou (1977) suggested that cerebral dysfunction gives rise to feelings of derealisation and depersonalisation which in turn, in the presence of paranoid ideation, *may* develop into Capgras' syndrome. However, clinical experience shows that the development of Capgras' syndrome is not always preceded by such phenomena.

The psychodynamic understanding of the Capgras' phenomenon, when reduced down to its essence, is basically a love-hate conflict that is resolved by projecting ambivalent feelings onto an imaginary double.

Within the patient there exist simultaneously two fundamentally opposing views about the same person, the object: love and hate. On the one hand there is the long-standing love and on the other hand an apparent "new" hatred. There is craving for reciprocation on the part of the object. In those cases where it occurs, it is very significant that before the onset of the delusion of doubles the patient exhibits increased affection and sexual craving towards the object. This excessive reaction results from a craving for reassurance regarding the love of the object and the simultaneous fear of losing it. The object not unnaturally instead of acquiescing to these demands becomes even more repulsed and is unable to cover up these feelings which obviously aggravate the situation, and a vicious circle is established.

The delusion of doubles is the solution to this problem of ambivalence. "The double," i.e. the bad object, can be met and confronted, and the patient reveals his hate and real aggressive feelings towards it without experiencing the guilt which would arise if such feelings were directed towards a loved and respected object. The good and real object is absent. This is well illustrated in the first case quoted. It was only after his efforts at gaining reassurance failed that the patient exhibited psychotic mechanisms.

Ambivalence creates doubt and uncertainties and a characteristic internal tension which serves to aggravate the situation which is already pregnant with suspiciousness and jealousy. This helps to explain the importance of the paranoid component which is often present, even in patients suffering with an affective disorder (Enoch, 1986). The affect is disturbed, and this leads to an impaired judgement and subsequent elaboration of the delusion of doubles. Courbon and Fail (1927) described this as a "disorder of coenaesthesia," i.e. the feeling of the function of life of the organism, or in other words of ego feeling, which accompanies all perception and of which the individual is normally unaware. Coleman (1933; 1934) stated that the feeling of coenaesthesia is only appreciated when it ceases to adhere to perceptive experiences. In healthy persons it only takes place during periods of fatigue and exhaustion. At such moments sensations no longer seem part of him and are no longer integrated within the personality, and a sense of depersonalisation results. In the next phase the condition is complicated by a disorder of affect, and the subjective experience is projected onto the outside world. The patient believes that it is the object that has changed and which no longer produces the effect on him.

This process of ambivalence followed by projection is the basic psychodynamic mechanism in the pathology of Capgras' syndrome. But it goes a stage further in that there is splitting, and the "bad feelings" are projected onto the present object, and the feelings of love and affection are projected onto the absent ideal object. Therefore, the patient deals with the problem of a fallen idol. A deterioration has occurred in the relationship with the object, and a "new" hate appears which is in conflict with the love that is already present. Of course, this "new" hate may well have been present unconsciously for some considerable time, but the changing relationship will have caused this hatred to become conscious, thus existing simultaneously with the love. The splitting process allows the patient to express the hatred and aggression, at the same time maintaining the love for the real person. Hence the explanation for the patient's belief that there has been no change in the external appearance of the object yet denying the object's existence. The true change is within his own feelings and in his relationship with the object. The real person is spared the hate of the patient and remains the "ideal," a model of virtue. The double, an impostor, is made the target for the hate that has now become overt.

Role of affect

In their above-mentioned review of explanatory aetiological models of Capgras' syndrome, Scholte-Stalenhoef and van den Bosch (2012) also concluded that these models converge in that they all assign a central role to a changed affect. Derombies (1935) attached great importance to the affective state of Capgras' patients, suggesting that the syndrome results from simultaneous cognitive recognition and affectively engendered non-recognition of faces. Anderson (1988) supported this contention, stating "that the Capgras' delusion results from lesions in the pathway for visual recognition at a stage when visual images are imbued with affective familiarity." This argument is supported by the extreme specificity of Capgras' syndrome, the fact that not all faces are duplicated but only faces of people close to the patient and especially emotionally close. In this respect some may argue that the Capgras' delusion sometimes extends to inanimate objects. But, neither objects nor places are affectively neutral, and so the very same mechanism may well apply to them.

In summary, a satisfactory model of Capgras' syndrome must be based on a combination of cognitive and perceptual impairments, organic disturbance, paranoid ideation and psychodynamic factors, although some antecedents may have a greater impact than others in particular cases. It is necessary to embrace both the organic and psychological aetiologies.

Nosology

In nosological terms, it is highly questionable whether Capgras' syndrome should be regarded as a clear-cut syndrome or merely a symptom occurring as part of a recognised psychosis. While the French have traditionally supported the former view, affording it a special place in psychiatric nosology, the English-speaking world has adopted the latter view. We believe that it should be regarded more accurately as a symptom. However, when it does occur, it has a tendency to colour the clinical state and usually dominates the symptomatology.

Munro (1994), while noting that the misidentification syndromes have no formal place in officially recognised diagnostic systems, emphasises that they are of great importance. He also made the point that the misidentification syndromes and delusional disorders hang together better than they do separately. Misidentification syndromes are best considered (based on the state of our present knowledge and understanding) as an essential link in the paranoid spectrum.

Management and treatment

There is little reported in the literature in respect of the treatment of Capgras' syndrome. No controlled studies have been carried out, and information is inevitably limited to retrospective and anecdotal reports. The principles underpinning the management and treatment of Capgras' syndrome are:

- Thorough investigation aimed at identifying an organic lesion or more widespread pathology
- Treatment of any underlying psychiatric condition whether organic or functional, such as a depressive psychosis
- Symptomatic treatment with antipsychotic medication
- Support for the spouse or partner (who may well be the "impostor")
- Risk assessment

Given that about one in three cases have an organic component or association, it is imperative to bear this possibility in mind when taking a detailed history, noting any relevant infections or traumas such as encephalitis or head injury. Furthermore, in a case of Capgras' delusion, it is essential to carry out detailed psychometric tests, EEG and CT or MRI neuroimaging. Such detailed examinations are now mandatory in spite of the fact that no specific location or lesion has been established as the primary cause of Capgras' syndrome.

There is no specific treatment for Capgras' syndrome. Antipsychotic drugs may be prescribed on a symptomatic basis, and remission has been reported for a wide range of neuroleptics (Enoch, 1963; Halsam, 1973; Sims and White, 1973; Todd et al., 1981). Some authors have reported trifluoperazine to be ineffective (Enoch, 1963; Lansky, 1974).

ECT has been reported as being both successful and ineffective (Enoch, 1963; Nilsson and Perris, 1971). Hay et al. (1974) have even reported a case where ECT precipitated Capgras' syndrome in a female patient already suffering from pseudohypoparathyroidism, but it is known that pseudohypoparathyroidism itself is associated with Capgras' syndrome (Prescorn and Reveley, 1978). In another patient suffering from an endocrine disorder, i.e. myxoedema, thyroid replacement therapy resulted in a dramatic improvement (Madakasira and Hall, 1981), while a more recent case with "myxoedema madness" and catatonic features responded to a combination of levothyroxine and olanzapine (Shlykov et al., 2016). Most cases of Capgras' syndrome occurring in a depressive setting respond to antidepressant drugs (Christodoulou, 1977; 1986). Mazzone et al. (2012) reported a case of Capgras' syndrome in an 11-year-old girl, accompanied by auditory hallucinations, persecutory delusions regarding her "impostor" parents and depressive symptoms which responded to a combination of risperidone and sertraline.

It is important to note that just as a deterioration in the interpersonal relationship between the patient and the object may occur before the onset of the delusion, an improvement in this relationship is an important factor in the amelioration of symptoms. Treatment, therefore, must include helping the spouse or person implicated to gain insight and perhaps change his or her attitude towards the patient (Christodoulou, 1978).

Forensic aspects

The anecdotal evidence that violence is a hazard in the delusional misidentification syndromes, including Capgras' syndrome, is now supported by empirical evidence. Victims of violence associated with Capgras' syndrome are usually misidentified family members who live with the patient (Bourget and Whitehurst, 2004).

More recently, Ahn et al. (2012) studied 88 patients with schizophrenia who had committed homicide and who were patients in the National Institute of Forensic Psychiatry, Seoul, between November and December 2007. Of these, 59 had committed parricide. Furthermore, 15% of those who committed parricide suffered from Capgras' syndrome at the time of the index offence, compared with none of the 29 patients who had killed strangers; that is, Capgras' syndrome was present at a significantly higher rate in the parricide group.

Prognosis

Systematic studies on the natural history of Capgras' syndrome (as is the case for most of the syndromes described in this book) are practically non-existent. In the authors' experience, the progress of the delusion of doubles does not necessarily follow the course of the associated psychosis. On some occasions the psychosis will clear as a result of treatment but the delusion of doubles persists and vice versa.

The long-term prognosis of Capgras' syndrome is usually dependent upon the nature of the associated (if any) psychosis or disorder. The majority of patients suffer from a functional psychosis, most frequently paranoid schizophrenia, and tend therefore to survive for many years. Surprisingly, many of these patients show little in the way of personality deterioration. Christodoulou (1986) has suggested that this phenomenon may be partially explained by the presence of a "dysrhythmic" component, revealed by EEG, akin to the observation of Pond (1957) that the affect of patients with psychosis associated with epilepsy tends to remain warm and appropriate with no typical "schizophrenic" deterioration.

In cases where the syndrome is associated with an underlying organic disorder, the long-term prognosis will depend upon the nature of the organic component and its response to the appropriate treatment.

References

Ahn, B.H., Kim, J.H., Oh, S., Choi, S.S., Ahn, S.H., Kim, S.B., (2012). *Australian and New Zealand Journal of Psychiatry, 46*, 621.

Anderson, D.N., (1988). *British Journal of Psychiatry, 153*, 699.

Ballard, C.G., (1995). *Psychotic Symptoms in Dementia Sufferers*. MD thesis, University of Leicester.

Ballard, C.G., Saad, K., Patel, A., Gahir, M., Solis, M., Coope, B., Wilcock, G., (1995). *International Journal of Geriatric Psychiatry, 10*, 447.

Berson, R.J., (1983). *American Journal of Psychiatry, 140*, 969.

Bidault, E., Luauté, J.P., Tzavaras, A. (1986). *Bibliotheca Psychiatrica, 164*, 80.

Bienenfeld, D., Brott, T. (1989). *Journal of Clinical Psychiatry, 50*, 68.

Bourget, D., Whitehurst, L. (2004). *Canadian Journal of Psychiatry, 49*, 719.

Bouvier, A. (1926). *Le Syndrome "Illusion des Sosies"*. Thesis, Paris.

Brochado, A. (1936). *Annals of Medical Psychology*, *15*, 706.

Capgras, J., Carette, J. (1924). *Annales Medico-Psychologiques*, *82*, 48.

Capgras, J., Reboul-Lachaux, J., (1923). *Bulletin de la Societé Clinique de Médecine Mentale*, *16*, 170.

Cecil, Lord David, (1943). *The Stricken Deer*. Constable, London.

Christodoulou, G.N., (1976). *Acta Psychiatrica Scandinavica*, *54*, 305.

Christodoulou, G.N., (1977). *British Journal of Psychiatry*, *130*, 556.

Christodoulou, G.N., (1978). *American Journal of Psychiatry*, *135*, 249.

Christodoulou, G.N., (1986). *Bibliotheca Psychiatrica*, *164*, 99.

Coleman, S.M., (1933). *J Ment Sci*, *79*, 42.

Coleman, S.M., (1934). *British Journal of Medical Psychology*, *14*, 3.

Courbon, P., Fail, G., (1927). *Bull. Soc. Cli. Med. Ment. 15*, 121.

Courbon, P., Tusques, J., (1932). *Annales Medico-Psychologiques*, *90*, 401.

Cutting, J., (1987). *British Journal of Psychiatry*, *151*, 324.

Cutting, J., (1994). *British Journal of Psychiatry*, *159*, 70.

Daniel, D.G., Swallows, A., Wolff, F. (1987). *Southern Medical Journal*, *80*, 1577.

Darby, R.R., Caplan, D., (2016). *Neurocase*, *22*, 251.

Derombies, M., (1935). *Annales Medico-Psychologiques*, *94*, 706.

Devinsky, O., (2009). *Neurology*, *72*, 80.

Dewhurst, K., (1954). *Irish Journal of Medical Sciences*, *1*, 263.

Disertori, B., Piazza, M., (1967). *Giornale di Psichiatra e di Neuropatologia*, *95*, 175.

Dostoevsky, F., (1871). *The Possessed*. Heinemann, London.

Dupouy, R., Montassut, M., (1924). *Annales Medico-Psychologiques*, *82*, 341.

Edelstyn, N.M.J., Oyebode, F., (1999). *International Journal of Geriatric Psychiatry*, *14*, 48.

Ellis, H.D., Sheperd, J.W., (1992). In *Aspects of Memory*, Eds. M. Gruneberg et al. Routledge, London.

Ellis, H.D., Young, A.W., (1990). *British Journal of Psychiatry*, *56*, 215.

Ellis, H.D., de Pauw, K.W., Christodoulou, G.N., Papageorgiou, L., Milne, A.B., Joseph, A.B., (1992). *Journal of Neurology Neurosurgery and Psychiatry*, *56*, 215.

Enoch, M.D., (1963). *Acta Psychiatrica Scandinavica*, *39*, 437.

Enoch, M.D., (1986). *Bibliotheca Psychiatrica*, *164*, 22.

Feinberg, T.E., Roane, D.M., (1997). *Neurocase*, *3*, 73.

Förstl, H., Almeida, O.P., Owen, A.M., Burns, A., Howard, R., (1991). *Psychological Medicine*, *21*, 905.

Förstl, H., Besthorn, C., Burns, A., Geiger-Kabisch, C., Levy, R., Sattel, A., (1994). *Psychopathology*, *27*, 194.

Frazer, F.J., Roberts, J.M., (1994). *British Journal of Psychiatry*, *164*, 557.

Gluckman, L.K., (1968). *Australian and New Zealand Psychiatry*, *2*, 39.

Halberstadt, G., (1923). *J. Psychol. Norm. Pathol. 20*, 728.

Halsam, M.T., (1973). *American Journal of Psychiatry*, *130*, 493.

Harciarek, M., Kertesz, A., (2008). *Alzheimer Disease and Associated Disorders*, *22*, 163.

Hay, G.G., Jolley, D.J., Jones, R.G., (1974). *Acta Psychiatrica Scandinavica*, *50*, 73.

Hillers Rodríguez, R., Madoz-Gúrpide, A., Tirapu Ustárroz, J., (2011). *Rev Esp Geriatr Gerontol*, *46*, 275.

Jackson, R.S., Naylor, M.W., Shain, B., King, C.A., (1992). *J. Acad. Child. Adolesc. Psych. 31*, 5.

Joseph, A.B., (1986). *Bibliotheca Psychiatrica*, *164*, 68.

Joseph, A.B., O'Leary, D.H., Kurland, R., Ellis, H.D., (1999). *Canadian Journal of Psychiatry*, *44*, 685.

Kirov, G., Jones, P., Lewis, S.W., (1994). *Psychopathology*, *27*, 148.

Koralus, P., Mascarenhas, S., (2013). *Philosophical Perspectives*, *27*, 312.

Lansky, M.R., (1974). *Bulletin of the Menninger Clinic*, *38*, 360.

Larrive, E., Jasiensky, J., (1931). *Annales Medico-Psychologiques*, *89*, 501.

Lebert, F., Pasquier, F., Steinling, M., Cabaret, M., Caparros-Lefebve, D., Petit, H., (1994). *Psychopathology*, *27*, 211.

Lévy-Valensi, J., (1939). *Gazette de Hopital Civil et Militaire, Paris.*, Paris.

MacCallum, W.A.G., (1973). *British Journal of Psychiatry*, *123*, 639.

Madakasira, S., Hall, T.B., (1981). *American Journal of Psychiatry*, *138*, 1506.

Mazzone, L., Armando, M., De Crescenzo, F., Demaria, F., Valeri, G., Vicari, S., (2012). *J Med Case Reports*, *6*, 406.

McKay, R., (2015). *Cognit Neuropsychiatry*, *20*, 456.

Munro, A., (1994). *Psychopathology*, *27*, 247.

Murray, J.R., (1936). *J Ment Sci*, *82*, 63.

Nilsson, R., Perris, C., (1971). *Acta Psychiatrica Scandinavica (suppl.)* *221*, 53.

Ohigashi, Y., (2006). *Seishin Shinkeigaku Zasshi*, *108*, 1009.

Oyebode, F., Sargeant, R., (1996). *Psychopathology*, *29*, 209.

Parrott, M., Koralus, P., (2015). *Cognit Neuropsychiatry*, *20*, 398.

Peña-Salazar, C., Cendrós, P., Escoté, S., Romero, T., García-Barrionuevo, J., Roura-Poch, P., Arrufat, F., (2014). *Journal of Neuropsychiatry and Clinical Neurosciences*, *26*, E23.

Pick, A., (1903). *Brain*, *26*, 260.

Politis, M., Loane, C., (2012). *Psychopathology*, *45*, 337.

Pond, D.A., (1957). *J Indian Med Prof*, *3*, 1441.

Potts, S.G., (1992). *Behavioural Neurology*, *5*, 19.

Prescorn, S.H., Reveley, A., (1978). *British Journal of Psychiatry*, *133*, 34.

Raschka, L.B., (1981). *Canadian Journal of Psychiatry*, *26*, 207.

Salvatore, P., Bhuvaneswar, C., Tohen, M., Khalsa, H.M., Maggini, C., Baldessarini, R.J., (2014). *Psychopathology*, *47*, 261.

Scholte-Stalenhoef, A.N., van den Bosch, R.J., (2012). *Tijdschr Psychiatr*, *54*, 1011.

Shiotsuki, H., Motoi, Y., Nakamura, S., Mizuno, Y., Hattori, N., (2010). *Journal of Neuropsychiatry and Clinical Neurosciences*, *22*, 352i.e14.

Shlykov, M.A., Rath, S., Badger, A., Winder, G.S., (2016). *BMJ Case Reports*, doi:10.1136/bcr-2016-215957.

Shraberg, D., Weitzel, W.D., (1979). *Journal of Clinical Psychiatry*, *40*, 313.

Signer, S., (1987). *Journal of Clinical Psychiatry*, *48*, 147.

Signer, S.F., (1994). *Psychopathology*, *27*(3–5), 168.

Silva, J.A., Leong, G.B., Lesser, I.M., Boone, K.B., (1995). *Canadian Journal of Psychiatry*, *40*, 498.

Sims, A., White, A., (1973). *British Journal of Psychiatry*, *123*, 635.

Simopolous, Goldsmith, (1985), *American Journal of Psychiatry*, *7*, 756–7.

Sno, H.N., (1994). *Psychopathology*, *27*, 144.

Staton, R.D., Brumback, R.A., Wilson, H., (1982). *Cortex*, *18*, 23.

Stern, K., MacNaughton, D., (1945). *Psychiatric Quarterly*, *19*, 139.

Tamam, L., Karatas, G., Zeren, T., Ozpoyraz, N., (2003). *Acta Neuropsychiatrica*, *15*, 290.

Thiel, C.M., Studte, S., Hildebrandt, H., Huster, R., Weerda, R., (2014). *Cortex*, *52*, 75.
Todd, J., (1957). *Psychiatric Quarterly*, *31*, 250.
Todd, J., Dewhurst, K., (1955). *Journal of Mental Diseases*, *122*, 47.
Todd, J., Dewhurst, K., Wallis, G., (1981). *British Journal of Psychiatry*, *139*, 319.
Vie, J., (1930). *Annales Medico-Psychologiques*, *88*, 214.
Vie, J., (1944). *Annales Medico-Psychologiques*, *100*, 273.
Wagner, E.E., (1966). *J. Prof. Tech. Pers. Assess.*, *30*, 394.
Wallis, G., (1986). *Bibliotheca Psychiatrica*, *164*, 40.
Young, G., (2011). *Cognit Neuropsychiatry*, *16*, 303.

Chapter 2

De Clérambault's syndrome

He hath, my lord, of late made many tenders
Of his affection to me.
...
My lord, he hath importuned me with love
In honourable fashion.

William Shakespeare, *Hamlet* (I, iii)

This disorder is a condition in which the patient, generally a woman, suddenly develops the delusional belief that a man, with whom she may have had little or virtually no contact, is in love with her.

Historical

In 1942, de Clérambault described the condition known as *psychose passionelle*. He endeavoured to differentiate the syndrome from the more generally accepted erotic paranoid state, referring to it as *erotomania*.

He regarded the condition as having certain special characteristics which he described in meticulous detail. The victim is usually of much higher social status – a public figure in politics, on the screen or television or is often a doctor or a priest for example, and is likely to be unobtainable on this account alone or perhaps for other reasons, such as already being married.

A further characteristic is the intensity of the morbid passion, and de Clérambault also formulated a "fundamental postulate" which he regarded as the essential basis of the whole syndrome: a conviction of being in amorous communication with a person of much higher rank, who has been the first to fall in love and was the first to make advances. He designated the two parties in this delusional amorous attachment as the *subject* and the *object*. He described five cases in detail and referred to one other patient:

A modiste, aged 53 years, with a paranoid psychosis of ten years duration, also believed that a sovereign, namely King George V, was in love with her. She was convinced that sailors and tourists she saw were his emissaries, sent by the King to proclaim his love for her. Previously she believed that King Edward VII was in love with her and that she had also been wooed by an American General. She persistently pursued King George V from 1918 onwards, paying several visits to England. She frequently waited for him outside Buckingham Palace. She once saw a curtain move in one of the palace windows and interpreted this as a signal from the King. She claimed that all Londoners knew of his love for her, but alleged that he prevented her from finding lodgings in London, made her miss her hotel bookings, and was responsible for the loss of her baggage containing money and portraits of him. Such doubts as she had never persisted for long. She vividly summarised her passion for him. "The King might hate me, but he can never forget. I could never be indifferent to him, nor he to me.... It is in vain that he hurts me. He is the most distinguished of men.... I was attracted to him from the depths of my heart. I wish to live under the same Heaven as he and in the midst of his subjects. If I have offended him I have suffered in my heart."

Another case described was as follows:

A promiscuous female, aged 50 years, believed that a much older Priest was in love with her. She claimed that he paid for her apartment and wanted to marry her but she also suffered from persecutory auditory hallucinations and had ideas of reference and influence. She repeatedly shouted abuse in the Church and once interrupted her Priest at a conference because she thought he was having her watched. Her behaviour led to action by the police. She believed the police were paid to treat her cruelly, but was always prepared to excuse the paradoxical behaviour of her lover. "The Priest has done nothing but evil to me, but I forgive him. He is always making suggestions to me."

De Clérambault described two other female patients aged 35 and 55 years, each with a chronic erotic delusion persisting unchanged for 7 and 37 years, respectively. The first patient did not regard her love-object's wife as a bar to his affection for her. She repeatedly waylaid him, struck him and was consequently often arrested. The other patient first met her love-object, a priest, when she was 17 years of age. She constantly pursued him and frequently caused scenes in public by trying to embrace him. She telephoned incessantly but rarely wrote to him. Her husband finally divorced her.

Only one of de Clérambault's cases was a male, and even in other respects he does not appear to be a typical example of the syndrome:

Aged 34 years, he had a morbid passion towards his ex-wife. Although she maintained that she did not love him, he claimed her attitude always belied her words. After her re-marriage he said she would once again become his mistress, and that when he had satisfied his pride he would again reject her. He said he would always be able to find her. He was constantly writing, ambushing her, and striking her in public. He carried a razor, threatening, "If you remarry I'll get you both." He alleged that her divorce from him was false and null and void.

It should be noted that, by modern standards, this male case might be considered to be a manifestation of a personality disordered individual with prominent narcissistic traits; indeed, this is a common clinical presentation in groups of stalkers.

De Clérambault essentially resurrected interest in a psychiatric concept, *erotomania*, which, even in his time had a long history dating back to ancient times:

- Hippocrates – who so diagnosed the ailment of Perdiccas (Rather, 1965).
- Plutarch – records a case treated by Erisistratus (Rather, 1965).
- Soranus – a Roman physician who commented on the delusional aspects of the condition, "Some have imagined themselves descending into Hades for the love of Proserpine; some have believed they were favoured by a promise of marriage to a Goddess, although she was the wife of another" (Zilboog, 1941).
- 1640 – Jacques Ferrand wrote the book *Erotomania or a Treatise, Discussing the Essence, Causes, Symptoms, Prognostiks and Cure of Lover or Erotique Melancholy* (Hunter and Macalpine, 1963).

From its inception, the term "erotomania" suffered from a lack of precise definition. For example, in the eighteenth-century medical lexicon erotomanics were defined as "those who engage in the furious pursuit of vagrant and illicit lust" (Rather, 1965). The terms "nymphomania" or, in the case of men, "satyriasis" more accurately describe these states. Esquirol (1772–1840) made this distinction between erotomania and nymphomania: "In the latter evil originates in the organs of reproduction, the irritation of which reacts upon the brain. In erotomania the sentiment which characterises it is in the head ... The subjects of erotomania never pass the limits of propriety, they remain chaste!"

Sir Alexander Morison (1848) defined erotomania as "monomania with love." He also commented on the forensic implications of this awkward complaint: "The fixed and permanent delusions of attending erotomania sometimes prompt those labouring under it to destroy themselves or others for although in general tranquil and respectful, the patient sometimes becomes irritable, passionate and jealous."

Other cases were described in the nineteenth century:

1863 – Winslow – "A young lady, subject for many years to violent hysteria, accompanied by occasional flightiness of manner, alternating with depression of spirits, suggestive of the possibility of insanity one day supervening, conceived an intense passion for a married clergyman whom she had never seen but on one occasion, and then only for a short period in the pulpit. Her family knew nothing of this circumstance until they received a visit from the gentleman, who had in his possession a number of epistles from the lady, couched in very high-flown and amatory language…. The prominent and salient feature of her mental melancholy was a vague unintelligible, morbid erotic feeling for the gentleman to whom she had so indiscreetly addressed the letters. Twelve months elapsed before the mind was restored to health. The cure was, apparently, a perfect one. After her recovery she often adverted to her insane passion for the clergyman, and said that she now fully realised that her penchant for him was only a symptom of insanity."

1887 – Clouston – "I will show you a one legged dressmaker of 40, with certainly no charms who went to her clergyman and asked him to 'proclaim' her and Mr – in Church. On enquiring he found the gentleman to be proclaimed had never spoken to her. He sat opposite her in Church and she said that he looked at her in such a significant way that she knew he wanted the banns proclaimed. She said it was all due to a scheming neighbour that she was not married to Mr –."

1899 – MacPherson wrote of *perverted insanity:* Under the title "erotomania" had been placed a large number of anomalous sexual peculiarities of a pathological nature. These range from an abnormal desire for coitus, or habits of masturbation up to indecent exposure of the penis, rape of children, connection with dead bodies, pederasty, sodomy and bestiality. Here we have to do with sexual obsession and impulse either exaggerated or grossly perverted. The underlying common factor in all of the groups and the one that distinguishes them from pertaining to the class of the degenerate is the besetment of the mind by the sexual idea.

This latter characterisation of erotomania is both reactionary and over-inclusive, perhaps heavily coloured by the strong moral overtones of the later Victorian era. It is also quite wrong!

At the turn of the nineteenth century, the term 'monomania' was on the wane, and those disorders formerly included under this heading reappeared in the guise of paranoia. In 1906, Bianchi used the term "paranoia erotica." This, he said, "occurred often in individuals of defective sexual life, not much inclined to copulation, sometimes in old maids who have never had an opportunity of marrying."

Bianchi considered that many cases of erotomania could be placed into the broader category of paranoid illnesses, whereas in other examples, it occurred as an isolated phenomenon without any other evidence of psychosis.

Emil Kraepelin (1921) classified erotomania as a form of *paranoiac megalomania*:

> The patient perceives that the person of the other sex, distinguished really or presumably by high position, is kindly disposed to him and shows him attention which cannot be understood. Sometimes it is an intercepted glance, a supposed promenade before the window, a chance meeting, which lets this hidden love become certainty to the patient. A female patient noticed that the reigning sovereign bowed with special respect to her in the theatre and made his children greet her.... Very soon the signs of the secret understanding increase in number. Every chance occurrence, clothing, meetings, reading, conversations acquire for the patient a relation to his imagined adventure. His love is an open secret and an object of universal interest, it is talked about everywhere, certainly never outspokenly, but always only in slight indications, the proposed meaning of which he understands very well.... The peculiar delusion may for a long time be further elaborated ... nourished especially by figurative advertisements in the newspapers without anything wrong appearing in the remaining activities of the patient who, indeed, tries to keep his affair secret.

In Hart, 1921, Bernard Hart redescribed a variety of paranoid erotomania, calling it *old maid's insanity*:

> An unmarried lady of considerable age and blameless reputation ... begins to complain of the undesirable attentions to which she is subjected by some male acquaintance. She explains that the man is obviously anxious to marry her, and persistently follows her about. Finally certain trifling incidents lead her to believe that he is scheming to abduct her by force, and on the strength of this she perhaps writes him an indignant letter, or lodges a complaint with the police. Investigation follows, and it is found that the man is not only entirely innocent of the charges levelled against him, but that he has never expressed the least interest in the lady and is probably hardly aware of her existence.

Over the next two or three decades, erotomania seems to have vanished into comparative obscurity, and if mentioned at all, it was regarded as no more than one of the several varieties of paranoia. Following de Clérambault's case descriptions, however, after a further quiescent period, psychiatric interest was revived. In Balduzzi, 1956, Balduzzi described a further case from Italy:

> An unhappily married female, aged 26 years, suddenly developed an ardent passion for a married doctor who attended her abortion. She constantly pestered him with telephone calls and almost daily messages, and frequently visited his home. She showed no concern whatsoever for her own daughter, and would talk of nothing but "him," alleging that he had "reciprocated several times with an ardour even more pronounced than her own." She maintained that when she first met Dr "P," "I felt changed into another person ... until then I had not lived'. Thereafter she ceased to feel alone and was convinced that everybody ... when they talk to me, inevitably ends by speaking about him." Finally the doctor's wife literally pushed her out of the door but threats and scenes only increased her love. "He acts like that only because, for reasons I am not yet able to understand, he is compelled to assume attitudes entirely contrary to his feelings, because he does not want others to understand his real passionate love: in fact, I have noticed that he has shown himself more aggressive to me verbally when that woman, who passes for his wife, is present. Dr P ... in fact, cannot be married; I do not know who that woman can be, but I know that she has been called to act a comedy which leaves me completely indifferent."

This patient also demonstrates the intensity of the morbid passion when referring to her object:

> No person or circumstance will be able to separate us, not even death, because this exists solely for those who love by the body; I will be united to him eternally because I love with my mind, as he loves me. He is part of me in so far as he integrates my personality; nevertheless he is much stronger, more powerful and more able to reason than me; I shall never be finally complete until I can live with him always.

The description of other cases in the literature soon followed (Arieti and Meth, 1959; Baruk, 1959).

An increasing number of cases (usually in the form of single case reports) have been described in association with other uncommon syndromes, such as *folie à deux* and the Capgras' and Fregoli syndromes (for example, Pearce, 1972; Sims and White, 1973; Drevets, 1987; Signer and Cummings, 1987;

Wright et al., 1993; Carter, 1995; Strip et al., 1996; Mann and Foreman, 1996; Singh et al., 2014; Grandstein et al., 2015).

Not surprisingly, in keeping with the changing sexual mores of Western cultures, cases have also been recorded in which the erotomanic process is homosexual or bisexual in nature, and even where the object was a child (Mannion and Carney, 1996; Michael et al., 1996; Remilagton, 1997; Holzer, 2017). In passing, it is worth noting that de Clérambault's syndrome is very well described in Ian McEwan's novel *Enduring Love* (McEwan, 1997; Rot, 2008).

Lerner et al. (2001) express their dissatisfaction with the use of eponymous syndromes, suggesting, for example, that de Clérambault's syndrome may be confused with Kandinsky-Clérambault's syndrome. Fortunately, the latter is relatively unknown in English-speaking countries, referring to a syndrome of mental automatism which was independently described by de Clérambault and the Russian psychiatrist Victor Kandinsky (Lerner et al., 2001).

Case reports

The following examples have been chosen to illustrate some variations on the theme of erotomania, some of which may fulfil de Clérambault's postulates, while others have features which suggest closer adherence to the concept of erotomania as part of a paranoid psychosis occurring either overtly or in an attenuated form. The first two cases which follow are examples of gross infatuation, which is different from erotomania (described in Cases 3 and 4).

Case 1

A well-spoken unmarried female, aged 20 years, whose mother died when she was four years old, brought up by an anxious over-protective father, whom she had always despised, and by a strict grandmother. Her first sexual experience at 17 years was with an elderly married man, and she had several short-lived affairs with other older men, which were bitterly opposed by her father. There were no obvious psychotic traits. She complained of excessive lethargy and was extremely untruthful.

For two years she had become infatuated with a bachelor aged 35 years, socially and intellectually her superior. He worked in the office where she was a clerk. "As soon as he spoke to me I felt I had known him all my life, and it frightened me … this was the man I was intended to love – from that moment to this I have never been the same." Her work suffered and she was dismissed. Before leaving she confronted her supposed lover and declared her feelings towards him. He was astonished, not realising how she felt, and became extremely embarrassed when she flung her arms around his neck and passionately kissed him in the office.

At interview he admitted being flattered by her attentions and was not, at first, averse to their association. He always emphasised the difference in their ages, however, and repeatedly assured her that there was no future for them and that marriage was impossible. Occasionally, he persuaded her to stop pestering him, but she soon telephoned again to arrange a further meeting.

He advised her to associate with a man of her own age. She then had intercourse with a youth, who did not attract her, and returned to her lover declaring triumphantly that the experiment had failed and that he was the only man for her.

On another occasion she presented him with contraceptives, which he declined. They both denied having intercourse although he undoubtedly encouraged her initially by "heavy petting." Frequently she telephoned him at the office several times a day or sent telegrams to his home, until in desperation he promised to see her "just one more time."

After admission, a meeting was arranged in hospital between the patient and her lover. He reiterated that there was no future for them. She explained that it was unfair that she had to suffer so much while he 'got off scot-free'. She then hit him smartly across the face, but at the same time, held his hand with her other one. She broke down and said that there was nothing left for her but suicide. While in hospital she continued to telephone him and write excessively, and her letters were mixed with love, abuse and threats of suicide. Drugs, ECT and insight-directed psychotherapy were all ineffective. Although she claimed to be overcoming her passion, on being pressed it was apparent that she still believed that he was attracted to her.

Case 2

A 19-year-old single girl first came under psychiatric care after attempting suicide by taking aspirin tablets. She said, "I'm in love with a priest, the reason why I tried to kill myself is that it would be better for him."

She was the fourth of a family of five. She described her father as moody, unstable and uninterested in his children, a man who worked seven days a week and came home drunk each night. When in drink he was at first merry, then stupid and, finally, aggressive. Despite this her childhood seems to have been relatively uneventful. She did well at school. During adolescence she became withdrawn and intensely religious. She toyed with the idea of becoming a nun, and in due course, of becoming a missionary. It was then that she fell in love with a priest 14 years older than herself. This was a crush at first, but after, so she claimed, he too had "confessed his love," her feelings strengthened and persisted.

What seems surprising was at the time of her suicidal attempt she had not seen or spoken to her priest for four years, having adored him only from afar. At the same time it seemed significant that, shortly before the event, a close friend had become pregnant with another priest with whom she subsequently lived as man and wife. It may have been this disturbing event which led her to describe her suicidal attempt not so much as an act of self-destruction but of self-sacrifice, "one that would solve the priest's problem." She claimed, furthermore, to have lost her faith completely, to see no meaning in life nor to understand why anyone else should find life meaningful.

A few months later, she said that the priest, having been told what had happened, wrote her "a rather cold, formal letter." Following this, and acting on the advice of a mutual friend, who she maintained "told her that the priest was still fond of her," she made contact with him. Whatever actually passed between them seems to have given her considerable emotional relief. She said she felt "much saner" and was able to view "the relationship" in a much more realistic way. Whereas she once used to believe "he was the only man there could ever be in my life," she now felt free to have "boyfriends" and indeed, during subsequent months, had a great many, once claiming that she went out with five different men in one week and was "getting quite a name for myself."

A year later there had been no return of her erotomanic attachment to the priest, although she remained an emotionally immature girl with a tendency to dramatise.

Case 3 differs from the previous ones as the patient was a male and there appears to have been a considerable affective element present. Despite the presence of some other psychotic manifestations and persistence in part of his original delusional belief, the outcome appears in the end to have been benign.

Case 3

A 41-year-old bachelor farmer was first seen on a domiciliary visit complaining of various physical symptoms for which no physical cause could be detected, together with a progressive preoccupation with feelings of guilt about masturbation. At the same time, he developed a passion for the local lady veterinary surgeon and believed that she reciprocated his feelings. She had visited his farm on a few occasions to attend to his stock, but apart from a few words of discussion about the animals, nothing else had passed between then. He, however, became obsessed with her, tried to visit her flat at night, telephoned and wrote passionate letters to her which sometimes had an obscene content, e.g. "What I would like to know is, is your mind the same as the day you did the bull?" In one such letter he stated also that he wanted to marry her and actually came to town on one occasion to see if she would do so at the Registry Office. He also made it clear that he believed she loved him. He admitted that she was above his station in life by reason of being vastly better educated (he himself was unable to read and write until eight years of age) and of having a profession. He referred to the fact that she had tried to discourage him and keep him away by remarking in another letter, "It is very annoying when we cannot speak to a person that means so much to life."

On occasions he had become severely depressed and allowed his farmhouse to deteriorate but did not, however, neglect his animals. His thoughts became muddled and confused, this being reflected in the content of some of his letters. He also believed that people in the area were talking about him, stating, in particular, that he should be married. He was also concerned about various "signs" which he had seen in paperback publications by Jehovah's Witnesses who had called on him fairly continuously during the previous months.

Treatment with psychotropic drugs was first begun at home, but because he did not co-operate but continued to pester the lady vet, he had to be compulsorily admitted to hospital. Following this he improved, and his *obsession* with the lady began to fade, although it did not entirely vanish.

Four years later he was referred again on account of having developed strange ideas and being worried about himself. However, by the time he was seen again, these symptoms had cleared. He then began to complain once again about numerous somatic symptoms. He was neither depressed on this occasion nor paranoid, and his condition improved when treated with a piperidine typical antipsychotic. Questioned again about the lady vet, he said that he had not seen her for several years as she had left the area, and he had made no further efforts to contact her. However, he maintained that he still believed that she had been in love with him, saying, "You can show feelings without saying anything."

When last seen he was without medication but had remained well.

Case 4

A 33-year-old divorcée presented believing that the songwriter Paul McCartney was in love with her. There was a family history of mental illness in that a maternal uncle had been a patient in a mental hospital for most of his life. Her parents were well, and she was the eldest of four children. A younger brother was apparently suffering from schizophrenia.

Her own personal history was rather chaotic in that she had had several relationships and had never kept a job for any length of time. She alleged that she had been forcibly seduced by her first boyfriend at the age of 16 years, then married an Iranian cook whom she divorced after nine months, alleging physical abuse. At present she was living with a lesbian. She had also had three therapeutic abortions for unwanted pregnancies.

She claimed that she had first met McCartney at the age of 18 years when she asked him for his autograph. Since that meeting she alleged that he had been besotted with her. A few days after the initial encounter an artist called on her to ask if he could sketch her portrait, saying that Paul McCartney had sent him. She said that she then had a short-lived affair with McCartney until she was 19 years of age. Her feelings towards him then changed because he had plagued and dominated her life. She stated that he did this because he is obsessed with her and wishes to marry her. She believed that he follows her wherever she goes and if unable to do this, he sends his entourage or "puppets" instead. She claimed that on several occasions she had been abducted by him, that he takes her to a hotel, shows her photographs that he has of her and forces her to have intercourse. McCartney's private physician then gives her an injection of some substance that makes her forget the experiences.

Mental state examination revealed a well-presented and attractive young woman with a central primary delusion. There was no disorder of form of thought, and hallucinations were absent while cognitive functioning was intact. However, she did have some ideas of reference.

Following several months' treatment, the delusions responded to perphenazine. However, after remaining asymptomatic for one year, the identical symptoms returned. For several months antipsychotic medication was necessary to reduce the intensity of the delusions and allow her to lead a fairly normal life.

Cases 3 and 4 seem to adhere fairly closely to de Clérambault's original description. In none was there any evidence of other symptoms that might have led the observer to believe that the patients were psychotic. The next case, however, is in a somewhat different category and follows rather more closely Hart's (1921) description of *old maid's insanity*.

Case 5

A university lecturer, a spinster of 41 years, fell in love with an unmarried professor, some 10 years her senior, in another faculty. Her passion emerged quite suddenly, although there had previously been one or two prodromal episodes with others. She developed an elaborate delusional system with ideas of reference which were centred around her erotomania.

She believed that the students knew of her passion for him and his for her and signalled to him news of her arrival in the university, saying that when she was not there "he is at his keenest." She plagued him periodically, not writing much, and maintained that his efforts to discourage her and his apparent antagonism really belied his underlying deep passionate feelings towards her.

She believed that persons outside the university knew of the relationship. She even interpreted the actions of tradesmen and others as meaningful in the light of her passion. "The butcher laughs when things are right, also my own doctor. The clergyman 'looks daggers' at me and cuts me dead." Apart from this mono-ideistic delusion and the ideas of reference, there was little evidence of psychosis, and she was able to continue working. She was observed for a period of three years, during which her morbid passion remained unchanged apart from minor fluctuations. She professed to have had several erotic experiences during childhood and had had a sexual affair with an elderly widower that persisted for several years and considerably antedated her passion for the university professor.

The next case is significant in revealing what occurs when the object of the delusion is, for some reason, removed from the scene.

Case 6

The subject of the case was a 50-year-old woman who was persistently mentally ill for over 20 years. She was the younger of a family of two children. She had never seen her mother, who had run away with another man when she was a baby. Her childhood was traumatic in that at the age of 5 years she was sexually interfered with by a man and at the age of 11 years was sexually interfered with by her father. She had three children, and one of her twin sons had been hospitalised for years with schizophrenia. She had been married for 24 years, but the marriage ended in divorce in 1976. Since then she had been living with a common-law husband and at the time of writing had been working as an auxiliary nurse and as a part-time saleswoman on a market stall. Since 1962, she had received various psychiatric treatments including antipsychotic medication and ECT. Although there had been periods of better functioning, she had remained psychotic throughout treatment. She became erotically preoccupied with a series of quantity surveyors. At the beginning of her illness, she implicated one quantity surveyor in a certain office and accused him of being the father of her twins. After a period of many years he died, but the patient then transferred her obsessive feelings onto another quantity surveyor from the same office. She would give a detailed description of how she met him and accused him of being the father of her third child. This man eventually retired and left the district, but then the patient began to have similar feelings about yet another quantity surveyor, again in the same office.

A mental state examination showed her to be a pleasant middle-aged woman. Her speech was spontaneous and her affect normal. However, she was psychotic in that she had a well-encapsulated delusional system. There were no hallucinations, and her cognitive functions were intact.

In contrast to the previous cases, of which the first four at least appear to adhere fairly closely to de Clérambault's concept, the next has been chosen as an example of frank paranoid schizophrenia having an erotomanic delusion as a focal point. Despite this seemingly primary feature, a marked disturbance of ego function was evident together with other unequivocally schizophrenic symptoms.

Case 7

Six years before first being seen, a 44-year-old divorced lady developed a sudden attraction for a highly respected married man who worked in the same firm. From then, she felt a "strong awareness" of his presence, strong rapport and occasional "accidental-on-purpose touching" for a month or so. She then became increasingly aware of "odd pressure" in her head and a "heavy, weighed-down pressure" on her shoulders which she had never experienced before, which she attributed to the man to whom she was so strongly attracted.

Eventually the point was reached when not only did she experience the pressure sensations in her head but, for the first time, heard a voice saying "We've made it, we've done it!" This she interpreted as meaning that some sort of barrier had been broken as a result of which she was now able to communicate with her *lover* via mental telepathy, he being a "transmitter" and she being the "receiver." It was, she said, like someone talking to her "via a mental wavelength." The next day when she and the man were sitting together at work, she heard him say, in her mind, as it were, "I love you." She replied in a similar vein, i.e. with her mind and with no words actually spoken. She felt as though she had had this form of contact continuously, right up to the time she was first seen, "sometimes willingly, sometimes most unwillingly." She also said that she had "an unignorable sexual heat and stimulation" in the pit of her stomach together with sensations in her vagina as if a man were entering into her in such a manner as might lead to orgasm. To her this was a way of experiencing a sexual relation without having an actual affair.

Throughout this time she heard the man's voice and sometimes someone else's also, clearly but quietly in her head. Sometimes what the voices said seemed to make sense; at others it would be all "mumble-jumble, completely incomprehensible!" One of the voices that she heard made derogatory remarks about her. Sometimes these consisted of a constant repetition of words which appeared to her to constitute a kind of lovemaking: "corn," "maize," "wheat," "engineering," "organisation," "pornography," "fuck," "lust," "cunt," "shit," "will," "John," "master-control," "fornication," "browned", "in," and so on. She said that for a 10-day period she had heard "shit" spoken almost continuously. She was so upset by this that she sent the man two packets of toilet paper through the post without attempting to disguise her handwriting! She also became increasingly aware of being made to see "sexual symbols" in quite ordinary things. At a later date this started what she believed the man concerned called "bunking," a kind of involuntary contraction of her pelvis over which she felt she had no control.

From the remarks made by the voices it seemed as though he knew all about her and her past. Sometimes the voice was more loving. On one occasion he said, "We are going to get married." Following this experience she started to knit baby clothes.

With drug treatment her condition improved considerably so that she soon began to feel so well as to have no need to take medication. Following this defection, and as might be expected, her florid psychotic symptoms returned, and thereafter she refused to co-operate in treatment.

Clinical features

De Clérambault's syndrome exists in a primary form where the delusion is the only psychopathology, when it can be referred to as *primary* or *pure* erotomania. This monodelusional state was termed "erotic monomania" by Esquirol (1845); other monomanias include pyromania, religious mania, reasoning mania and homicidal mania (Mullen et al., 2000).

When, however, the condition is merely part of a more generalised paranoid psychosis or other psychotic disorder, it is better termed *secondary* erotomania.

The clinical features of the primary syndrome, which need not all occur simultaneously, are:

- A delusional conviction of being in amorous communication with another person.
- This person is of a much higher rank.
- This person was the first to fall in love and to make advances.
- The object of the amorous delusion remains unchanged.
- The patient gives an explanation of the loved one's paradoxical behaviour.
- The course is chronic.
- Hallucinations and other psychotic features are absent.
- The onset is often sudden.

As has been shown, not all of de Clérambault's own cases were of the pure type, some suffering apparently from other possibly related paranoid psychoses. However, some of these other cases together with Balduzzi's (1956) case and another cited by Baruk (1959) do appear, at least at first sight, to fall within the former category. It is of historical interest to note that, in contrast to the above, Krafft-Ebing (1893) observed that hallucinations may indeed be a feature of erotomania, while Kraeplin (1921) agreed and further suggested that paramnesias might be a feature (see also Berrios and Kennedy, 2002; Marková and Berrios, 2000).

Of the cases we ourselves have reported, the first appears to be an example of pure erotomania. It is, however, atypical in that although there were no ideas of reference and the morbid passion had a precise onset, the patient did not openly proclaim her "lover's" affections towards her unless pressed to do so, and even then freely admitted that she did most of the chasing, not, as is more usually the case, that he was in amorous pursuit of her. There were no unequivocal psychotic features in her case, although much of her behaviour had a "psychopathic" tinge.

Our second case is one which some might choose to regard as an exaggerated adolescent *crush*. There were, nevertheless, other features that seem to justify inclusion of her condition under the heading of de Clérambault syndrome. Of particular interest was her apparent *cure by confrontation*, which, it should be noted, is an exceptional occurrence.

Our third case also appears to fulfil de Clérambault's postulates, although some ideas of reference were, for a time, apparent. While he later lost these, his delusion that the lady to whom he was so strongly attracted also loved him still persisted, although the strength of this notion appears to have waned sufficiently as to compel him no longer to take any action on this account.

Our fourth and fifth cases show more extensive ideas of reference and appear, on this account, to be closer to an overt paranoid psychosis. Nevertheless, there were no hallucinations or unequivocal symptoms of schizophrenia. Their conditions may therefore be regarded as *encapsulated*, a state of affairs that persisted during the several years both were kept under observation.

Our last case, in contrast to the previous six, suffered extensively not only from persistent auditory hallucinations but also, as has already been noted, from other obviously schizophrenic symptoms, and on this account falls quite clearly outside of de Clérambault's category.

The *subject* is likely to be a woman; many of the reported male cases are in fact examples of secondary erotomania (Magner, 1992; Durson et al., 1994). There is no evidence to support the claim of Arieti and Meth (1959) that the affected women are generally married. An examination of de Clérambault's cases not only fails to demonstrate this, but it should also be noted that five of our seven cases were unmarried, and two were divorcées. In Brüne's (2001) review of 246 published cases of erotomania gleaned from the whole of the twentieth century, the majority (69%) were women; 76% of the women were unmarried, as were 95% of the men; women were older (mean age at onset 33.5 years) and of higher social status (5% high, 59% average) than men (mean age at onset 28 years; 55% of low social status).

The *object*, usually a man, is typically someone with whom the subject has had only a brief acquaintance. He is often intellectually and socially superior and generally much older than the patient. It is not unusual, in today's age of mass communication and heavy media reporting, for the object to be a well-known public figure. The age of the love object was available in 107 cases in Brüne's (2001) review; there was a marked sex difference, with the object being older for women with erotomania (74% older, 7% the same, 19% younger) and younger for men with erotomania (21% older, 13% the same, 67% younger). In 206 cases, the social status of the love object was also estimated to be higher for women with erotomania (87% high, 13% low) compared with affected men (72% high, 28% low) (Brüne, 2001). The perceived sexual attractiveness of the love object was available in 42 cases and again showed a marked sex difference, with the object being rated as sexually attractive in just over half the cases for women with erotomania (10/18 or 56%) but in nearly all cases for men with erotomania (23/24 or 96%) (Brüne, 2001). The number of love objects was similar for women and men, being reported, in 246 cases, as usually being "one" (82% for women with erotomania, 80% for men), less often as "consecutive" (14% for women, 16% for men) and least often as "simultaneous" (6% for women, 4% for men) (Brüne, 2001).

Cases in which the pathological interest in the object is of a homosexual or homoerotic nature have been infrequently reported (Peterson and Davis, 1985; Urbach et al., 1992; Boast and Coid, 1994), including examples of female homosexual erotomania (Dunlop, 1988). Michael et al. (1996) described a case of homosexual erotomania that at a later stage developed into heterosexual erotomania.

Some patients may bring chaos to the lives of their victims. They may bombard them with text messages, letters (including e-mail) and telephone calls, and via social media, without respite, both at home and at work and for long periods of time. The psychological stress and personal strain experienced by victims can be immense and exacting. Faden et al. (2017) reported the case of a 24-year-old male college student who repeatedly sent unwanted Twitter messages to a female student. After she gave a printout of his reams of messages to both the police and the college administration, he continued to send her messages, changing his Twitter username on each occasion. Following admission, he was diagnosed with erotomania (delusional disorder, erotomanic type) and treated with risperidone, to which he appeared to show little response; he was subsequently lost to follow-up (Faden et al., 2017).

Some patients have been arrested for *stalking* or even perpetrating assaults on the objects of their delusions. The latter phenomenon is particularly liable to occur when the patient reaches the stage of resentment or hatred that often replaces the love after repeated advances are unrequited. The forensic aspects of the condition are covered in a later section of this chapter.

The prevalence of suicidal attempts by sufferers is uncertain. Kovács et al. (2005) reported the case of a suicide attempt by a 35-year-old male sufferer whose erotomania was associated with depression. Two months following the start of antidepressant treatment, he became euthymic, and within a further three months his erotomania resolved (Kovács et al., 2005).

Aetiology and psychopathology

A great debate continues concerning the nosological status of de Clérambault's syndrome: Is its occurrence always seen as part of another psychotic disorder/ process, or can it develop and exist in a pure, primary form? The arguments underpinning each point of view are not restricted to de Clérambault syndrome and have been applied to many eponymous conditions.

To some extent the wheel of history has turned full circle, and conditions which in former times would have been classed as paranoia or as a monomania once again are categorised as disorders distinct from the schizophrenias in modern classificatory systems. The term "delusional disorder" is found in both *ICD-10* and *DSM-5* and refers to a group of conditions characterised by a single delusion (said to be "non-bizarre" in the previous *DSM-IV*) or set of related delusions of a highly variable content and in which hallucinations, although sometimes present, are not prominent. In the case of *DSM-IV* and *DSM-5*, a separate, distinct subtype – *erotomanic type* – is recognised. At the time of writing, it appears likely that the forthcoming *ICD-11* will include delusional disorder within the block on "schizophrenia or other primary psychotic disorders" (Gaebel, 2012).

The aetiology of the condition is not clearly understood. Although it has been described in association with cases of clear organic pathology, its causation and psychopathology is almost certainly that of a functional psychosis. Particularly in examples of the primary syndrome, the disorder can often be understood as arising from psychopathological processes superimposed upon pre-existing prominent personality traits. Kelly (2005) has expressed the hope that future genetic and neuroimaging studies, together with insights from evolutionary psychopathology, will deepen and broaden our understanding.

Nosology

Ellis and Mellsop (1985) reviewed 53 cases described in the English literature between 1966 and 1985 along with five cases of their own and as a result questioned the existence of the primary syndrome. They argued that under close examination the majority of cases simply do not fulfil all of de Clérambault's postulates and can adequately be classified, therefore, as examples of other disorders such as schizophrenia.

Alternatively, however, Mullen and Pathé (1984) described 16 cases, and on dividing their sample into the primary (5 cases) and secondary (11 cases) syndromes, observed some factors to distinguish between the two groups. For example, the primary group all fulfilled *DSM-III-R* criteria for personality disorder, and in the second group the erotic focus tended to shift from one object to another. These authors argued that the concept of primary erotomania as a distinct diagnostic entity should remain. A similar view was later expounded by Garland and McGennis (1998), at least on pragmatic grounds.

It is the authors' view, therefore, no doubt to the chagrin of those who dislike eponymous syndromes, that there is some justification for the retention of de Clérambault's syndrome as a nosological entity.

Biology

Cases have been recorded in the literature in which erotomanic symptomatology and syndromes have occurred in association with such coarse brain diseases as Alzheimer's disease, HIV infection, brain damage and a left frontal lobe tumour (Drevets, 1987; Boast and Coid, 1994; John and Ovsiew, 1996; Stupinski et al., 2017). A useful review of the several reported cases of erotomania associated with neurological and medical conditions has been conducted by Anderson et al. (1998). Such examples, however, form a small minority of all cases recorded and, in aetiological terms, de Clérambault syndrome behaves like a functional psychosis.

Michael et al. (1996) described an interesting case of bisexual erotomania associated with polycystic ovary disease. These authors, in the light of the condition having also been observed following the ingestion of oral contraceptives and steroids and following abortion, postulated that a disturbance in the balance of central monoamines may provide an organic substrate for the psychosis. Further, Wijeratne et al. (1997) reported a case of primary erotomania in which structural and functional neuroimaging revealed left medial temporal lobe damage due to childhood radiotherapy administered for a tumour. The authors discussed this case in the setting of contemporary ideas about the relationship between psychotic symptoms and brain function and, in particular, how connections between the medial temporal lobe and the frontal cortex may be impaired in psychotic patients. Delusions subsequently result because of a failure of internal cognitive monitoring.

It is interesting to note that, of the 15 patients with erotomania studied by Kennedy et al. (2002), almost half (seven) had a positive psychiatric history in a first-degree relative. Of these, three (20% of the total) had a parental history of a monodelusional disorder, suggesting the possibility of a genetic component to monodelusional disorders (Kennedy et al., 2002).

Psychodynamics

An ambivalent sexual attitude often lies at the heart of the psychopathology of erotomania. Erotomania is certainly not founded upon platonic love. On the contrary, de Clérambault showed that most patients craved for a sexual relationship. The writings of some of them surpassed the imagination in terms of sensual crudity. There certainly appears to have been nothing platonic in the association of our first case with her lover, whom she attempted to seduce by providing contraceptives. And yet, despite this, and taking into account the fact that the patients are themselves so frequently unmarried and that the love object is usually unattainable, not only because of differing social status but by virtue of being married or unmarriageable for other reasons, the observer may be forced to the conclusion that however overtly sexual the patient's behaviour, a need exists to avoid sexual fulfilment. It is this that may lead in some cases to the patient developing a notion that she is being persecuted so that she fears that sexual advances may be thrust upon her.

Unfortunately, de Clérambault devoted very little attention to the previous histories or personalities of the patients he otherwise described in meticulous detail. Consequently, he made little reference to the psychopathology of the condition. An attempt at understanding the psychopathology can be made with reference to our own cases.

Our first case was an only child. Her mother died when she was 4 years of age and probably when she was well into the Oedipal situation. She was then left to the attentions of her overpowering father, whom she resented from the time she was 9 years old, although she obtained comfort from an uncle, "a quiet, passive type", whom she much preferred to her father. Thereafter she sought the company of older men, resulting in further paternal disapproval. She admitted that her lover, a mother-bound individual, reminded her very much of her uncle but maintained that both he and her uncle had completely opposite temperaments to her father.

Our second patient also had a disturbed relationship with her father, whom she despised on account of his behaviour when drunk. This might well have led her to transfer her affection to her love object, a priest, who, to her, clearly represented an *ideal* father, one who could not only be loved on this account but, furthermore, loved safely, i.e. without any danger of sexual reciprocity. The likely truth of this seems to be shown by the fact that when she learned that a friend had actually had a sexual relationship with another priest, the "safeness" of her own fantasy relationship fell into doubt. Hence her suicidal attempt, together with the psychological projection that this would "solve the priest's problem."

The affective element and hypochondriacal features apparent in our third patient have already been noted. However, a more striking feature from the point of view of his underlying psychopathology may have been his strong feelings of sexual guilt, overtly about masturbation, but possibly more likely over latent homosexual tendencies. This may have accounted for the transient emergence of mild ideas of reference at one stage, particularly his belief that people in his locality were stating that he ought to be married.

Our fifth patient, whose condition has been likened to Hart's (1921) *old maid's insanity*, differs from those so far considered in that she had actually had several previous sexual experiences, in particular, when she was much younger, a prolonged affair with a much older man. She, however, felt persistently guilty over this affair, especially on account of the remonstrations of her overpowering mother. It should be noted furthermore that her love object, an unmarried middle-aged university professor, may well have been homosexual, though this could not be proven. Indeed, the selected love objects in many instances of the erotomanic syndrome merit further study. In addition to Case 5, the supposed "lover" in Case 1 was also an unmarried middle-aged bachelor, who once again could well have had covert, if not overt, homosexual tendencies and like the priest in Case 2 may have been regarded as unattainable on this as well as other counts and therefore "safe" as a love object.

This theme may be worth further pursuit. Thus Arieti and Meth (1959) suggested that in erotomania the love involved may be self-love, denied or projected onto another person, or alternatively may be a defensive manoeuvre which substitutes a delusional heterosexual attachment for denied unconscious homoerotic trends not altogether dissimilar to the psychogenic mechanisms in the delusional jealousy syndrome. Freud's representation of this defensive manoeuvre is contained in the formulation, "I don't love *him*; I love *her*, because *she* loves *me*." Reik (1963), however, considered that Freud's formulation did not pay sufficient attention to the role of narcissism in erotomania and saw this illness as representing a self-rescue attempt by the patient, "from the depth of contempt and humiliation" which derived from insignificance.

Narcissism there is indeed in these cases, and in plenty. For example, Marie Bashkirtseff, a young Russian girl who developed an overwhelming passion for the Duke of Hamilton (which, although she had never actually met him, lasted seven years and filled very many of the pages of the 84 volumes of her diary) was, according to her biographer, Doris Langley Moore, even more narcissistic than is usual for an adolescent. Thus, in addition to complaining that she did not enjoy a performance at the opera because there was no one there to admire her, she wrote, "I am capable of remaining for hours together in my dressing room quite naked in front of the glass. Never has anyone seen such whiteness, fineness and elegance of modelling" (Moore, 1966).

Perhaps Balduzzi (1956), although he did not specifically refer to his patients as having marked narcissistic tendencies, nevertheless concluded that her desire for affection reached obsessional proportions as a result of losing the attentions of her relations. Her husband, a harsh man with a paranoid jealous disposition who was much older than herself, seemed to reproduce the paternal image. However, there existed these two which led

Balduzzi to speculate as to whether the patient's psychosis might have been induced by her husband's own morbid mentality. Furthermore, her husband and father were psychologically similar, so that while under the influence of a "negative infantile repressive phase" she was neurotically motivated to an absurd marriage. During the course of her matrimonial life, this neurosis steadily asserted itself, only to erupt suddenly into an "expansive and positive phase" when she first encountered her lover. At the same time she rationalised her conviction of certainty by emphasising her past suffering and stated that until that moment she had never lived. In her psychosis, however, she had not escaped from her Oedipal conflict but showed instead a tendency to strengthen it, in so far as she sought refuge and shelter in her delusions. Such observations suggest that in this psychosis, as in others, there is a persistence into adult life of infantile modes of thinking. On this basis, delusional reasoning, which may so readily be superimposed, becomes more meaningful.

The "ideo affective knot" tantamount to the development of *psychose passionelle* rests upon a basis of unsatisfied affection on the one hand and the necessity for rebellion on the other. Furthermore, de Clérambault himself emphasised that the principal source of erotomania is really sexual *pride* rather than love: "Pride predominates over passion, for never has thwarted passion been able to produce such durable results." Erotomania then evolves from pride, leading to desire and then to hope. If hope is repeatedly spurned, it may readily be replaced by a phase of spite and grievance, depending on the personality of the patient and the circumstances of the *affaire de coeur*. This is often illustrated in the writings of these patients and in the otherwise unprovoked attacks that they have been known to make upon their lovers and those associated with them. When this phase is reached, however, it may completely overshadow the original erotomania, readily leading to misdiagnosis of the condition and an erroneous tendency on behalf of clinicians to classify all these cases as paranoid or examples of paranoid schizophrenia.

Erotomania and love

Erotomania is fundamentally about being loved, and not loving, and is certainly not, therefore, a variant of the aspect of the human condition understood by laypeople as romantic or erotic love. The two concepts do, however, share some common characteristics.

Erotic love is undoubtedly a powerful force, often of passionate intensity, whose presence may so influence an individual's behaviour as to lead others to conclude that in such a condition reason becomes impaired. This phenomenon finds its expression in many commonly quoted terms, such as 'head over heels in love' and "starry eyed." In the popular mind, therefore, where madness and rationality are intimately related, intense erotic love can be viewed as a form of madness. This opinion was expressed even in ancient times by Cicero: "Of all the emotions there is none more violent than love" and "Love is madness" (Rather, 1965).

Furthermore, it is known that love, particularly if unrequited, can have adverse consequences for an individual's physical, mental and spiritual health. Thus did Jerome Gaub write in 1763, in his essay 'De Regimene Mentis': "How often do beautiful maidens and handsome youths, caught in the toils of love, grow ghastly pale and waste away, consumed by melancholy green sickness or erotomania" (Mayer, 1921).

Likewise in his *Decameron*, Boccacio wrote of Lisa, daughter of an apothecary, who fell deeply in love with King Pietro of Aragon, whom she saw riding by: "Her love continued to increase and one melancholy mood followed another until the girl could endure it no longer and fell ill, plainly wasting away from day to day like snow in the sun."

At the turn of the eighteenth century, Sir Alexander Crichton (1798) speculated on the dynamics of falling in love:

> A curious question arises which is, upon what principle is this sudden and romantic admiration to be explained? Those who fall in love have not for any personal acquaintance had any proof of the moral qualities of the person they love and yet their love is as much founded on a supposed moral beauty as on personal charms. The true explanation seems to be this. Every person is endowed to a certain degree with physiognomical science, founded on the cast of features of those who have been our associates through life. We think that experience has uniformly shewn us, that a certain cast of moral features belongs to a certain moral character, and this kind of judgement becomes so habitual to us that we all form prepossessions either in favour or against other people at first sight.

Crichton referred to Shakespeare's acknowledgement of this principle in making some of his most exulted lovers, for example, Romeo and Juliet and Rosalind and Orlando, fall in love *suddenly*. His ideas seem very far ahead of his time and pre-empt the psychoanalytic concept of transference and the ethologic paradigm of imprinting.

Berrios and Kennedy (2002) argued that:

> Erotomania is a construct, a mirror reflecting Western views on spiritual and physical love, sex, and gender inequality and abuse. On account of this, it is unlikely that there will ever be a final, "scientific" definition rendering erotomania into a "natural kind" and making it susceptible to brain localization and biological treatment.

Perhaps the application of empathic psychology, therefore, allows some understanding of the forces driving the behaviour of some erotomanic patients and the persistence displayed in their attempts to make contact with the love object.

Management and treatment

The essential components of the treatment of erotomania, particularly the primary syndrome, are:

* Admission to hospital, if necessary under the provisions of mental health legislation
* Antipsychotic medication
* Long-term supportive psychotherapy

Treatment of primary erotomania (de Clérambault's syndrome) is first and foremost medication in the form of antipsychotic drugs in low to moderate doses combined with counselling and psychotherapy. Historically, *pimozide* has been noted to have a specific anti-erotomanic action, particularly in primary erotomania (Mullen and Pathé, 1984; Munro et al., 1985; Durson et al., 1994). More recently, atypical antipsychotics such as *clozapine, risperidone* and *olanzapine* have been reported to be useful as a first-line treatment (Kelly, 2005; Grandstein et al., 2015; Alao et al., 2000).

The psychotherapeutic approach should consist of confronting the cognitive distortions which help sustain erotomanic fixations, and an attempt should be made to move the patient on so as to engage more successfully with other people. The treatment process is often protracted and frustrating with frequent reverses and slow progress, the real therapeutic gains only occurring if the patient can be persuaded to remain in regular long-term treatment.

Since patients often do require considerable psychotherapeutic support over a long period, there is the inherent danger of the erotic focus shifting onto the therapist. Therefore, it is imperative that the therapeutic relationship develops within the setting of adequate clinical supervision, especially if the patient and practitioner are of different genders.

In secondary (symptomatic) erotomania, treatment should be aimed at the underlying disorder, e.g. often mania or schizophrenia, augmented where appropriate with antipsychotic agents and psychotherapeutic interventions directed at the erotomanic element. A few cases have been reported in the literature in which an amelioration of symptoms occurred following the use of electroconvulsive therapy (ECT), not only in secondary erotomania but also in the primary syndrome (Munro et al., 1985; Remington and Jeffries, 1994).

Admission to hospital informally or compulsorily under the powers provided by mental health legislation may become necessary in some cases because of the real danger of the erotomanic patient causing harm to the object. In the case of the erotomanic stalker, it may be inappropriate to deal with him or her under the criminal legislation, e.g. the Protection from Harassment Act 1997 and the Protection of Freedoms Act 2012 (Sections 111 and 112 in relation to stalking). (Interestingly, the first anti-stalking legislation was passed in California in 1990 [Davis and Chipman, 1997].) Recourse to this method of disposal, perhaps with accompanying imprisonment, can sometimes aggravate the condition, causing greater resentment and so reinforcing the delusion. It is important to emphasise this point at a time when mental health professionals are increasingly approached for their opinions by courts and others about the appropriate disposal of erotomanic patients and especially stalkers driven by erotomanic delusions. For, in spite of an ongoing debate about the efficacy of the treatment described above, it can be emphasised that it is, at present, the only possible effective treatment capable of freeing the patient from an all-encompassing delusional preoccupation and the victim from a harrowing and dangerous pursuit. We disagree with Leong (1994), who proclaims that courts and social policy makers "should not place much emphasis on psychiatry and other mental health disciplines in diminishing the erotomanic delusion" and that criminal and civil sanctions are more appropriate in managing cases of erotomania.

Psychosocial factors must also be taken into consideration in the management of both primary and secondary erotomania. Social support groups and specific networks of patients can give effective support in reducing isolation and helping to create new relationships, thus helping to loosen the pathological relationship that dominates their lives.

Prognosis

Traditionally it has been considered that the prognosis of primary erotomania is poor and that it does not respond well to any form of treatment and usually follows a chronic course. The prognosis of secondary erotomania is regarded as being dependent upon the response to treatment of the underlying psychosis.

Published reports used to support this view; for example Segal (1989), in reviewing the literature and his own experience, noted the persistence of erotomanic delusions, except in a rare instance. Gillet et al. 1990 described a poor response in their four cases with an underlying schizophrenia and a surprisingly poor response in a case with an underlying mania – both the mania and the erotomanic delusions being refractory. Leong (1994) also emphasised the poor response to treatment, which led him to doubt the value of psychiatry in the management of this particular condition.

However, more recent reports appear to adopt a more optimistic view. Retterstol and Opjordsmoen 1991 reported a good response in two cases, fair in one and poor or uncertain in three others. Munro et al. (1985) have consistently advocated the use of the antipsychotic drug *pimozide* as being effective in the treatment of delusional disorders in general, including de Clérambault's syndrome. Stein 1986 has also supported the use of antipsychotic medication in this condition.

Mullen and Pathé 1994 clearly emphasised that the therapeutic pessimism of the past, regarding erotomania, was misplaced. In their experience four out of five pure erotomanic patients made a full recovery or showed a significant amelioration of symptoms with a combination of low-dose neuroleptics and supportive psychotherapy. The need for the persistence of the treatment over a long period of time was emphasised. The authors also noted that the response in secondary or symptomatic erotomania reflected the nature and severity of the underlying psychosis. For example, three cases secondary to a manic illness made a complete recovery, whereas those patients with an underlying schizophrenia tended to maintain their erotomanic delusions, albeit in a less florid and preoccupying form.

Jordan et al. (2006) have published two case reports of women suffering from erotomania, one who had been studied for 37 years and the other for over 30 years, making these amongst the longest single case longitudinal reported studies. The first, whose case was published by the same group in 1980 (Jordan and Howe, 1980), had continued to hold essentially unchanged erotomanic delusions over almost four decades in spite of treatment, including antipsychotic pharmacotherapy; there was only a two-to-three-week period of relative freedom from the delusions immediately following a course of ECT (12 shocks administered over four weeks). Similarly, in the second case, the erotomanic delusions have not responded to antipsychotic medication (Jordan et al., 2006).

There is some cause for optimism, however Kennedy et al. (2002) reported that, of three cases of primary erotomania, delusions eased but did not completely resolve with depot antipsychotic treatment in one case, while complete resolution occurred in association with pharmacotherapy with risperidone in one case and with trifluoperazine in the other. Of 12 cases of secondary erotomania, four out of nine subjects with schizophrenia or schizoaffective disorder did not respond to antipsychotic treatment, while all three cases of bipolar disorder only manifested erotomanic symptomology while manic, which completely resolved with treatment of these episodes (Kennedy et al., 2002).

It can be concluded, therefore, that the general therapeutic pessimism associated with the management of the erotomanic syndromes is misplaced. Unfortunately, in clinical practice, it becomes a self-fulfilling prophecy made prior to any substantial trials of treatment. However, a sea-change is occurring, and therapeutic pessimism is giving way to some therapeutic optimism in the light of recent research. We wish to endorse this positive shift in opinion while agreeing that there is a need for more long-term follow-up studies designed to establish more firmly the typology of erotomania, which should have clear therapeutic implications.

Forensic aspects

In recent years erotomania has attracted widespread public attention and renewed psychiatric interest on the grounds of its association with well-publicised examples of acts of violence, particularly when the victim has been of celebrity status, and because of the suggestion of a possible specific link with dangerousness. In 1848, Morison wrote, "Erotomania sometimes prompts those labouring under it to destroy themselves or others, for although in general tranquil and respectful, the patient sometimes becomes irritable, passionate and jealous." De Clérambault's (1942) believed that although erotomania began in pride, love and hope, it all too easily degenerated into resentment and anger.

Stalking – which can be defined as repeated attempts to establish intrusive and unwanted contact or other forms of communication with the object of the stalker's attention – is one potential behavioural consequence of the erotomanic syndromes. People in the public eye who have been stalked have included Catherine Zeta-Jones, Madonna, Steven Spielberg, Ken Dodd, Vanessa Mae and Andrew Murray. The majority (80–90%) of stalkers are male, while the majority of victims (around 80%) are female (James and MacKenzie, 2018). It should be noted, however, that earlier studies show that only about 10% of samples of stalkers suffer with erotomania (Melroy, 1994; Davis and Chipman, 1997). More recently, in a study of 211 stalkers referred to a community forensic mental health service, McEwan et al. (2009) found just six cases (3%) of erotomania. A study of 299 juvenile (aged 18 years or less) stalkers found essentially no evidence of erotomania in this age group (Purcell et al., 2009).

Some studies containing small samples of erotomanic offender patients have been published (Taylor et al., 1983; Noone and Cockhill, 1987; Leong, 1994). In their retrospective study, Menzies et al. (1995) reported the prevalence of erotomanic delusions in male forensic admissions to a secure psychiatric hospital with a diagnosis of psychosis to be nearly 2%, while for male patients admitted to a community psychiatric hospital with a diagnosis of delusional disorder it was a little over 3% (see also Menzies, 2017). Unlike the case in civil situations, most of the reported patients in a forensic setting are male, and the object tends to be female. This is consistent with the pattern of violent offences in general, where perpetrators tend to be predominantly male. In diagnostic terms, most of the patients in such samples are reported as suffering with schizophrenia (the secondary syndrome) or delusional disorder (primary erotomania).

The issue of whether the presence of erotomanic delusions *per se* necessarily results in an increase in the risk that the patient poses to others is unclear. The retrospective study of male erotomania by Menzies and colleagues pointed to two variables which discriminated dangerous from non-dangerous patients: a history of antisocial behaviour outside of the erotomanic attachment and the development of attachments to multiple objects (Menzies et al., 1995; Menzies, 2017). Leong (1994), in his sample, reported cases with no previous history of violent offending, possibly suggesting that erotomanic delusions were associated with a degree of inherent dangerousness. Taylor et al. (1983) support the view that de Clérambault syndrome should be considered a distinct clinical disorder because of the important advantages this approach brings, in particular that of being able to predict behaviour. This view is not shared, however, by Bowden (1990), who refers to the "spectre of dangerousness" which, in this condition, in reality, amounts to little more than an "apparition."

In cases where violence is perpetrated, the victim may not invariably be the love object. Melroy (1994) introduced the term (albeit predominantly with respect to the broader category of stalkers) "triangulation" to describe the phenomenon whereby the target of violence is a third party who is perceived by the subject as impeding access to the object. This author also discusses in some detail the psychodynamics of that particular process.

In the study of Leong (1994), in two out of the five cases the victims (and objects) were healthcare workers. Leong suggested that healthcare workers may be at special risk of becoming the objects of erotomanic attachments and that psychotherapists were at an even greater risk because of the processes of transference. In this regard, Pathe and Mullen (1993) refer to the "Hippocratic curse."

In summary, de Clérambault's syndrome may be taken to refer to pure erotomania and is an illness which requires medical treatment. The authors very much share Kelly's (2005) hope that future genetic and neuroimaging studies, with insights from evolutionary psychopathology, will deepen and broaden our understanding.

References

Alao, A.O., Armenta, W., Yolles, J.C., (2000). *Annals of Pharmacotherapy, 34,* 266.

Anderson, C.A., Camp, J., Filley, C.M., (1998). *Journal of Neuropsychiatry, 10/3,* 330.

Arieti, S., Meth, M. (eds), (1959). *American Handbook of Psychiatry,* Vol. 1. Basic Books, New York.

Balduzzi, E., (1956). *Rivista Sperimentale di Freniatria e Medicina Legale delle Alienazioni Mentali, 80,* 407.

Baruk, H., (1959). In *Traite de Psychiatre,* Vol. 1. Masson, Paris. See also Hirsch, S.R., Shepherd, M. (eds) (1974) *Themes and Variations in European Psychiatry.* Wright, Bristol.

Berrios, G.E.,Kennedy, N., (2002). *History of Psychiatry, 13,* 381.

Bianchi, L., (1906). *A Textbook of Psychiatry,* Trans. J.H. MacDonald. Baillière, Tindall and Cox, London.

Boast, N. and Coid, J., (1994). *British Journal of Psychiatry, 164,* 842.

Boccacio, G., (1349–1351). *The Decameron, The Tenth Day, Seventh Tale,* Trans. R. Aldington (1958), Vol. 2. Elek, London.

Bowden, P., (1990). In *Principles and Practice of Forensic Psychiatry,* Eds. R. Bluglass, P. Bowden. Churchill Livingstone, London.

Brüne, M., (2001). *Evolution and Human Behavior, 22,* 409.

Carter, S.M., (1995). *Clinical Gerontologist, 15/3,* 45.

Clérambault, C.G. de, (1942). *Les Psychoses Passionelles,* Oeuvre Psychiatrique. Presses Universitaires,Paris.

Clouston, T.S., (1887). *Clinical Lectures on Mental Diseases,* 2nd edn. Churchill, London.

Crichton, A., (1798). *An Enquiry into the Nature and Origen of Mental Derangement,* Vol. 2. Cadell and Davies, London,312.

Davis, J.A., Chipman, M.A., (1997). *Journal of Clinical Forensic Medicine, 4,* 166.

Drevets, W.C., (1987). *British Journal of Psychiatry, 151,* 400.

Dunlop, J.L., (1988). *British Journal of Psychiatry, 153,* 830.

Durson, S.M., Mathew, V.M., Reveley, M.A., (1994). *Journal of Psychopharmacology, 8/3,* 185.

Ellis, P., Mellsop, G., (1985). *British Journal of Psychiatry, 146,* 90.

Esquirol, E., (1845). *Mental Maladies. Treatise on Insanity,* Trans. E.K. Hunt. Lea and Blanchard, Philadelphia.

Faden, J., Levin, J., Mistry, R., Wang, J., (2017). *Case Reports in Psychiatry,* 10.1155/2017/8652524.

Feder, S., (1973). *International Journal of Psychoanalytic Psychotherapy, 2,* 240.

Gaebel, W., (2012). *Schizophrenia Bulletin, 38,* 895.

Garland, M., McGennis, A., (1998). *Irish Journal of Psychological Medicine, 15/1,* 22.

Gillet, T., Eminson, S.R., & Hassanyeh, F. (1990). *Acta Psychiatrica Scandinavica, 82/1,* 65, 10.1111/acp.1990.82.issue-1.

Grandstein, J., Strimbu, K., Francois, D., Kahn, D., (2015). *Journal of Psychiatric Practice, 21,* 306.

Hart, B., (1921). *The Psychology of Insanity.* Cambridge University Press, Cambridge.

Holzer, L., (2017). *Acta Psychopathologica, 3,* 3.

Hunter, R., Macalpine, I., (1963). *Three Hundred Years of Psychiatry.* Oxford University Press, London.

James, D.V., MacKenzie, R.D. (2018). In *Forensic Psychiatry: Fundamentals and Clinical Practice,* Eds. B.K. Puri, I.H. Treasaden. CRC Press, Boca Raton.

John, S., Ovsiew, F., (1996). *Journal of Intellectual Disability Research, 40/3,* 279.

Jordan, H.W., Howe, G., (1980). *Journal of the National Medical Association, 72,* 979.

Jordan, H.W., Lockert, E.W., Johnson-Warren, M., Cabell, C., Cooke, T., Greer, W., Howe, G., (2006). *Journal of the National Medical Association, 98,* 787.

Kelly, B.D., (2005). *CNS Drugs, 19,* 657.

Kennedy, N., McDonough, M., Kelly, B., Berrios, G.E., (2002). *Comprehensive Psychiatry, 43,* 1.

Kovács, A., Vörös, V., Fekete, S., (2005). *Archives of Suicide Research, 9,* 369.

Kraepelin, E., (1921). *Manic Depressive Insanity and Paranoia,* Trans. M. Barclay, Ed. E. Robertson. Livingstone, Edinburgh.

Krafft-Ebing, R. von, (1893). *Lehrbuch der Psychiatrie,* 5th edn. Ferdinand Enke, Stuttgart.

Leong, G.B., (1994). *Journal of Forensic Sciences*, *39/2*, 378.
Lerner, V., Kaptsan, A., Witztum, E., (2001). *Canadian Journal of Psychiatry*, *46*, 441.
Macpherson, J., (1889). *An Introduction to the Study of Insanity*. Macmillan, London.
Magner, M.B., (1992). *South African Medical Journal*, *81*, 167.
Mann, J., Foreman, D.M., (1996). *Journal of Intellectual Disability Research*, *40/3*, 275.
Mannion, L., Carney, P.A., (1996). *European Psychiatry*, *11/7*, 378.
Marková, I.S., Berrios, G.E., (2000). In *Memory Disorders in Psychiatric Practice*, Eds. G.E. Berrios, J.H. Hodges. Cambridge University Press, Cambridge.
Mayer, W., (1921). *Zeitschrift Gesamte Neurologie und Psychiatrie*, *71*, 187.
McEwan, I., (1997). *Enduring Love*. Jonathan Cape, London.
McEwan, T.E., Mullen, P.E., MacKenzie, R.D., Ogloff, J.R.P., (2009). *Psychological Medicine*, *39*, 1469.
Melroy, J.R., (1994). *Journal of Forensic Science*, *44/2*, 421.
Menzies, R.P.D., (2017). *Forensic Psychiatry: Fundamentals and Clinical Practice*, Eds. B.K. Puri, I.H. Treasaden. CRC Press, Boca Raton
Menzies, R.P., Fedoroff, J.P., Green, C.M., Isaacson, K., (1995). *British Journal of Psychiatry*, *166*, 529.
Michael, A., Zolese, G., Dinan, T.G., (1996). *Psychopathology*, *29/3*, 181.
Moore, D.L., (1966). *Marie and the Duke of H.* Cassell, London.
Mullen, P.E., Pathé, M., (1984). *British Journal of Psychiatry*, *146*, 90.
Mullen, P.E., Pathe, M., (1994). *British Journal of Psychiatry*, *165*, 614–23.
Mullen, P.E., Pathé, M.,Purcell, R., (2000). *Stalkers and Their Victims*. Cambridge University Press, Cambridge.
Munro, A., O'Brien, J.V., Ross, D., (1985). *Canadian Journal of Psychiatry*, *30*, 619.
Noone, J.A., Cockhill, L., (1987). *American Journal of Psychiatry*, *8*, 23.
Pathe, M., Mullen, P.E., (1993). *Medical Journal of Australia*, *159/9*, 632.
Pearce, A., (1972). *British Journal of Psychiatry*, *121*, 116.
Peterson, G.A., Davis, D.L., (1985). *Journal of Clinical Psychiatry*, *46*, 448.
Purcell, R., Moller, B., Flower, T., Mullen, P.E., (2009). *British Journal of Psychiatry*, *194*, 451.
Rather, L.J., (1965). *Mind and Body in Eighteenth Century Medicine*. The Wellcome Historical Medical Library, London.
Reik, T., (1963). *The Need to Be Loved*. Farrer, Straus, New York.
Remilagton, G.I., (1997). *Journal of Clinical Psychiatry*, *58/9*, 406.
Remington, G.J., Jeffries, J.J., (1994). *Journal of Clinical Psychiatry*, *55*, 306.
Retterstol, N., & Opjordsmoen, S. (1991). *Psychopathology*, *24*, 388–97.
Rot, U., (2008). *European Neurology*, *60*, 12.
Signer, S.F., Cummings, J.L., (1987). *British Journal of Psychiatry*, *151*, 404.
Segal, J.H. (1989). *American Journal of Psychiatry*, *146*, 1261, 10.1176/ajp.146.10.1261.
Sims, A., White, A., (1973). *British Journal of Psychiatry*, *123*, 635.
Singh, H., Ganjekar, S., Ghandhi, P.B., Thyloth, M., (2014). *Journal of Mental Health and Human Behaviour*, *19*, 83.
Stein, M. (1986). *Canadian Journal of Psychiatry*, *31/3*, 289, 10.1177/070674378603100326.
Strip, E., Lecomte, T., Debruille, J.B., (1996). *Australian and New Zealand Journal of Psychiatry*, *30/2*, 299.
Stupinski, J., Kim, J. Francois, D., (2017). *Journal of Neuropsychiatry and Clinical Neurosciences*, *29*, 186.

Taylor, P., Mahendra, B., Gunn, J., (1983). *Psychological Medicine, 13*, 645.

Urbach, J.R., Khalily, C., Mitchell, P.P., (1992). *Journal of Adolescence, 15*, 231.

Wijeratne, C., Hickie, I., Schwartz, R. (1997). *Australia and New Zealand Journal of Psychiatry, 31*, 765.

Wright, S., Young, A.W., Hellawell, D.J., (1993). *Journal of Neurology, Neurosurgery and Psychiatry, 56/3*, 322.

Zilboog, G., (1941). *A History of Medical Psychology.* Norton, London and New York.

Chapter 3

Othello syndrome

> But jealous souls will not be answer'd so;
> They are not ever jealous for the cause,
> But jealous for they are jealous: 'tis a monster,
> Begot upon itself, born on itself.
>
> William Shakespeare, Othello (III, iv)

Othello syndrome is an illness in which a delusion of infidelity of the spouse is the central denominating symptom. The delusion of infidelity can occur in pure form or in a setting of an already established psychosis. In the latter case, there is some doubt as to whether the term "Othello syndrome" is appropriate, but if the delusion is constant, central and dominates the symptomatology, then its use may be justified. If, however, delusion is merely one minor, inconstant feature of another psychotic process, the term is not applicable.

- Other suggestive titles given to this condition include sexual jealousy (Kraepelin, 1910), the erotic jealousy syndrome (Langfeldt, 1961; 1962), morbid jealousy (Ey, 1950; Shepherd, 1961; Mowat, 1966) and, perhaps most apt of all, psychotic jealously, paranoid jealousy or delusional jealousy.
- When it does occur in pure form, it may be regarded as a special variety of paranoia, in particular Kraepelin's "true paranoia," or as one example of the monosymptomatic delusional states (Kraepelin, 1910; 1921; Riding and Munro, 1975; Kenyon, 1976), similar to de Clérambault's syndrome described in Chapter 2.

Historical

Fiction abounds in descriptions of morbid jealousy. In Roman mythology, Juno, chief goddess, was known for her intense jealousy, and she persistently harassed her husband Jupiter. Over 2,000 years ago, Euripides related the story of Medea, who, having been rejected by Jason in favour of Creusa, developed a jealous rage in which she murdered her rival and wrought vengeance on Jason by murdering his children.

A Greek myth forms the basis of the modern play *Amphitryon 38* by Jean Giraudoux (1929/1938). Jupiter falls in love with Alcmene, faithful wife of the mortal Amphitryon, and longs to be loved in return as a mortal. He expresses doubts whether this would ever be possible to the god Mercury. Thus, "Faithful to herself or faithful to her husband.... You know, Mercury, most faithful wives are unfaithful to their husbands with everything except ... The difference with these virtuous wives is not to seduce them, but to persuade them that they may be seduced confidentially."

Jupiter appears in the guise of Amphitryon and descends to Earth with Mercury for this purpose. The latter arranges a war so that Amphitryon is called away to duty, allowing Jupiter to approach Alcmene's chambers. Although she proclaims her ability to see through this disguise, Jupiter is ambivalent about his apparent conquest, feeling triumphant yet dissatisfied, saying, "What do I want? What every man wants! A thousand contradictory desires! That Alcmene should remain faithful to her husband and also give herself to me. That she should remain chaste under my caresses and yet that desire should flare up under my very sight. That she should know nothing of this intrigue and yet she should commune at it with all her might."

Seidenberg (1952) also indicated this element of ambivalence and doubt leading to the need for testing the partner in another modern play, *The Guardsman* by Franz Molnar (1910/1924). A newly married old actor with a promiscuous past, believing he has found his true love, is compelled to test his wife's fidelity, yet realising that proof of her infidelity would be unbearable. "I have never really been in love until now," he states, "this time it is the last, greatest ... love that exhausts my innermost power of feeling." He disguises himself as a guardsman and is partially successful in his advances. But on revealing himself, his wife is adamant that she never doubted his true identity. However, neither the husband nor the audience is convinced of this.

The characteristic situation in which the delusion of jealousy occurs is the "eternal triangle," which is the basis of some of the greatest works of famous writers. In the fourteenth century, Boccaccio, in *The Decameron*, relates the story of a merchant, Bernarbo, who although at first vehemently opposing even the possibility of his wife ever being unfaithful to him was later tricked into believing that she had betrayed him. Ambroginolo, who persistently taunted him about this, gave him the facts which, although in themselves not conclusive were accepted by Bernarbo as proof of his wife's infidelity. In *Othello* Shakespeare describes a classic case of the syndrome. Often Othello has been portrayed as a majestic figure, wrongly duped by Iago. The truth, however, is that Iago merely fanned the flame of jealousy which was already embedded in Othello's personality. It has been further suggested that it was after he had realised that he could be jealous that Othello became mad (Tynan, 1965). The fact is that his jealousy was the central symptom of his psychosis, and his behaviour, including the killing of his wife, resulted directly from this. There are early signs of this jealousy reaction long before it becomes pronounced and obvious. When, for example, Othello is interrogated by Iago in Act III (Scene iii), over relatively trivial matters, he explodes in outrage until even Iago is surprised by the ferocity of the reaction and observes, "O, beware, my lord, of jealousy;/ It is the green-ey'd monster, which doth mock/ The meat it feeds on."

Shakespeare again described psychotic jealousy in *A Winter's Tale*. Here we have a man who initially resembled Boccaccio's Bernabo in believing explicitly in his wife's fidelity, and indeed he lived happily with her for years. His jealousy exploded rather suddenly and inexplicably, with no precipitating circumstances. He had himself encouraged his own friend to become his wife's as well.

Tolstoy's description of the psychotic jealousy mechanism in *The Kreutzer Sonata* is cruder than Shakespeare's and obviously coloured by his new attitude towards the female sex, which has undergone a complete reversal in his own time. But it is a useful description of how jealousy progresses into insatiable, consuming fury leading to Pozdnyshev murdering his wife. He was promiscuous in his youth, but at the same time he expected his wife to be completely chaste. The doubt regarding her fidelity, which arose in his mind early in the marriage, resulted in frequent quarrelling. It was significant that when he was happier about this then his outward relationship with her improved. He renounced leisure and all worldly pleasures as he regarded them as sexually stimulating. He became suspicious even of the doctors who examined his wife. His jealousy became particularly focussed on the wife's music teacher, in spite of the latter's unattractiveness. He believed that the first *Adagio sostenuto - Presto* movement of Beethoven's *Kreutzer Sonata* was particularly sexually stimulating to his wife, and this music haunted him. On returning home unexpectedly, he found the musician with his wife and believed that all his fantasies and doubts were thus confirmed. His rage was unbounded and, refusing to accept any rational explanation for their being together, he killed his wife. There have been numerous adaptations of this novella, for example, the 2008 film by the same name directed by Bernard Rose.

- Accounts of morbid jealousy now abound in the psychiatric literature and in standard psychiatric textbooks.
- Up to the turn of the nineteenth century, the condition was always regarded as being associated with alcohol. Then Von Krafft-Ebing (1903)

and Kretschmer (1942) claimed that sexual jealousy of a paranoid type could occur in other mental illnesses, both functional and organic.

• More recently there have been several detailed accounts of psychotic jealousy (Jasper, 1910; Langfeldt, 1951; Mooney, 1965; Mullen, 1990; Seeman, 2016).

Case reports

Three cases are now described in some detail to illustrate the main features of Othello syndrome.

Case 1

A 50-year-old man was referred by his own doctor in 1963 because he was accusing his wife of infidelity. There had been a similar episode in 1956–57. Then he had been suspicious for a few months, but he suddenly developed the frank systematised delusion of his wife's infidelity. Eight years later he was able to recount this episode in detail. He stated that his wife had been on a day trip alone, with members of a public house club. On returning, the barmaid made insinuating remarks to him about his wife's behaviour; at that moment the local butcher entered, and the patient instinctively "knew" that this was the man with whom his wife had been associating. This belief became more firmly focussed in his mind, and he "went to pieces," became agitated and unable to carry on with his work. He believed that "he knew" that his wife met the alleged paramour at certain times. Minimal clues were misinterpreted as providing definite proof of the liaison, e.g. the change in the appearance of his wife's clothing or behaviour and attitude. He responded well to treatment with chemotherapy and outpatient psychotherapy; his agitation cleared, and within 18 months he believed the affair was over.

The delusion recurred suddenly in 1963. At first he had vague suspicions about his wife's relationship with her own nephew, a much younger man, and this later blossomed into a frank delusion. He claimed that he found a skirt which his wife had hidden, which he alleged had seminal stains on it which "proved his wife's misbehaviour with his nephew." Although there was no evidence whatsoever for his belief, he continued to harbour this delusion. He misinterpreted many small clues as "proving" that she was meeting her "lover." When she bought new things for the house, he stated that she was able to do so with the money given to her by her lover. Later when she demanded more housekeeping money from him, and he knew that the nephew was unemployed, he believed that she was now giving money to him. Underclothes given to her by a neighbour as a Christmas present he believed came indirectly from her lover. Again he believed that she sent sheets to the laundry without his knowledge because "she wanted to cover up her own misdeeds."

All this time he was physically ill and had not been able to leave the house at all. Although he suffered from cor pulmonale, he never showed signs of organic confusion. There was no evidence of any other delusion or hallucination, or any evidence of any other psychosis. Indeed, he was a most pleasant man, sociable and most appreciative of all the help he received.

His wife nursed him effectively, and it was only when she could tolerate the situation no longer that he was admitted to hospital. He has had three readmissions since 1963 and always improves in hospital with medication. Usually after a short period both he and his wife demand his discharge.

This is a case of delusional jealousy occurring in a pure form, "true paranoia." It is ironic that the wife's own sister was killed by her husband, who also suffered the delusion that his wife was unfaithful.

Case 2

A young French woman married to a British officer was referred because she was jealous of her husband and in particular accused him of gaining sexual satisfaction from looking at pornographic pictures of sexy women. She would interrogate him for hours, trying to get him to admit his true feelings. His non-committal replies would only aggravate the situation. Sometimes his answers would satisfy her, but later she would return to the subject. She even attacked her husband physically. These episodes usually occurred when her husband was forced to go away for a few days in the course of his duty. During the acute attacks, she was completely deluded about her husband's infidelity. In between the attacks, however, she had doubts about the validity of her accusations. There were no other signs of any psychotic illness.

She did get periodic episodes of depression, which responded to drugs. During the two-and-a-half years' psychotherapy, she verbalised a great deal of her aggression towards her sister and mother, towards whom she revealed marked ambivalence. She was able to modify her attitudes and feelings and able to control her jealousy much better, the attacks of jealousy becoming less frequent and intense. In the course of therapy, she realised that she was herself sexually stimulated by these pornographic pictures, thus revealing her own homoerotic tendencies.

Case 3

A 28-year-old plumber was referred because of marital disharmony which resulted in his young wife threatening separation. The illness started abruptly when their baby was 13 months old. He disapproved of his wife working, although their financial state made this necessary. The baby had come rather earlier than planned and had aggravated their difficulties. He began to accuse his wife openly of being unfaithful and of carrying on with men at her place of work. If she were five minutes late at night in returning home he would interpret this as "proving" that she was spending her time with other men. He interrogated her for hours, sometimes well into the night. He would check her clothing for any clues to prove his contention. This resulted in intense, frequent quarrels.

Their real sexual problems aggravated the situation. The young wife had always been frigid, and having conceived very early in the marriage she feared another pregnancy. At this time she betrayed these feelings to her husband, who probably began to blame himself for her difficulties and lack of libido. Later he believed that the reason for this was that she was receiving sexual satisfaction elsewhere. He became extremely irritable, moody and unable to concentrate on his work, which became a burden to him. He became quite depressed with diurnal variation and early morning waking as well as having feelings of guilt.

He had always been a shy, sensitive, rigid and obsessional personality. He felt acutely the fact that his wife, unlike himself, had a grammar school education and was obviously more intelligent than he was. He responded well to out-patient psychotherapy and antidepressant drugs. Later, difficulties with his young daughter exacerbated his depressive symptoms, but there was no recurrence of the Othello delusion.

This is an example of Othello syndrome occurring with an underlying depressive illness with biological features.

Epidemiology

Whereas scant mention of this syndrome in textbooks suggested that it was a rare condition, now it is not uncommon in clinical practice and is often encountered not only in the patients themselves but also in their relatives. This is reflected in increasing numbers of accounts of morbid jealousy appearing in the psychiatric literature including psychiatric textbooks.

Soyka et al. (1991), in studying a large series of 8,134 patients admitted to the University Hospital of Munich between 1981 and 1985, identified 93 patients with delusions of infidelity, i.e. 1.1% of all admissions. From her study of 40 cases, selected from 600 published reports, Seeman (2016) concluded that the prevalence of delusional jealousy appears to be equal between men and women and greater in the elderly, perhaps as a result of the higher prevalence of neurological disorders and cognitive and/or sensory difficulties in this age group.

Modern classification systems may miss cases. Easton et al. (2008) found that, of 398 case histories of jealousy disorder (including delusional, morbid and pathological jealousy, Othello syndrome and conjugal paranoia) published between 1940 and 2002, just 4% met the *DSM-IV-TR* criteria for delusional disorder – jealous type.

Clinical features

The condition, which can occur in isolation or as a symptom of another psychotic disorder, shows the following clinical features:

- The core feature is the delusion of infidelity of the sexual partner. The importance of the sexual component is obvious in the nature of the delusion and the fact that it is always focussed on the sexual partner.
- Associated features include irritability and despondency as well as aggression.
- Either sex may be implicated, although it appears that males are more often implicated than females in clinical practice.
- It usually presents in the fourth decade with no previous history of any mental illness, although there may be a history of prodromal minor episodes of jealousy.
- The onset is usually seemingly sudden, but on closer examination the history of a few months of increasing suspicion is often elicited.
- Minimal clues are used to confirm the delusion. The patient takes great pains to test the partner and to "catch her out", indeed, checking is the hallmark of the jealousy, checking, rechecking, cross-checking and always checking.
- Psychotic jealousy is an exception to the rule that most psychiatric illnesses do not necessarily lead to violence. There is a high risk of violence directed towards the partner.

The checking behaviour can be so intense as to completely dominate the clinical picture. One husband used to take full details of the exact order of the overcoats in the cloakroom at his home, which he checked on returning at the end of the day to see whether they had altered their position. A change in the order was regarded as proof that "someone" had entered the house in his absence with the expressed purpose of being unfaithful with his wife. Another man checked the barcodes on goods bought by his wife to ensure that she had visited the specific supermarket that she had claimed. Many of the patients continually check their spouse's clothing for seminal stains, the bed linen for the marks of illicit love. Other activities may include inspecting clothes for tell-tale hairs, searching through pockets and watching and following. The patients often give involved explanations of how certain events confirm their beliefs, yet on close questioning they cannot sustain these arguments. It is striking that the imaginary lover is often unidentified, and not even the simplest of details of the imaginary lover can be given, e.g. the name, address or description. He usually remains a shadowy figure removed from the main encounter. Rarely, however, the rival is identified and so then may be at risk.

The patient's own so-called evidence is often contradictory and does not hang together, but neither this nor the flimsiness of the evidence prevents him proceeding to more intensive investigations. Hours will be spent in interrogation in an attempt to extort a confession from the spouse. Even if the patient is temporarily satisfied with the answers and explanations, he returns later to the same theme of interrogation, and the suspected partner is subject to constant inquisitions on every detail of her present and past behaviour. As a result of this, there is increased conflict and quarrelling and sometimes violence. The incessant demand is for a confession, which will put jealousy's mind at rest, but even if a confession is made it merely results at best in only temporary respite and usually in an explosive and potentially violent response and more accusations. One patient who confessed never had a moment's peace for the rest of his married life and was himself driven to a mental illness.

Quite paradoxically, the patient often evades rather than seeks unequivocal proof. For example, he may state that his wife is having an affair at a particular time with the imagined lover, at a particular place, and yet he will not intervene to seek certain proof. On questioning he is usually evasive and will proceed to describe another situation which is suggestive of his wife's infidelity. Morbid jealousy in general engenders contradictory behaviour and feelings. The jealous desire is to expose and to punish the supposed infidelity yet at the same time wanting to retain or to restore the relationship. The jealous person desires both to be justified in his suspicious accusations and yet be reassured that his lover is faithful. His desire is to hurt but also to love and be loved. He fears loss but pursues a course of action which inevitably leads to division and separation. Often accompanied with the delusion is an excessive sexual zeal and increased sexual activity. This usually causes repulsion on the part of a partner, and this in turn is interpreted as proving that she is gaining satisfaction elsewhere.

Since he is so preoccupied with the delusion and is irritable, tense and depressed, he is often unable to cope with routine tasks such as his job. Life becomes a veritable hell for him and also for his family. His desires, feelings and behaviour are controlled by his delusions of infidelity.

There is often a discrepancy in the intellectual, educational or social spheres of the patient and the spouse. The latter may have more outside interests and friends. The patient being unable to fit in with his life hence feels the odd man out and inferior. In some cases the spouse is aware of the jealous nature of the partner before the marriage, but this does not prevent the marriage taking place.

Not infrequently one of the parents of the patient has been subjected to rages of jealousy if not suffering from a frank delusion. The father is often rather feelingless, showing little interest in his children, while the mother is submissive and over-protective. The patient's own personality may exhibit marked obsessional traits, frigidity and a tendency to be suspicious.

Symptomatic morbid jealousy

The condition can be found as a symptom of another established psychotic illness. The most common psychosis in which it occurs is a paranoid state, although it can also be a feature of an affective psychosis, psychopathy and certain organic conditions such as epilepsy, dementia and alcoholism.

There is an established association with alcohol abuse. However, Shepherd (1961) found only six cases among his 81 patients (7%). Glatt (1961; 1982) reported that over 20% of his alcoholics listed jealousy as a major problem, and in their systematic study of sexual jealousy in alcohol abuse, Shrestha et al. (1985) found a prevalence of morbid jealousy of 27% in the men and 15% in the women. A similar male prevalence was reported by Michael et al. (1995), who found 71 cases of morbid jealousy in 207 male patients with DSM-III R alcohol dependence (34%). In larger series of morbid jealousy, alcohol abuse is reported in 6–20% of the patients. Soyka et al. (1989), in studying 15 inpatients with persistent alcoholic delusional jealousy, were able to distinguish two types, the more frequently occurring mono-symptomatic form with a gradual onset and a second type with an acute onset with hallucinations. They found that the prognosis, especially of the second type, was very poor.

If the delusions of infidelity occur in association with another mental disorder such as schizophrenia, depressive illness or an organic psychosyndrome the symptoms of the co-existing illness will be present. In the case of schizophrenic disorders, the morbid jealousy may be one of its manifestations and in some cases its most prominent feature. The jealousy complex may be the initial presentation, with a late progression to frank schizophrenia involving other symptoms.

In Shepherd's (1961) series of patients admitted over a three-year period, 14% who were diagnosed with schizophrenia or paranoid illness had jealousy as a prominent feature. In Langfeldt's (1961) series of morbid jealousy patients, 5 of 66 were diagnosed as suffering with schizophrenia. Shepherd (1961) reported 5 of 81. Mullen and Maack (1985) reported 15 of 138, and Soyka et al. (1991) found that 52 (56%) out of 93 patients with delusions of jealousy had schizophrenia.

A range of organic conditions have been described as occurring in association with morbid jealousy. These include diabetes mellitus, tabes dorsalis, cerebral tumours, lead poisoning, panhypopituitarism, multiple sclerosis, Parkinson's disease, Alzheimer's disease and presenile dementias.

The abuse of substances other than alcohol, such as amphetamines and cocaine, can also lead to morbid jealousy, when delusional ideas can rapidly become intense and not infrequently lead to violence. The delusional ideas may persist for some time after the drugs have been withdrawn.

Neurotic jealousy

Some authors have differentiated so-called neurotic jealousy from delusional jealousy (Mairet, 1908; Freud, 1911; 1922; Mooney, 1965). Although neurotic and delusional jealousy overlap, and the nature and the intensity of the jealousy fluctuate at different times, this distinction is valid. However, the syndrome is equally malignant in whatever form it occurs. Indeed, even the borderline between normal and pathological jealousy is ill-defined, and in those said to be exhibiting normal jealousy, that which is considered typical of the mental state and behaviour of pathological jealousy may occur. The distinction, however, for all its difficulties between formal and pathological jealousy, has considerable practical implications both clinically and legally.

The category of thoughts referred to as overvalued ideas has been considered to have particular relevance to morbid jealousy (McKenna, 1984). Overvalued ideas are convictions of overriding personal significance out of all proportion to their overt content. They differ from the strongly held beliefs of the commonality in the degree of emotional investment and the central place they occupy in the mental life of the individual (Fish, 1962; Mullen et al. 1985). They are regarded as sitting on a continuum between the deeply held convictions of normal individuals and delusional beliefs. They are similar to strongly held religious and political beliefs, differing largely in their highly personalised (not to say egocentric) quality.

Aetiology and psychopathology

- Traditionally pathological jealousy has been understood as arising within a psychodynamic framework with particular emphasis placed upon the presence of a core feeling of inadequacy and an associated sense of insecurity.
- More recently attention has focussed upon a possible organic basis for the delusion, and cognitive-behavioural approaches have been adopted with the intention of developing an understanding of the psychopathology.

Normal jealousy

Before considering the aetiology and psychopathology of morbid jealousy, some understanding of the nature and purpose of what can be called normal jealousy is desirable. Jealousy for one's spouse or partner – and even a desired but as yet unreciprocating love object – is an emotion experienced and recognised by the vast majority of human beings in a myriad of cultural settings and historical eras. Indeed, the complete absence of jealousy in certain conditions, which the French call *unaesthetique jalousie,* may be regarded as pathological. The loss of a partner to another is much more than the loss of a prized possession. The emotional response to such an incident in most individuals far outweighs that associated with the loss of even one's most treasured chattel. The persistence of such potentially destructive emotions throughout human history indicates that they must have some useful purpose.

Provided they are not too intense and disruptive, jealous feelings probably contribute to the long-term maintenance of established interpersonal relationships. A view from a socio-cultural perspective would emphasise the benefits that stable relationships endow upon the wider community. In evolutionary terms, strong feelings of jealousy may ensure the survival of one's genes into the next generation and beyond. David M. Buss (2000), in his *The Dangerous Passion: Why Jealousy Is as Necessary as Love and Sex*, emphasises that jealousy has evolved to protect love and yet it can rip a relationship apart. Thus, it arises in response to a threat to a valued relationship in which a person has invested heavily. It is usually a transient and episodic experience and not a permanent affliction.

Indeed jealousy, paradoxically, flows from deep and abiding love but can shatter the most harmonious of relationships. The paradox was reflected in O. J. Simpson's statement: "Let's say I committed this crime [the slaying of his estranged wife, Nicole Brown Simpson]. Even if I did do this it would have to have been because I loved her very much, right?" This emotion of jealousy, designed to shelter a relationship from intruders, turns homes that might be sanctuaries of love into hells of discord and hate.

Humans can typically interpret a partner's jealousy as a sign of the depth of their love and a partner's absence of jealousy as lack of love. Augustine noted this link when he declared that "he that is not jealous, is not in love." Shakespeare's tormented Othello "dotes, yet doubts, suspects, yet strongly loves."

Biology

As described, many organic conditions have been reported as being associated with pathological jealousy. However, most of the objective data refer to single case reports, and the nature of the organic conditions is such that either the disinhibition of pre- existing jealous characteristics or some adverse effects upon sexual function are likely to be the key aetiological influences in such examples. A large series of 3,552 brain-damaged servicemen revealed that only 42 had developed jealous paranoia (Achté et al., 1967; 1969).

More recently, a number of cases have been described of delusional jealousy and Othello syndrome occurring secondary to right-sided (nondominant) cerebral infarcts (Richardson et al., 1991; Wong and Meier, 1997; Westlake and Weeks, 1999; Rocha et al., 2014). Rocha et al.

(2014) reported the cases of two men in their sixties who each developed Othello syndrome following a right-sided cerebrovascular infarction. In one case, the patient had a sudden onset of left hemianopia, mild left hemiparesis and euphoria. His MRI scan revealed a right-sided temporoparietoinsular ischaemic lesion. The following day, he began manifesting symptoms of Othello syndrome, believing that his wife was being sexually unfaithful with others – first with other patients in the hospital ward and then with her stepson (his biological son); following antidepressant and antipsychotic treatment, he fully recovered from these delusional beliefs within four months (Rocha et al., 2014). In their literature review of cases, published between 1964 and 2008, of neurological disorders associated with the onset of jealousy, Ortigue and Bianchi-Demicheli (2011) reported 10 cases, mostly of delusional jealousy, four of which involved right-sided brain lesions. These case reports lie very easily with contemporary discussions concerning "content-specific delusions" and the role of the right cerebral hemisphere and frontal lobe in their genesis.

In their study of 103 consecutive attendees to a neurology clinic, of patients with Alzheimer's disease, Migliorelli et al. (1995) found that four (4%) suffered from Othello syndrome; all believed that their spouses were being sexually unfaithful to them, and one had exhibited violence towards the spouse because of this.

In many cases a constitutional factor is suspected and thus is raised the possibility of a genetic component to aetiology. However, in none of the relevant studies is it possible to distinguish between the inherited and environmental influences; for example, 20 of Vauhkonen's 1968 patients had parents who were reported to have exhibited jealous behaviour. This could be explained on a genetic basis, but equally the behaviour might have been learnt from modelling, for the family backgrounds of both patients and spouses showed little significant differences.

Cognitive-behavioural influences

A cognitive-behavioural formulation of pathological jealousy is based on the concept of an affected individual possessing a schema consisting of a persistent anticipated threat of loss of his sexual partner. Intili and Tarrier (1998) demonstrated that jealous subjects, as compared with non-jealous controls, were particularly prone to detect jealousy-related stimuli presented in a dichotic listening task. The authors concluded that in cases of pathological jealousy, there may be an attentional bias towards jealousy-related information. Maggini et al. (2006) distinguish carefully between morbid jealousy and jealous love. The latter, in their view, may be considered to be a trait, providing the behavioural and cognitive-affective precondition of the former, which is considered to be a state.

Psychodynamic aspects

The core of the problem is one of inadequacy, arising from a discrepancy between what the patient wants to be and what he considers he actually is (Boccaccio, 1958). It does not mean that the patient thinks little of himself, on the contrary he is usually narcissistic and egocentric, but "realises" albeit unconsciously, that he has important weaknesses. Kretschmer's (1942) schema of morbid jealously is classified among "his expansive" reactions. The patients displaying "a spot in the core of their being, a hyposensitive, nervous vulnerability, a buried focus and an old inferiority feeling."

A certain event or events may activate these feelings of inferiority, which in turn are always accompanied by anxiety, insecurity and hypersensitiveness. The threat to the ego becomes real, it must be defended at all costs, and jealousy tends to manifest itself. This in turn is dealt with by the mechanism of projection and the "inadequacy" projected onto the spouse who is accused of infidelity (Parant, 1902; Sjobring, 1947; Revitch, 1954; Ovesey, 1955; Stauffacher, 1958). The feelings of inadequacy may specifically be linked with:

- Feelings of a threat to the patient's position and prestige
- His own unfaithfulness
- Homosexuality
- Inability to love

First, if any of the patient's possessions are threatened from outside, e.g. loss of position, power or prestige, feelings of inadequacy and inferiority may be released. Any real or imaginary threat to the husband-wife relationship at this time considerably enhances these feelings. The reason for this is that in our society's ideology, the spouse is looked upon as the property of the other. Descartes emphasised that jealousy feelings arise from the possession instinct and hence any threat to the possession, especially one so greatly valued as the spouse, leads to increased jealousy. Indeed, such a threat results in the patient craving for even greater or more complete possession, for, as Ley and Wauthier (1946) indicate, jealousy is a desire to have complete and exclusive possession of the object. Any interest shown by others therefore constitutes a threat.

It would appear that in order for jealousy to exist, a person must have become self-conscious of his possession and the world, which he can legitimately expect to control (Boeuff, 1938). A child, therefore, could not be jealous before such a measure of self-consciousness developed, with a power to distinguish his inner world from the world outside, i.e. that which belongs to the "I" and that which is alien to it (Seidenberg, 1952). Having realised that the "I" and "thou" words exist, the relationship depends on the amount of self-surrender and self-assertion which is present. Lagache (1947; 1950; 1955) describes the polarity by using the terms *amour captatif* and *amour oblatatif,* which he borrowed from Pichon. In the former the person demands complete possession of the partner even without reciprocation; in the latter he wants to give himself completely to the object. Most relationships, however, operate along a spectrum between these two extremes, but the more the love is shifted in the direction of *amour captatif* the greater the tendency towards jealousy.

The question remains why some people have a greater propensity towards jealousy, for there is continual threat to the "I" in everybody's life. This may well be explained by constitutional factors. Shakespeare was well aware of such a constitutional factor, which was expressed by Desdemona thus: "Alas, the day! I never gave him cause," and through Emilia's significant rejoinder quoted at the head of this chapter.

Second, the central inadequacy may be linked with the patient's own illicit desires to be unfaithful, which in turn are projected onto the spouse. In other words, these unconscious impulses or tendencies towards infidelity exist in the patients. One of our patients during the course of prolonged psychotherapy revealed clearly and spontaneously that during sexual intercourse with her husband she had fantasies of having relations with various other men. Jones (1929a,b) considers that impulses towards unfaithfulness are themselves neurotic traits, showing a lack of self-confidence. The tendency towards a restless flight from object to object, he points out, is the outcome of anxiety resulting from narcissistic dependence of the jealous person on his object. He further states, "Marital infidelity has more equally the one believes, a neurotic origin. It is not a sign of liberty and potency, but of the opposite."

These Don Juan activities of the patients themselves only tend to make them more likely to develop delusions of infidelity regarding the partner. Indeed, the greater the success of his own past illicit affairs the greater his doubts regarding his own wife's faithfulness. Tolstoy's *Kreutzer Sonata* clearly illustrates this. Pozdnyshev was very promiscuous before marriage and later, believing that his wife was unfaithful with the music master Troukhatchevsky, he states, "He is what all men are, what I was when a bachelor. For him it is a pleasure, he even smiles when he looks at me as though saying, 'What can you do about it? It is my turn now.'" In the case of the old actor in *The Guardsman* described above, his urge to test his young wife's fidelity was enhanced by his own earlier promiscuity. Burton emphasises this point in his *Anatomy of Melancholy:*

> There is none jealous, I durst pawn my life,
> But he that hath defiled another's wife,
> And for that he himself hath gone astray,
> He straightway thinks his wife will treat that way.

Third, the inadequacy which is projected may reveal itself as a propensity towards homosexuality. We have had two very striking examples of young wives who, while accusing their husbands of erotic stimulation from pornographic pictures and sexy women, themselves revealed that they were sexually stimulated by those very pictures and those very women. Freud (1911; 1922; 1938) was strongly of the opinion that psychotic jealousy had a homosexual basis. Fenichel (1945) points out, "Freud led the way through his understanding of jealousy paranoia. He emphasised that jealousy was used not only to ward off an impulse towards unfaithfulness but also towards homosexuality. The delusion of infidelity arising from psychotic jealousy serves the purpose of hiding the patient's own 'denied' repressed homosexuality." This is a variant of Freud's formulation of the persecutory paranoid patient, as it were, who defends himself by a denial, "I do not love him" and a projection onto the woman, "She loves him and not me." In the course of analysis, it becomes evident that the patient, when suspecting his wife, is actually interested in the other man but strives to rid himself of his homosexuality by means of projection.

Fenichel (1953), while supporting this view, that the jealous patient strives to rid himself of impulses towards unfaithfulness and homosexuality by means of projection, further referred to the frustration inherent in the Oedipus complex as being "the basis of all jealousy." Melanie Klein (1957) expressed views that are substantially similar, although coloured by her own theoretical standpoint: "Jealousy is based on the suspicions of a rivalry with a father, who is accused of taking away the mother's breast, and the mother. The rivalry marks the early stages of the direct and inverted Oedipus complex, which normally arises concurrently with a depressive position in the second quarter of the first year."

Fourth, the importance of the Oedipus complex is also emphasised by Schmidberg (1953), who believed that a significant factor is the lack of ability to love. Fenichel also emphasised this, believing that an inability to love was in turn "based on a deep ambivalence." Those with ever-present delusional jealousy are those who are unable to develop genuine love because all their relationships are intermingled with a narcissistic need. Such jealousy is strikingly not most intense when hitherto love and gratification have been most intense; on the contrary, patients disposed to jealousy are those who change their love objects continually and regularly.

Sexual dysfunction

Sexual dysfunction, particularly impotence, becomes an important factor in the psychopathology of morbid sexual jealousy in some cases. Indeed, some authors regard the impotence itself as being of a primary, paramount importance (Bleuler, 1911; 1923; 1926; Campbell, 1953; Noyes and Kolb, 1963). Impotence occurring commonly in alcohol abuse plays a part in the production of delusions of infidelity in such cases. This impotence has been explained as being the direct result of toxic effects of the alcohol on the related nervous and endocrine mechanisms.

Since morbid jealousy inevitably involves two people in sexual contact, the sexual function of the partner is also of crucial importance. Vauhkonen (1968) found that in his group of subjects, 7 of the 16 husbands reported sexual dysfunction (2 with loss of libido, 1 with erectile difficulties and 4 with premature ejaculation), while 32 out of 37 wives reported difficulties (15 with total frigidity and 17 with orgasmic difficulties). Thus a failure in the sexual sphere appears to be frequently associated with morbid jealousy, although whether it is primary or secondary is difficult to say. Certainly morbid jealousy is often closely followed by sexual dysfunction in the wife. In the case of examples associated with alcohol abuse, other factors are present which exacerbate the condition. Even at a comparatively early stage, i.e. before the appearance of impotence, the drunken husband's behaviour repulses the wife, and he in turn interprets this as a lack of desire on her part to have sexual relations with him, and this means that she must be obtaining satisfaction elsewhere.

Equally, marked disparity in the sexuality of married partners can also be an important factor in the psychogenesis. Such disparity appears to render both partners as equally vulnerable to the Othello phenomenon. This disparity may occur in other spheres as already indicated, such as intellectual ability, educational background and social status. Disparity in ages is an important factor, and an elderly husband married to a young wife is particularly vulnerable. Burton refers to old men married to young women thus: 'With old doting Janivere in Chaucer, they begin to mistrust all is not well:

> She was young and he was old,
> And therefore he feared to be a cuckold'.

The plain wife is likewise prone and vulnerable to jealousy. It is noteworthy that a number of our cases had partners who were particularly attractive and provocative. Oscar Wilde, in *A Woman of No Importance*, illustrates the point as follows: "Curious thing, plain women are always jealous of their husbands, beautiful women never are!"

Management and treatment

The principles of managing and treating this condition are:

- Establish a precise diagnosis, i.e. primary syndrome or features that are secondary to another condition, and initiate the appropriate medical treatment.
- Assess the degree of risk to the partner and any other parties such as dependent children, and take appropriate action, e.g. formal detention

under mental health legislation, advise geographical separation or initiate child care proceedings.

- Provide psychological support to both parties; specific psychological treatments may be indicated.
- Treat any aggravating factors, e.g. alcohol abuse, sexual dysfunction or any other organic factor.

When delusions of jealousy occur as a secondary phenomenon, the treatment is that of the underlying condition. In the case of schizophrenia, for example, antipsychotic medication is prescribed, and in the case of a depressive psychosis antidepressants are the treatment of choice. When the setting is that of an organic psychosyndrome, the underlying infection, neoplasm, etc. must be the target of the treatment. Even if the illness cannot be treated, as in the example of Huntingtons' disease (chorea), neuroleptics may nevertheless lead to a resolution of the delusions without modifying the basic pathophysiology. It is noteworthy that in both cases reported by Rocha et al. (2014), of the onset of Othello syndrome following a right-sided cerebrovascular infarction, a combination of antidepressant and antipsychotic medication (sertraline plus quetiapine in one case; fluvoxamine plus chlorpromazine in the other) was associated with successful treatment of the psychiatric symptomology in one case and partial improvement in the other. Similarly, following the onset of pathological jealousy in a 25-year-old woman after a right cerebrovascular infarction, antidepressant treatment with a selective serotonin reuptake inhibitor for six weeks was associated with almost complete resolution (Westlake and Weeks, 1999).

When delusions of infidelity occur in pure form as a monosymptomatic delusional disorder or where the delusional jealousy is the cardinal dominant feature of a more extensive psychotic state, the administration of antipsychotic medication is essential. In practice, modest dosage of neuroleptics can often be successful in removing the delusions, whilst at other times much larger doses are required. There has been a strong advocacy for *pimozide* as the drug of choice in monosymptomatic delusional disorders including paranoid jealousy, with Byrne and Yatham (1989) describing a successful treatment with the drug in a 39-year-old man with pathological jealousy. In some cases when adequate control of the delusions has been established and the relevant relationship conflict resolves efficiently, it may be possible to reduce the dosage and eventually discontinue it altogether. There is, however, a group of patients who rapidly relapse without antipsychotic medication, and in this group long-term maintenance is the only solution.

Behavioural psychotherapy

Behavioural psychotherapy has been advocated as the treatment of choice. Cobb and Marks (1979) reported using a broad spectrum of behavioural techniques to treat four cases of excessive jealously which did not reach delusional intensity. The therapeutic strategy used included self-regulating exposure in fantasy and in real life, response prevention for jealous rituals, thought-stopping for jealous ruminations and social skills training. The package of measures was beneficial in three of the cases, although significantly, direct stimulation of jealous thoughts was reported to be more anxiety provoking than helpful.

Cognitive behaviour therapy

Cognitive behaviour therapy for the treatment of morbid jealousy was first reported in 1989 by Bishay et al. They also described a significant im-provement in 10 of their 13 patients treated by this method. Further reports have since been provided suggesting that the approach does have much potential, particularly for non-psychotic cases (Dolan and Bishay, 1996a,b).

Intense suspicions of infidelity have been reported in the context of an obsessive-compulsive disorder (Cobb and Marks, 1979; Mullen, 1990; Stein, 1994). Indeed, Parker and Barrett (1997) have suggested that morbid jealousy be considered a variant of obsessive-compulsive disorder, while morbid jealousy has been found to respond to therapeutic strategies developed primarily for the management of obsessive-compulsive dis-order (Cobb and Marks, 1979; Bishay et al., 1989; Stein et al., 1994). Curling et al. (2018) have recently provided evidence, from a single case study, that cognitive analytic therapy may be helpful in the treatment of obsessive morbid jealousy.

As sexual problems are common in relationships plagued by jealousy either pre-dating the jealousy or arising during the course of the disorder, and given their presence as potent factors in maintaining the morbid jea-lousy, therapy should be focussed upon them. The exact management of these sexual problems depends upon their specific nature, their severity and their role in maintaining the pathological jealously. The opinion of a col-league who specialises in the treatment of sexual disorders may be sought.

The relationship between the patient and partner must become a focus of treatment. For couples where the jealousy is obviously groundless, a process of clarification and reassurance may assist. The reframing of the relationship and the clarification of its boundaries also has a place. In cases where infidelity has actually occurred, the patient's reaction to the disclosure is crucial and can have important implications for the progress of the jealousy. Confessions, far from leading to a resolution of the conflict, often lead to more intensive interrogation and an outburst of further accusations and threats.

Once established, morbid jealousy becomes a part of the relationship system that is perpetuated by the very reaction and attempted solution of the partners. One form of management is directed to the disruption of the pathological relationship patterns and to substituting methods of coping likely to produce a resolution of the jealousy. Role-play has been used to encourage effective strategies of jealousy management. Jealousy workshops to promote joint understanding and insight have been described (Blood and Blood, 1977; Marolin, 1979; Im and Breit, 1983; Constatine, 1986).

Conjoint therapy

Conjoint therapy, which is aimed at clarifying and modifying areas of judgement and redefining the boundaries and expectations in the relationship and improving communications between the partners, is increasingly used. This has resulted from the fact that increasing numbers of non-delusional jealousy cases are now being referred to outpatient practices as relationship or marital problems. This strategy usually reduces the intensity and frequency of the jealous behaviour but does not necessarily lead to a "cure" (Purdey and Nickle, 1981).

Treatment on an individual basis may range from supportive psychotherapy, where the minimum aim is encouragement of compliance and monitoring of response, to deep insight-producing psychotherapy with the purpose of changing behaviour and dealing with a patient's deep personality problems such as his inadequacy. It is rare for patients to be taken on for psychoanalytic treatment. Freeman (1990) describes four cases of morbid jealousy including two non-psychotic women who were in psychoanalytic treatment.

A risk assessment is essential in all cases, and where marital domestic violence becomes a practical issue it must be managed in its own right. It has been established that the condition of morbid jealousy has been associated with a number of repeat homicides following release from prison or hospital (Scott, 1977). If physical abuse is occurring, the victim should be informed of the legal remedies, and if any children are at risk, they must be referred to the appropriate child support services. The severity and chronicity of violence is often such that a separation, temporary or permanent, becomes the only solution. With the considerable increase in the elderly population, there is an accompanying significant increase in people suffering from dementia. Delusional jealousy is a frequent problem in dementia and often leads to violence. This violence in demented patients suffering from delusional jealousy is well documented and the forensic aspects highlighted by Cipriani et al. (2012).

Prognosis

Traditionally, the prognosis has been considered to be very doubtful. The purer the form the more lasting is the illness. If it occurs in association with another psychosis, it often follows the pattern of this illness. Sometimes, however, when the other symptoms clear, the Othello delusion becomes more obvious. This development is unlike that of de Clérambault's syndrome but resembles that of Capgras' syndrome.

Langfeldt (1951) reported that 56% of the patients in his series improved after treatment. Following up a group of 50 patients after a 17-year interval, he found that 6 had died and 17 were untraceable. Of the remaining, only 12 were fully recovered, 6 were periodically improved and 9 showed no improvement. Patients with severe personality disorder or psychotic illness had a particularly poor prognosis.

Mooney (1965), reporting his treatment results, concluded that, "about one third of the patients seem to be much improved, one third slightly improved and one third unchanged," and again the psychotic cases did worse.

Clinical experience demonstrates that morbid jealousy has a tendency to recur following resolution. This is shown even when the original relationship has been replaced by a new partnership. The new partner then becomes the focus of the morbid jealousy.

Postscript

When we first wrote about delusions of infidelity, it was appropriate to place Othello syndrome among the curiosities of the rare or uncommon psychiatric syndromes. Since then it has been realised that morbid jealousy is a common phenomenon frequently seen in clinical practice. However, this condition's position in contemporary psychiatry remains ambiguous. But, the suffering it generates in the patient and in others can be so great that the condition should not be neglected. Although morbid jealousy remains a complex challenge to the psychiatrist, the present state of knowledge suggests that, with an eclectic approach involving pharmacotherapy, behavioural techniques, psychotherapy and conjoint marital/relationship therapy, the outlook may not be as pessimistic as has been traditionally believed.

References

Achté, K.A., Hillbom, E., Aalberg, V., (1967). *Reports of the Rehabilitation Institute for Brain Injured Veterans in Finland, Vol. 1.*

Achté, K.A., Hillbom, E., Aalberg, V., (1969). *Acta Psychiatrica Scandinavica, 45,* 1.

Bishay, N.R., Peterson, N., Tarrier, N., (1989). *British Journal of Psychiatry, 154,* 386.

Bleuler, E., (1911). *Dementia Praecox or the Group of Schizophrenias (1950),* Trans. J. Zinken. International University Press, New York.

Bleuler, E., (1923). *Textbook of Psychiatry,* 4th edn., Trans. A.A. Brill. Macmillan,New York.

Bleuler, E., (1926). *Affektivitat, Suggestbilitat, Paranoia,* 2nd edn. Halle Marholz,Marhold, Germany.

Blood, R., Blood, M., (1977). In *Jealousy,* Eds. G. Clanton, L. G. Smith. Prentice Hall, New York.

Boccaccio, G., (1958). *The Decameron.* Elek, London.

Boeuff, C.W. du, (1938). *Over Jolverschbeidswan.* Zutphen, Ruys.

Buss, D.M., (2000). *The Dangerous Passion: Why Jealousy Is as Necessary as Love and Sex.* The Free Press, New York.

Byrne, A., Yatham, L.N., (1989). *British Journal of Psychiatry, 155,* 249.

Campbell, J.D., (1953). *Manic-Depressive Disease.* Lippincott, Philadelphia.

Cipriani, G., Vedovello, M., Nuti, A., di Fiorino, A., (2012). *Psychiatry and Clinical Neurosciences, 66,* 467.

Cobb, H., Marks, I.M., (1979). *British Journal of Psychiatry, 14,* 395.

Constatine, L.L. (1986). In *Clinical Handbook of Marital Therapy,* Eds. N.S. Jacobson, A.S. Gurman. Guildford Press, New York.

Curling, L., Kellett, S., Totterdell, P., Parry, G., Hardy, G., Berry, K., (2018). *Psychology and Psychotherapy, 91,* 95.

Dolan, M., Bishay, N.R., (1996a). *Journal of Cognitive Psychotherapy: An International Quarterly, 10/1,* 35.

Dolan, M., Bishay, N.R., (1996b). *British Journal of Psychiatry, 168,* 588.

Easton, J.A., Shackelford, T.K., Schipper, L.D., (2008). *Journal of Clinical Psychology, 64,* 264.

Ey, M , (1950). Jalousie morbide, In *Etudes Psychiatriques, Vol. 2.* de Bronwen, Paris.

Fenichel, O., (1945). *The Psychoanalytic Theory of Neuroses.* Norton, New York

Fenichel, O., (1953). *A Contribution to the Psychology of Jealousy.* In *The Collected Papers of Otto Fenichel.* Norton, New York.

Fish, E.J. (1962). *Schizophrenia,* Bristol, Wright.

Freeman, T., (1990). *British Journal of Psychiatry, 156,* 68.

Freud, S., (1911). *Psychoanalytic Notes upon an Autobiographical Account of a Case of Paranoia (Dementia Paranoides).* In Collected Papers, 1959, Vol. 3. Basic Books, New York.

Freud, S., (1922). *Certain Neurotic Mechanisms in Jealousy, Paranoia, and Homosexuality.* Collected Papers, 1922, Vol. 2. Hogarth, London.

Freud, S., (1938). *The Basic Writings of Sigmund Freud,* Trans. A.A. Brill. Modern Library, New York.

Giraudoux, J., (1929/1938). *Amphitryon 38,* Adapted by S.N. Behrman. Random House, New York.

Glatt, M.M., (1961). *Acta Psychiatrica Scandinavica, 3,* 788.

Glatt, M.M., (1982). *Alcoholism.* Hodder and Stoughtan, Sevenoaks, UK.

Im, W., Breit, M., (1983). *Family Process, 22,* 211.

Intili, R., Tarrier, N., (1998). *Behavioural and Cognitive Psychotherapy, 26/4,* 323.

Jasper, K., (1910). *Zeitschrift Gesamte Neurologie Psychiatrie, 1,* 567.

Jones, E., (1929a). *Revue Francaise Psychoanalytique, 3,* 228.

Jones, E., (1929b). *Jealousy.* In Papers on Psych-analysis (1948), 5th edn. Bailliere, Tindall and Cox, London.

Kenyon, F.E., (1976). *British Journal of Psychiatry, 1,* 291.

Klein, M., (1957). *Envy and Gratitude.* Tavistock Publications, London.

Kraepelin, E., (1910). *Psychiatrie,* 8th edn. Barth, Leipzig.

Kraepelin, E., (1921). *Manic-Depressive Insanity and Paranoia,* Ed. E. Robertson, Trans. M. Barclay. Livingstone, Edinburgh.

Krafft-Ebing, R., (1903). *Lehrbuch der Psychiatrie.* Enke, Stuttgart.

Kretschmer, E., (1942). *A Textbook of Medical Psychology.* Hogarth, London.

Lagache, D., (1947). *La Jalousie Amoureuse.* Presses Universitaires de France, Paris.

Lagache, D., (1950). *International Journal of Psychoanalysis, 31,* 24.

Lagache, D., (1955). *Discussion* In *L'Evolution Psychiatrique,* Paris.

Langfeldt, G., (1951). *Acta Psychiatrica Scandinavica, 26*(Suppl. 73), 3.

Langfeldt, G., (1961). *Acta Psychiatriac Scandinavica, 36*(Suppl. 151), 7.

Langfeldt, G., (1962). *Journal of Neuropsychiatry, 3,* 317.

Ley, L., Wauthier, M.L., (1946). *Etudes de Psychologie Instinctive et Affective.* Presses Universitaites de France, Paris.

Maggini, C., Lundgren, E., Leuci, E., (2006). *Acta Biomedica, 77,* 137.

Mairet, A., (1908). *La Jalousie: Etude Psycho-physiocoque.* Clinique et Medico-Legale, Montpellier.

Marolin, G., (1979). *American Journal of Family Therapy, 7,* 13.

McKenna, P.J., (1984), Disorders with Overvalued ideas. *The British Journal of Psychiatry, 145,* 579–585.

Michael, A., Mirza, S., Mirza, K.A.H., Babu, V.S., Vithayathil, E., (1995). *British Journal of Psychiatry, 167,* 668.

Migliorelli, R., Petracca, G., Tesón, A., Sabe, L., Leiguarda, R., Starkstein, S.E., (1995). *Psychological Medicine, 25,* 505.

Molnar, F., (1924). *The Guardsman.* Boni and Liveright, New York.

Mooney, H.B., (1965). *British Journal of Psychiatry, 111,* 1023.

Mowat, R.R., (1966). *Morbid Jealousy and Murder.* Tavistock Publications, London.

Mullen, P.E., (1990). In *Principles and Practice of Forensic Psychiatry,* Eds. R. Bluglass, P. Bowden. Churchill Livingstone, London.

Mullen, P.E., Maack, L.H., (1985). In *Jealousy, Pathological Jealousy and Violence,* Eds. D.P. Farringdon, J. Gunn. Wiley, London.

Noyes, A.P., Kolb, L.C., (1963). *Modern Clinical Psychiatry,* 6th edn. Saunders, Philadelphia.

Ortega, M.J., (1959). *Psychoanalytic Review, 46,* 102.

Ortigue, S., Bianchi-Demicheli, F., (2011). *Medical Science Monitor, 17,* RA1.

Ovesey, L., (1955). *Psychiatry, 18, 163.*

Parant, V., (1902). *Journal of Mental Science, 48,* 133.

Parker, G., Barrett, E., (1997). *Australian and New Zealand Journal of Psychiatry, 31,* 133.

Purdey, F., Nickle, N., (1981). *Social Work and Groups, 4,* 111.

Revitch, E., (1954). *Diseases of the Nervous System, 15,* 271.

Richardson, E.D., Malloy, P.F., Grace, J., (1991). *Journal of Geriatric Psychiatry and Neurology, 4/3,* 160.

Riding, J., Munro, A., (1975). *Acta Psychiatrica Scandinavica, 52,* 23.

Rocha, S., Pinho, J., Ferreira, C., Machado, A., (2014). *Journal of Neuropsychiatry and Clinical Neurosciences, 26,* E1.

Schmidberg, M., (1953). *Psychoanalytic Quarterly, 40,* 1.

Scott, P.D., (1977). *British Journal of Psychiatry, 131,* 127.

Seeman, M.V., (2016). *Psychiatry, 79,* 379.

Seidenberg, R., (1952). *Psychoanalytic Review, 39,* 345.

Shepherd, M., (1961). *Journal of Mental Science, 107,* 687.

Shrestha, K., Rees, D.W., Rix, K.J.B., Hobe, B.D., Faragher, E.B., (1985). *Acta Psychiatrica Scandinavica, 72,* 283.

Sjobring, H., (1947). *Acta Psychiatrica Scandinavica, 47*(Suppl.), 74.

Soyka, M., Naber, G., Völcker, A., (1991). *British Journal of Psychiatry, 158,* 549.

Soyka, M., Sass, H., Völcker, A., (1989). *Psychaitrische Praxis*, *16*, 189.
Stauffacher, J.C., (1958). *Journal of Clinical Psychology*, *14*, 99.
Stein, O.J., Hollander, E., & Josephson, S.C. (1994). *Journal of Clinical Psychiatry*, *55*, 30.
Tynan, K., (1965). *Olivier by Tynan, The Observer Magazine*, 12 December.
Vauhkonen, K., (1968). *Acta Psychiatrica Scandinavica*, Supplement 202.
Westlake, R.J., Weeks, S.M., (1999). *Australian and New Zealand Journal of Psychiatry*, *33/1*, 105.
Wong, A.H.C., Meier, H.M.R., (1997). *Neurocase*, *3/5*, 391.

Chapter 4

Ganser's syndrome

Polonius: Though this be madness, yet there is method in 't.

II, ii, 207

King: Nor what he spake, though it lacked form a little,
Was not like madness. There's something in his soul.

William Shakespeare, *Hamlet* (III, i, 171)

This is a condition, the basis of which is not well understood, that was first described in 1897 in a classic lecture by Sigbert Ganser. It is characterised by the giving of approximate answers to simple and unfamiliar questions, in a setting of disturbed or clouded consciousness.

Historical

Ganser gave an account of the syndrome being exhibited in four prisoners. He saw this as a form of hysterical twilight state, having as its other main features impairment of grasp, attention and concentration; anxiety; perplexity; hallucinations; and manifestly hysterical sensory and motor symptoms, all terminating abruptly with amnesia for the whole episode (Ganser, 1898). Various synonyms have since been applied to this condition (although none is satisfactory as they all fail to do justice to the full breadth of the symptomatology):

- Nonsense syndrome
- Balderdash syndrome
- Pseudodementia syndrome
- Prison psychosis

The syndrome has endured, albeit controversially, with its status as a distinct nosological entity and even its very existence questioned (Debeyne et al., 2016; Wirtz et al., 2008). It is, nevertheless, recognised in the World Health Organisation's tenth edition of the *Classification of Mental and Behavioural Disorders* (*ICD-10*) under "Other dissociative [conversion] disorders" (F44.8). At the time of writing, it also occurs in the beta draft of *ICD-11* under "Other specified dissociative disorders" (6B8Y).

The real significance of the disorder resides in the insight it provides into certain psychopathological processes, skirting as it does the hinterlands of schizophrenic illnesses, affective disorders, organic states, hysteria and malingering. Its relationship with the last state in particular reveals much about the workings of the human mind when facing an intolerable, confining situation – physical or otherwise – from which there is no easy escape.

Case reports

Case 1

A man of 55 years of age was first seen at home at the request of his GP in mid-December 1961. He had been treated for low backache for a few months. Although this had improved, he had become increasingly disturbed and confused. He had also taken to wandering away from home. Because of this, and as examination revealed some vague neurological signs in his lower limbs, he was immediately admitted to hospital for observation and investigation.

The patient's father, who died at the age of 56 years, was described as an easy-going friendly man; his mother aged 86 years was well. He was the eldest of eight children, and there was no family history of mental disorder. Born in Ireland, where he lived as a child, he had had no serious illnesses or any neurotic traits in childhood. After a council-school education until aged 14 years, he worked as a gardener and later became a plate-layer on the railway.

After living with a woman for 30 years, together with her illegitimate son, he eventually married her in October 1961.

He was a conscientious man with some obsessional traits. He tended to be moody, was affectionate at times and quick tempered at others. He readily became anxious, especially when things went wrong at work. Despite these personality traits, he had never suffered from any mental disorder. He had also been physically fit until June 1958, when he fell between two railway tracks at work. No bony injury or neurological abnormalities were detected, and he returned to work the following February. In June 1961, he was seen at an orthopaedic clinic and because some limitation in straight-leg raising was found, he was considered to be suffering possibly from a prolapsed intervertebral disc. He was admitted to hospital for pelvic traction and was discharged again in September 1961.

A few days before seeing the orthopaedic surgeon again, he himself cut off his plaster jacket but then became distressed at having done so.

On examination his back condition was found to be satisfactory, but he was noted to be mentally disturbed. On returning home that evening, he left the house to buy cigarettes but did not return for three days and could give little or no account of himself. He continued to behave in a strange manner, wandering off for hours and appearing confused.

On admission he appeared to be an old-looking man of 55 years, though well built and well nourished. Apart from brisk reflexes in both lower limbs and limitation of straight-leg raising, more so on the right side, no abnormal physical signs were detected. He was obviously perplexed, anxious, confused and appeared to be in pain. He was not then hallucinated but stated that he had heard voices a month ago. He showed poverty of speech, limited spontaneity and considerable sensorial impairment. He was disorientated for time and place. On being asked what month it was (December) he answered, "November." On being asked what place he was in, he answered "I forget where I am at times." Attention and concentration were poor. Asked to subtract serial sevens from one hundred, he gave the answers: $100 - 7 = 83$; $83 - 7 = 76$; $76 - 7 = 63$; $63 - 7 = 46$. There was obviously a patchy memory loss present which seemed to confirm his assertion that he forgot things. He was particularly vague about the circumstances of his marriage which had occurred only two months previously. It was noted that he answered questions with great deliberation and took them very seriously.

He was extensively investigated because the clinical picture was at first suggestive of an organic state, although at the same time the history of fluctuation in his condition, the oddities in his behaviour, and the pattern of the sensorial defect strongly suggested that he was suffering from pseudodementia. Apart from some osteoarthritic changes and narrowing of the lumbosacral articulation, all physical investigations were within normal limits.

Further mental testing confirmed the diagnosis of a Ganser's state. His responses to arithmetical tests and to a lesser extent to vocabulary and agnosia tests showed them to come within the category of "approximate answers." For example, when asked to do six simple arithmetical calculations four were wrong, but only very narrowly so, viz: $4 + 2 = 7$; $3 + 4 = 8$; $5 + 5 = 10$; $6 - 3 = 3$; $5 - 2 = 2$; $7 - 4 = 2$. When asked to count the number of fingers the examiner was extending he gave the wrong answer each time, either one more or one fewer. On being asked how many legs a dog had, he responded very seriously, giving a considered and correct reply, but only after counting slowly on his fingers. Shown the picture of a crab, having three legs on one side and two on the other, he insisted that a leg was missing from the side which had three legs. Pointing to this he counted four legs and contrasted it with the other side, which he said had three. Many other inconsistencies were apparent. There was also a variation in the performance of similar tasks within a short time-span, with failure to cope with easy items in contrast to success in more difficult ones. Overall, there was a mixture of correct, approximate and clearly wrong answers. His complete lack of surprise or resentment at being asked such simple questions as "How many legs has a dog?" was noteworthy.

One month later there was a vast difference in his performance. Whereas his full-scale IQ (WAIS) had originally appeared to be 72, it was now found to be 94, and although some variation between subtest scores remained, this was certainly less marked. No approximate answers or unusual features of the kind observed on first testing were noted on this occasion. When asked to perform simple arithmetical calculations, his answers were completely accurate. Likewise he made no error when asked to count the number of fingers the examiner was extending. Indeed, he now expressed surprise at being asked such simple questions and said he found it hard to believe that he had previously failed to answer them successfully.

This improvement began within five days of his admission. Although he still complained of pain in his back and right thigh, this did not appear to be anything like so severe or incapacitating as before. Indeed, his attitude towards whatever pain he did experience was considerably changed. Whereas at home he stayed in bed, apparently writhing in agony, in hospital he was soon able to get up every day and walk around the hospital grounds. He did not then refer to his pain except when directly questioned. He no longer appeared confused, although for a time he still complained of some periodic patchy memory loss. In the course of psychotherapy, he began to talk more freely about his anxiety, and in particular of his wife's attitude towards him. She seemed to be more closely attached to her illegitimate son than to the patient so that he felt he had to take second place. He felt that he had married under some duress so that he would not be forced to leave home. He also expressed some worries about his work and financial situation.

As a result of being able to ventilate these anxieties there was an immediate and considerable improvement in his clinical state. This continued, and after two months in hospital he was discharged, his symptoms almost completely cleared. At this time there was no evidence whatsoever of any clouding of consciousness or of memory impairment. His answers were clear, direct and almost always correct. He said that while he had periodic twinges of backache he was not particularly worried about this. He stated that he knew what it was, that he could tolerate it and that it certainly would not cripple him. He left hospital optimistic about the future and remained well over the next two years during which he was followed up.

Case 2

A widow of 35 years of age was also first seen at home at the request of her GP. During the previous few days she had taken to her bed, being no longer able to cope with her house, farm and two sons as well as holding down a job.

When first seen she showed a stupid listlessness, lay prostrate in bed, eyes closed, generally flabby and flaccid as if she could not sit up or stand (although she could do both on request). At times she grunted and mumbled irrelevantly; at others she spoke sensibly. Although after a while her concentration and attention improved and she took an interest in the proceedings, she still appeared confused. Correct replies to questions were interspersed with approximate ones, obviously ridiculous ones and sometimes "I don't know" answers. Asked "How many legs has a cow?" she replied, "I do not keep cows, only pigs." Asked to name the first day of the week, she answered, "Friday." A deep red flower on the wallpaper was said to be pink. In addition she would say, "I don't know" when asked to do simple calculations such as 3 + 2. She tended to go off at a tangent and talk a mixture of sense and nonsense. Some obviously emotionally charged questions she did not seem to hear at all, for example those relating to the death of her husband and her future. Even during the course of a single interview, her condition fluctuated so that she appeared less confused at one time and more so at another. She seemed unable to give a clear account of her past life.

On being questioned about the possibility of admission, she was adamant that she would not go into a mental hospital but would consider going into a general hospital. She then referred to the general hospital to which she had recently been admitted for an operation but could not remember its name or location. She insisted that all she needed was a rest, that she could have this at home and that a friend would look after her. She could give no details of how this could be carried out successfully and did not seem to comprehend that for the past two days her own mother had been running the house and looking after her and her boys. There seemed to be a definite degree of dissociation present.

She also appeared to be hallucinated. She stated she could "see" and "hear" her GP at the foot of the bed while in fact he was silent and to the side and behind the interviewer. She also said she had heard and seen him a few weeks previously when she was in hospital for her hysterectomy.

No neurological signs were present or any other physical abnormality, but in view of her condition, her obvious inability to cope, her mental state and the concern of her family and GP, she was admitted immediately to hospital.

During the first 24 hours, her condition remained very much the same. She lay listlessly in bed, showing no interest in her surroundings. When she did speak she appeared to be confused. The following day she started to take more interest in her surroundings and protested that she wanted to go home and again that all she needed was a rest. She spoke more clearly, showing more spontaneity of both speech and action. She complained of pain in the left side and of great weakness all over her body, saying, "My legs can't hold me." She then admitted she was very worried, that she had been lonely and depressed and had had difficulty in sleeping. On the third day there was a further improvement in her condition so that her confusion became very much less. Indeed, she now answered most questions correctly, there being no evidence whatsoever of the approximate and ridiculous answers she had given before. She laughed when she was told about them, having apparently forgotten what she had done. She began to dress and to get up, although maintaining that she still felt weak.

When first admitted she clearly exhibited all the manifestations of Ganser's syndrome; it was also apparent that this was superimposed upon a depressive state. Accordingly, anti-depressive therapy (amitriptyline) was begun. She continued to show marked improvement daily and within 10 days became quite bright and cheerful. At the end of a fortnight all evidence of depression had disappeared.

In the course of psychotherapy she became able to verbalise her anxieties. She made up her mind to tackle her problems realistically one by one, becoming resigned to the fact that she could not cope with everything at once. As she became more optimistic about the future, she also became more amenable to advice and patient enough to remain longer in hospital to consolidate her improvement.

The above cases demonstrate the core clinical features of the syndrome – confusion, hallucinations, somatic symptoms and the giving of approximate answers. In the first case the precipitating aetiological factor was an emotionally charged and psychologically confining social situation, whereas in the second case the condition was superimposed upon a depressive illness.

The following case is interesting as, unlike the previous examples, it developed within a penal setting, again in response to overwhelming stress associated with confinement.

Case 3

A 23-year-old serving prisoner was facing fresh charges of riot following a serious disturbance in an English prison. He was born into a family with no history of mental disorder, brought up in an inner-city environment, attended mainstream schools and started offending (mostly in an acquisitive fashion) in his early teenage years. He had been previously healthy with no history of contact with psychiatric services, but there was a history of illicit drug abuse.

He reported sustaining a head injury during the prison disturbance resulting in unconsciousness for a period of several minutes. There was, however, no independent evidence to confirm that this event had happened.

Following the disturbances he initially co-operated with the investigating police but then had criminal charges of riot made out against him. He then found himself in the quandary of having to give more information about fellow prisoners in order to successfully defend himself and avoid a substantial prison sentence. In addition, however, he had received a number of threats of violence from co-defendants demanding his silence. Likewise his family had also been subjected to harassment from the families of co-defendants.

Several months after the prison disturbance, he developed problems with his health and had a brief admission to a medical ward for breathing problems and what was thought to be an epileptic convulsion. A number of investigations were performed including a series of EEGs and an isotope brain scan. All were normal apart from a proportion of the EEG traces. Prison staff observed a change in behaviour; at times he appeared confused and complained of hearing voices. His symptoms, however, responded quickly when he was removed from ordinary prison location onto the hospital wing. Prison staff, after observing the thrashing and flailing of limbs during a convulsion, doubted how genuine the symptoms were and considered him to be malingering. His condition worsened as the trial date approached.

When psychiatrically examined some 20 months after the prison disturbance, he proved a difficult person to interview, unwilling to divulge information although he was otherwise co-operative. He was vague, evasive with seemingly poor concentration and grasp. He described hearing whispering voices talking to him, originating from other prisoners, and, over a number of interviews, he gave approximate answers. He refused or was unable to co-operate with formal psychometric tests, but a clinical estimation revealed him to be functioning at the lower end of the normal intellectual range.

Following transfer to a psychiatric ward, his demeanour and behaviour rapidly settled, although he remained anxious and tense about his trial and predicament. Strangely, he demonstrated some insight into his condition, stating that doctors could only help him if they could "perform miracles," and he described his experience as being like "an animal in a cage."

He was considered to be suffering with Ganser's syndrome, exhibiting all the core features, and was managed conservatively with support and occasional doses of anxiolytic drugs. His disturbed mental state settled sufficiently to allow him to complete his trial. One year later he was living in the community and was mentally healthy.

The following case is newly reported, arising in an Australian jurisdiction. The patient displayed all of the core features of Ganser's syndrome: the underlying nature of the presentation was considered to be a combination of classic Ganserism along with an element of malingering.

All of the details reported have already been recorded within the public domain (State of Tasmania v Lokendra Singh 11/11/16).

Case 4

A 30-year-old man who originated from India was convicted of the attempted murder of his wife. He cut her throat with a knife as she was sleeping. There had been a background of marital disharmony, particularly (although not exclusively) centred round financial matters. He had previously been the victim of an assault when at work and had subsequently been treated for a variety of vague somatic and affective symptoms.

He underwent a psychiatric examination when in custody awaiting sentence. At this time the most prominent aspect of the presentation was a paranoid syndrome; he complained of being hunted and persecuted by the alleged assailant of the previous assault. He was then transferred to a secure hospital for further observation and detailed assessment.

During the course of the several-months-long admission, he presented in a consistent manner with an air of perplexity. He complained of seeing and hearing his supposed persecutor on the ward. He reported a variety of somatic complaints and at times would walk with a limp. When observed he would display unusual behaviours, such as attempting to dress himself by placing his underwear on his head.

When interviewed, although he could readily articulate his concerns about his supposed persecutor, he would start to ramble and become hard to follow when asked further questions, such as about the offence. In response to direct questions, he provided a series of approximate answers: for instance, when asked to count three upright fingers on the hand of the examiner, he counted four; when asked to give his age, he said 7; and when asked to put forward his right limb, he would proffer his left.

The gross disturbances in behaviour resolved immediately on return to prison. However, the complaints of hallucinations and the approximate answers would reappear whenever the patient was reinterviewed.

Epidemiology

The rarity of the syndrome has been commented upon by virtually all authors who have written on the subject. Indeed, Goldin and MacDonald (1955) in an extensive review found that up until 1955 only 14 cases had been reported in the English medical literature. This, perhaps, partly explains the paucity of epidemiological studies and hence the almost complete absence of data concerning the incidence and prevalence of the disorder.

Cases have been infrequently reported (surprisingly perhaps given the disorder's probable hysterical basis) more so in the European than the North American literature. In 1987, Carney et al. (1987), following a useful literature review, concluded that probably fewer than 50 cases of the complete syndrome were recorded. Since that date fewer than 50 further cases have been reported, not all of which have all, or even the majority, of the features originally described by Ganser. It appears fair to conclude, therefore, that in terms of the English medical literature, under 100 cases had been reported in the 120 years following Ganser original description. Although the infrequent reporting may have been contributed to by the syndrome having been seldom recognised, it remains likely that it is genuinely uncommon.

The closest there is to a full-scale epidemiological survey is the work of Tsoi who, in 1973, surveyed 1,200 admissions to a mental hospital in Singapore serving a population of 2 million, and in this sample reported 10 cases of the syndrome. This is a somewhat surprisingly high figure, amounting to slightly less than 1% of all of the hospital's admissions, although not all of the sample exhibited the complete syndrome. A further numerical hint of incidence was provided by Tyndel (1956) who, between the years 1950 to 1954, examined "several thousand" individuals for social insurance purposes and reported finding 25 cases with Ganserian features.

In terms of sex incidence, the syndrome when it occurs seems to be almost always confined to males. Whitlock (1967) considered that this difference may be more apparent than real, perhaps being related to a higher frequency of reporting in prisoners – both military and civilian. However, many of the reported studies do consist of male-only samples, and case reports of females remain few and far between.

Ganser's original patients were criminal prisoners, but subsequent writings have implied that the syndrome can be equally seen in non-forensic settings. Jolly (quoted by Weiner and Braiman, 1955) reported that one-third of his cases were non-criminal civilians and, of the six cases in the sample of Weiner and Braiman (1955), only one was a prisoner. More recently, in a study of the incidence of Ganser's syndrome following mild traumatic brain injury (TBI), Dalfen and Feinstein (2000) found that, of 513 mild TBI cases assessed in a tertiary care outpatient clinic, just four (0.8%) developed Ganser's syndrome; of these four, there was an absence of litigation in three cases. These findings, together with published case reports, suggest that the view that the syndrome only occurs in civilian or military prisoners, and in persons seeking compensation for accident, is erroneous (see also Cases 1 and 2).

One interesting observation has been that of some association with an ethnic minority status. For example, of Tsoi's (1973) sample, 60% were from the Indian minority of Singapore; at the time of the study, those of Indian origin made up just 7% of the island city's population. More recently, Sigal et al. (1992) reported a study of 15 cases from Israel, in which over 50% of the sample was of Arab origin, whereas at the time Arabs made up 19% of Israel's population.

Traditionally, it has always been believed that the syndrome is restricted to the realm of adult psychiatry. Indeed, Scott (1965) could find not one instance in the 8,000 juvenile delinquents he personally examined. However, in recent years 10 case reports have been published indicating its occurrence in adolescents and prepubescent children, some within a forensic setting. While not all the cases exhibited the full syndrome, in nine (90%) of the cases co-morbidity was present, as shown in Table 4.1.

Clinical features

The four essential clinical features of Ganser's syndrome are:

- Approximate answers
- Clouding of consciousness
- Somatic conversion features
- Hallucinations

The complete syndrome, exhibiting all of the core symptoms, is rare. Within the medical literature, however, there are several case reports which demonstrate two or three of the features, and these more frequently encountered examples, therefore, probably represent *formes frustes* of the full syndrome.

The central and constant symptom, the approximate answer, has hitherto been referred to as *vorbeireden*, "talking past or beside the point." A study of the original shows that this word was not used by Ganser himself. Instead he employed the word *vorbeigehen*, "to pass by," which appears to describe the symptom more accurately, i.e. the patient "passes by" the correct answer to the question and gives one near to it (Ganser, 1898; 1904).

Table 4.1 Co-morbidity in published case reports of Ganser's syndrome in children and adolescents

Case report	Co-morbidity
Whitlock (1967)	Schizophrenia
Nardi and Di Scipio (1977)	Psychosis
Adler (1981); Adler and Touyz (1989)	Head injury
Burd and Kerbeshian (1985)	Gilles de la Tourette's syndrome and atypical pervasive developmental disorder
Dabholkar (1987)	None
Apter et al. (1993) – two adolescent brothers	Mood disorder (in both cases)
Miller et al. (1997)	Head injury
Refaat et al. (2002)	Gilles de la Tourette's syndrome
Spodenkiewicz et al. (2012)	Depression

For example, he may answer that the sum of two plus two equals five, that he has 11 fingers, and that there are eight days in a week. Answers such as these may be interspersed with correct responses, with some that are obviously ridiculous, and "I don't know" answers requiring but the simplest knowledge of everyday facts. Absurd though some of these answers are, each is given with deliberation and apparently serious intent. For example, when asked the time of day, the patient may say that it is midnight although it is to be seen that the sun is shining.

A wide variety of ridiculous and approximate answers may be given. Colours may be incorrectly named. One of our patients, when given a block design test, insisted that the red areas on the blocks were white and the white areas were red. Asked how many legs a dog had, he arrived at the correct answer only after considerable deliberation and counting on his fingers. Attention must be given not only to the absurdity of the answers but also to the manner in which they are given. Inconsistency is a hallmark of the performance; the tendency to give approximate answers may alter dramatically during an examination and can be radically influenced by the responses and attitude of the interviewer. As the suspicions of the examiner are aroused and questions pressed more ardently, "I don't know" responses tend to become more frequent, the degree of dissociation tends to increase and the subject may show increasing lack of interest in the proceedings or lapse into sullen silence.

The state of clouded consciousness that occurs is reflected in the patient's general appearance and demeanour. The expression may be one of apathetic indifference or of anxious bewilderment. The subject appears lethargic and may be semi-stuporous so that attention is difficult both to gain and sustain. Grasp is impaired, disorientation is evident and in particular a disturbance of memory is apparent. This deficit of memory resembles psychogenic rather than organic amnesia in that it is most constant and striking in relation to matters pertaining to the core of the problem. Away from these, less impairment is obvious and there is a much greater degree of fluctuation. As with other forms of psychogenic amnesia, it clears completely when the problem is resolved, and at this time the patient may express surprise at being so confused. Associated with this confusion is a state of perplexity which is characteristic. Ganser himself described it at times as cloudiness (*benommenheit*) and at others as entanglement (*verwirrtheit*) (Citterio and Della Rovere, 1962).

A large variety of somatic symptoms can occur involving both motor and sensory systems. These cover the whole range of pseudoneurological symptoms familiar in hysterical states. Ataxia and a disorder of balance appear to be particularly common. There may be difficulty in moving the limbs either spontaneously or on request. The posture may be characterised by flaccidity while lying in bed or on other occasions by unnatural rigidity. Those unfamiliar with the clinical picture may mistake it at first for a catatonic state or regard it as the outcome of some organic disorder of the nervous system. Together with these a variety of sensory symptoms can occur. Complaints of headache, backache or other pains or bodily discomforts are common. A case has been reported in which a patient was said to have demonstrated the symptom of prosopagnosia as a hysterical feature (Mahadevappa, 1990).

Physical examination is likely to reveal signs of high autonomic arousal such as a mildly elevated blood pressure and brisk tendon jerks. On sensory testing, analgesia or areas of anaesthesia may be evident.

If hallucinations are present, these may be auditory or visual in nature; reports of abnormal perceptions in other modalities are unknown to the authors. They can be of a rather fantastic nature, and their content tends to bear a general relationship to the patient's life situation and may suggest a re-enactment of emotionally charged episodes. The second patient in the case reports saw a vision of her general practitioner standing at the foot of her bed. From what she said, she had a strong need for him in that she felt he was the only one who could help in her present circumstances. The nature of these perceptual disturbances and their integration into the patient's current situation indicate that they are not true but pseudohallucinations, such as are characteristic of some other varieties of hysterical twilight state.

The patient's general behaviour may be chaotic and disturbed, fluctuating between stupor and violence. Such a presentation, when it occurs, adds to the diagnostic difficulty by masking the more subtle core features.

The differential diagnosis includes:

- *Organic dementia* – characterised by "hard-core" cognitive deficit; usually presents few problems.
- *Organic twilight state* – responses are slow and, although may be wrong *vorbeireden* is not present.
- *Depressive pseudodementia* – can present great difficulty; inpatient observations necessary.
- *Hysterical pseudodementia* – no clouding of consciousness.
- *Schizophrenia* – look for thought disorder and affective incongruity.
- *Malingering* – rare, difficult to sustain such a role over a long period of time.

Aetiology and psychopathology

Technically speaking the aetiology and psychopathological interpretation of Ganser's syndrome is unproven and remains obscure. Many writers have argued that the condition is really a non-specific manifestation of psychotic processes, either organic or functional. Such a hypothesis was extensively explored by Whitlock (1967). It is the authors' shared view, however, that the bulk of evidence currently available continues to support Ganser's original opinion, that the disorder has its origins in psychoneurotic mechanisms. Careful consideration does, nevertheless, have to be given to other, not necessarily mutually exclusive, themes such as organicity, psychosis, affective disorder and malingering.

Biology

The clouding of consciousness and pseudodementia features of the clinical picture are initially suggestive of an organic brain syndrome. Furthermore, some of Ganser's original cases followed cerebral trauma, as have other subsequently recorded cases. Similarly, the restricted consciousness and perplexed affective responses can be clinically indistinguishable from a complex partial seizure or post-epileptic twilight state.

Few studies have been performed specifically focussing on a potential organic substrate, and those that have been are patchy and fail to provide strong evidence in its favour. Cocores et al. (1986) reviewed 50 cases from various sources in the literature, including a single case report of their own. Only 18 of the cases had reported EEG results ,and of those 11 (61%) were normal, two (11%) "questionably abnormal" and five (28%) definitely abnormal. In addition, CT scans performed on reported cases are usually normal, and psychometric examinations either provide evidence of psychoneurotic mechanisms or organic-like results, which nevertheless return to their pre-morbid normal level following resolution of the disorder.

While emphasising that the Ganser's syndrome was classified as a dissociative disorder in *DSM-IV*, Ouyang et al. (2003) have pointed out that the syndrome does occur in association with organic states such as head trauma or strokes. The mechanism by which these cerebral insults lead to Ganser's syndrome remains an intriguing question; Ouyang et al. (2003) hypothesise that there may be merit in considering the role of hyperglutamatergic neurotransmission, as glutamate surges are associated with both cerebral infarcts and dissociative symptoms (as in posttraumatic stress disorder) (Moghaddam et al., 1997; Chambers et al., 1999; Berthier et al., 2001; Duggal, 2003). Interestingly, in line with the above-mentioned review by Cocores et al. (1986), the EEG of the case of Ganser's syndrome reported by Ouyang et al. (2003) was normal, while his CT scan "revealed a few scattered punctate foci of decreased attenuation in both frontal lobes ... most consistent with old lacunar infarcts." Wirtz et al. (2008) also suggest that Ganser's syndrome may be associated with brain injury and illustrate this with the case of a right-handed 43-year-old woman who developed this syndrome following large left middle cerebral artery infarction that was revealed by CT scan.

However, as mentioned above, Dalfen and Feinstein (2000) reported that less than 1% of 513 patients who had suffered mild TBI went on to develop Ganser's syndrome. Nevertheless, Dalfen and Feinstein (2000) advise clinicians to be alert to the possibility of patients presenting with Ganser's syndrome following mild TBI.

Ladowsky-Brooks and Fischer (2003) also referred to the many reported cases of Ganser's syndrome having a history of head injury while reporting on a patient presenting with core symptoms of this syndrome in the early stages of frontal-temporal lobe dementia. This raises the further question as to whether a reported symptom of Ganser's syndrome may be accounted for by frontal-temporal lobe dysfunction.

Psychosis

Some of the behavioural and verbal responses of Ganser's patients can be strongly reminiscent of certain psychotic disorders, especially the buffoonery state and negativistic syndromes of catatonic schizophrenia. Ganserian answers do seem to share some of the characteristics of what Cameron (1944) referred to as "metonymic distortions," which form one basis of schizophrenic thought disorder.

A great dispute surrounds the possible relationship between Ganser's syndrome and schizophrenia. The term "buffoonery state" has been used to describe the bizarre behaviour of certain catatonic patients whose replies to questions and general attitude are such as to merit no less a description. There is also a resemblance here to so-called hysterical puerilism, but both occur in a setting of clear consciousness and, in the former instance, together with gross thought disorder and affective incongruity. In addition, Sim (1963) has made a very useful point in differential diagnosis. Referring to the schizophrenic "buffoonery syndrome," he stated, "In this condition there is an air of defiance about the patient, his behaviour is incongruous rather than ridiculous and the approximate answers which may be offered are never so crude." Atypical schizophrenic psychoses with clouding of consciousness, so-called oneirophrenic states, may also have to be considered in the differential diagnosis, although the schizophrenic nature of these is usually readily apparent.

Underlying affective disturbance

The occurrence of pseudodementia in the setting of an affective disturbance presents both clinical and theoretical difficulties. Indeed, there are some grounds for believing that Ganser's syndrome, together with some other disorders which present in hysterical guise, is not infrequently a manifestation of a depressive illness in which some clouding of consciousness occurs (Anderson et al., 1959). Thus a 29-year-old woman suffered a series of episodes of pseudodementia and stupor which responded strikingly to ECT and which were apparently caused by recurrent attacks of depressive illness. Another somewhat different example was provided by a 33-year-old university student who, having failed his final BA examination, suddenly developed a paranoid depressive reaction accompanied by episodes of stupor and pseudodementia.

Malingering

The view that Ganser's syndrome is little more than a manifestation of malingering is commented upon by Szasz (1961):

> It is astonishing how well persons exhibiting the typical features of the Ganser's syndrome ... have succeeded in convincing both themselves and those around them that they are, in fact, sick (meaning by this, disabled, not responsible, perhaps even bodily ill) ... But in so doing, nevertheless both they and we are misled and confused.

This view brings Ganser's syndrome and malingering closer together than those with less radical views about the nature of mental illness than Szasz might care to accept. Perhaps insufficient regard is given to the heightened emotional tone of the situation in which the patient is enmeshed and which leads, among other things, to the occurrence of pseudohallucinations which, in turn, emerge on the basis of clouded consciousness. Szasz's opinion is, by contemporary standards, unsophisticated and confuses the form of the psychopathological process with the underlying motivation, and hence fails to distinguish between dissociative/conversion disorder, factitious disorder and true malingering.

Psychopathology

It can be seen, therefore, that the overwhelming evidence continues to support the view that Ganser's syndrome is, in its pure form, a hysterical dissociative reaction that occurs as a result of an unconscious effort by the subject to escape from a confining intolerable situation, but in a limited way. There is little doubt whatsoever that the syndrome, although unconsciously motivated, does serve a gainful purpose – the adoption of the sick role. This is reflected in the fact that when efforts are made to approach the central core of the problem, repression is enhanced and the flight from reality becomes more obvious. In addition to an attempt to evade responsibility or of having to face a seemingly intolerable life situation, there is a simultaneous desire to keep in touch with reality and thereby limit the degree of withdrawal. This compromise is reflected in the symptomatology. This, too, as Leiberman (1954) and Weiner and Braiman (1955) have pointed out, explains the central symptom of *vorbeireden* (or Ganser's *vorbeigehen*), why the answer to a question is not merely a shot in the dark but a near miss.

Owing to the amnesia which follows recovery, patients with this syndrome are later unable to explain why they originally gave approximate or ridiculous answers, or even that they ever did so. Indeed, when reminded of some of the questions asked on initial examination, they may laugh at their absurdity, let alone that of their own responses. Some idea of the underlying process may, however, be gained by the study of those who are asked to simulate mental disorder for experimental purposes (Anderson et al., 1959). Like patients with Ganser's syndrome, quite a proportion of these tend to give approximate answers, but not being amnesic are later able to throw some light on their mental activity during the experimental period. It has to be appreciated, however, that the circumstances under which the experimental simulations are carried out are not strictly analogous to those which pertain to the Ganser's state, motivation in the two instances being of a different order. One experimental subject, who produced a whole series of approximate and near approximate answers to mental arithmetic questions during examination, later explained his reasoning process at the time thus: "Supposing I am asked to add two and two. The answer comes four! What shall I do? Give an approximate answer, five? No! That's not good enough, say six!"

Another subject rearranged or transposed numbers in a given series of digits he was asked to repeat. He explained that, while he at first made a conscious effort to do so, he later withdrew his attention to help him in giving wrong or near right answers. Most experimental simulants who are able to produce these kinds of responses admit that the pull of reality makes the exercise difficult to perform, particularly if the examination is at all prolonged. This points to the fact that it is the clouding of consciousness, the second principal feature of Ganser's syndrome, which is conducive to sustaining the role. As Anderson et al. (1959) have pointed out, "The Ganser's patient who can exercise a selective apprehension of an experience, can or will attend only to certain aspects and thus his answer is perverse. Since wholes are not grasped, the total sphere of relevant experience is not drawn upon, in some way access to this is blocked."

As hysterical symptoms are usually an imperfect representation of the condition they resemble and correspond to the mental image the patient expects to have of the illness or emotional state which is resembled, then, given the fact that the disorder has almost always been reported in individuals of less than superior intelligence, the apparently crude nature of much of the symptomatology is readily understandable.

Management and treatment

Hospital admission

Although the natural history of the condition is towards recovery, the acute phase of the disorder causes so many problems, including much distress for the patient and diagnostic difficulties for clinicians, that admission to hospital is often inevitable. Indeed, in many instances hospital admission with or without compulsory detention becomes essential to allow for a detailed assessment in order to exclude co-morbid conditions such as depressive illness and, of course, malingering.

In certain settings (e.g. remand prisoners) medico-legal issues are raised, and transfer to hospital may be necessary to ensure fitness to plead and to stand trial.

General treatment

General treatment approaches include sympathetic nursing care, the provision of a safe and structured environment and a supportive expectant attitude on the part of the attending physician. The aim is to help the patient return to normality, and this is aided by overlooking the ridiculous answers, providing gentle encouragement and by not imparting to the patient a sense of disbelief or any suspicion of malingering.

Specific therapies

Ganser's syndrome has been reported to make an excellent response to a brief course of ECT (Goldin and MacDonald, 1955; Tyndel, 1956). This should, however, be reserved for exceptional cases with severe or potentially life-threatening features. Co-morbid depression must of course be treated vigorously. Improvement has also been reported following administration of neuroleptic medication, but again it must be stressed that the vast majority of patients will respond to the general measures outlined earlier in this section without recourse to drugs or ECT.

It is not known whether any form of treatment, including drug, cognitive or other form of psychotherapy, has a prophylactic effect in reducing the risk of future occurrences.

Prognosis

The tendency towards a natural complete resolution has already been commented upon, and the *short-term* prognosis of the disorder is excellent, despite the continuing presence of stressful factors, such as impending trial or litigation.

It is generally accepted that the disorder can re-emerge in the form of a *relapse* when the patient is stressfully challenged at a later date and, indeed, such recurrences are said to be common. There are no studies, however, to support this anecdotal clinical impression or to provide a numerical expression of relapse rates. This is not surprising given the rarity of the disorder. Again, clinical impression is that recurrences following new stresses are usually transient and resolution is complete.

Malingering

Malingering is frequently suspected in prisoners awaiting trial. Such suspicions are not only reserved for those with no clear previous psychiatric history but are increasingly applied to individuals who have previously attracted a diagnosis of genuine mental disorder. For example, in the authors' experience prisoners who present with psychotic symptoms such as auditory hallucinations may have these dismissed by their civilian psychiatrist as being "unconvincing" or "put on," apparently in an attempt to evade punishment by the courts. Chiswick and Dooley (1995) claim that "inexperienced practitioners imagine that all prisoners are malingerers unless proved otherwise." These authors also emphasise that "in practice malingering is unusual in prisoners and is usually easily detected." This situation often becomes increasingly confused as other concepts are introduced in order to provide an explanation for the symptoms. These include co-morbid personality disorder and a so-called drug-induced psychosis. Such attitudes are not only erroneous but also potentially dangerous and can deny patients appropriate treatment. This diagnostic tendency is contributed to by a fundamental confusion which fails to distinguish a syndrome described in terms of its clinical features from its underlying motivation. In short, there is a lack of definitional clarity.

Malingering is the false reporting of symptoms with the intention to deceive, in order to achieve some goal (ethical or otherwise) – usually the avoidance of an unpleasant situation. The mechanism is essentially one of conscious lying, and the individual responsible is aware of the untruthful nature of the symptoms. The concept of malingering cannot, therefore, be applied to a case in which the patient is unaware of the mechanism of symptom production, as, whatever the psychopathological basis, the symptoms by definition are genuine.

Cases are on record in which mental illness has been successfully simulated in order to avoid a difficult or unpleasant situation. One of the best documented is that of Jones (1955), who in his book *The Road to En-Dor*, recounted how he simulated mental disorder in order to escape from a Turkish prisoner-of-war camp in World War I. Further examples have come to light more recently, including the case of Winston Thomas, who, after evading a prison sentence by simulating schizophrenia, was subsequently successfully prosecuted for perverting the course of justice (*Daily Express*, November 18, 1992). Such instances must, however, be considered highly unusual, and it is generally accepted that to consistently and successfully deceive an experienced psychiatrist is a difficult and exceptional feat.

Some idea of the rarity of malingering is provided by the work of Hay (1983), who, in a review of 12,000 new admissions to a psychiatric unit in South Manchester over a 10-year period, reported only five cases. Furthermore, malingering as a phenomenon has some special inherent features, strongly suggesting a pathological nature in its own right. This is nowhere more so than in the way feigned mental illness often subsequently develops into genuine psychosis, as in the fictional literature of Andreyev's *The Dilemma*. Such a tendency, and the caution it generates in psychiatrists, has been reflected throughout much of the classical psychiatric literature:

• Bleuler (1924) – "Simulation of insanity is not nearly so common as the layman supposes. Those who simulate insanity with some cleverness are nearly all psychopaths and some are actually insane. Demonstration of simulation, therefore, does not at all prove that the patient is mentally sound and responsible for his actions."

• Kraepelin (1919) – "In this domain the utmost caution is necessary. In several such cases, in which I believed with certainty that I had to do with undoubted dissimulation, I nevertheless saw dementia praecox develop later."

• Maudsley (1867) – "When a man feigns madness so perfectly as to deceive an experienced observer, we may hold, I think, that he is not far from being the character which he represents; for, unless there be a foundation of real madness beneath the feigned phenomena, there will be some want of coherence in them as a whole, and an incongruity with any known form of mental disease."

The emerging themes of malingering in a psychiatric setting – its rarity, its status as a manifestation of underlying genuine mental disorder and the caution with which retrospective confessions of simulation should be accepted – were additionally commented upon by Jung (1903). With this in mind, the case of Bucknill and Tuke (1862), quoted in earlier editions of *Uncommon Psychiatric Syndromes*, can now be seen as most likely representing an erroneous diagnosis of simulation.

Follow-up studies conducted on cases of initially diagnosed simulated mental illness have confirmed the views of earlier writers in demonstrating either co-existing mental disorder or the subsequent development of social disability or frank mental illness, often in the guise of schizophrenia (Hay, 1983; Humphreys and Ogilvie, 1996). This mechanism was well described by Schneck (1970), who used the term "pseudomalingering." This concept implies that the phenomenon of malingering, in a psychiatric setting, is often a symptom of disorder – a prodromal feature of genuine psychosis – which can be interpreted dynamically as an ego-supporting mechanism or, as Berney (1973) described, a "last-ditch attempt" to compensate for personality disintegration. It seems clear, therefore, that pure malingering, in a psychiatric setting, is rare; it should only be diagnosed after other possibilities have been exhaustively explored and excluded, never as a first-line diagnosis. If elements of it are suspected, then the eventual development of psychosis should be anticipated.

References

Adler, R. (1981). *Australian and New Zealand Journal of Psychiatry, 15,* 339.

Adler, R., Touyz, S. (1989). *Australian and New Zealand Journal of Psychiatry, 23,* 124.

Anderson, E.W., Trethowan, W.H., Kenna, J. (1959). *Acta Psychiatrica Scandinavica, 34* (suppl.), 1.

Apter, A., Ratzoni, G., Iancu, I., Weizman, R., Tyano, S. (1993). *Journal of the American Academy of Child and Adolescent Psychiatry, 32,* 582.

Berney, T.P. (1973). *South African Medical Journal, 47,* 1429.

Berthier, M.L., Posada, A., Puentes, C. (2001). *Journal of Neuropsychiatry and Clinical Neurosciences, 13,* 101.

Bleuler, E. (1924). *Textbook of Psychiatry.* The MacMillan Company, New York.

Bucknill, J.C., Tuke, D.H. (1862). *A Manual of Psychological Medicine.* Churchill, London.

Burd, L., Kerbeshian, J. (1985). *Canadian Journal of Psychiatry, 30,* 74.

Cameron, N. (1944). Experimental Analysis of Schizophrenic Thinking. In *Language and Thought in Schizophrenia.* University of California Press, Berkley.

Carney, M.W.P., Chary, T.K.N., Robotis, P., Childs, A. (1987). *British Journal of Psychiatry, 151,* 697.

Chambers, R.A., Bremner, J.D., Moghaddam, B., Southwick, S.M., Charney, D.S., Krystal, J.H. (1999). *Seminars in Clinical Neuropsychiatry, 4,* 274.

Chiswick, D., Dooley, E. (1995). In *Seminars in Practical Forensic Psychiatry,* Eds D. Chiswick and R. Cope. Gaskell, London.

Citterio, C., Della Rovere, M. (1962). *Archivio di Psicologia, Neurologia e Psichiatria, 23,* 19.

Cocores, J.A., Schlesinger, L.B., Gold, M.S. (1986). *International Journal of Psychiatry in Medicine, 16,* 59.

Dabholkar, P.D. (1987). *British Journal of Psychiatry, 151,* 256.

Dalfen, A.K., & Feinstein, A. (2000). *Brain Injury, 14,* 1101.

Debeyne, M., Haekens, A., Peuskens, H. (2016). *Tijdschrift voor Psychiatrie, 58,* 659.

Daily Express, November 18, 1992.

Duggal, H.S. (2003). *Journal of Neuropsychiatry and Clinical Neurosciences, 15,* 245.

Ganser, S.J. (1898). *Archiv für Psychiatrie und Nervenkrankheiten, 30,* 633.

Ganser, S.J. (1904). *Archiv für Psychiatrie und Nervenkrankheiten, 38,* 34.

Goldin, S., MacDonald, J.E. (1955). *Journal of Mental Science, 101,* 268.

Hay, G.G. (1983). *British Journal of Psychiatry, 143,* 8.

Humphreys, M., Ogilvie, A. (1996). *Psychiatric Bulletin, 20,* 666.

Jones, E.H. (1955). *The Road to En-Dor.* Pan Books, London.

Jung, C.G. (1903). On simulated insanity. In *Collected Works of C.G. Jung,* Vol. 1 (1957). Routledge and Kegan Paul, London.

Kraepelin, E. (1919). *Dementia Praecox and Paraphrenia.* E. & S. Livingstone, Edinburgh.

Ladowsky-Brooks, R.L., Fischer, C.E. (2003). *Journal of Clinical and Experimental Neuropsychology, 25*, 761.

Leiberman, A.A. (1954). *Journal of Nervous and Mental Disease, 120*, 10.

Mahadevappa, H. (1990). *Journal of Clinical Psychiatry, 51*, 167.

Maudsley, M. (1867). *The Philosophy and Pathology of the Mind.* Macmillan, London.

Miller, P., Bramble, D., Buxton, N. (1997). *Journal of the American Academy of Child and Adolescent Psychiatry, 36*, 112.

Moghaddam, B., Adams, B., Verma, A., Daly, D. (1997). *Journal of Neuroscience, 17*, 2921.

Nardi, T.J., Di Scipio, W.J. (1977). *American Journal of Psychiatry, 134*, 453.

Ouyang, D., Duggal, H.S., Jacob, N.J. (2003). *Indian J Psychiatry, 45*, 255.

Refaat, R., Firth, D.A., Robertson, M.M. (2002). *European Child and Adolescent Psychiatry, 11*, 234.

Schneck, J.N. (1970). *Psychiatric Quarterly, 44*, 49.

Scott, P.D. (1965). *British Journal of Criminology, 5*, 127.

Sigal, M., Altmark, D., Alfici, S., Gelkopf, M. (1992). *Comprehensive Psychiatry, 33*, 134.

Sim, M. (1963). *Guide to Psychiatry.* E. & S. Livingstone, London.

Spodenkiewicz, M., Taïeb, O., Speranza, M., Moro, M.-R., Révah-Levy, A. (2012). *Child and Adolescent Psychiatry and Mental Health, 6*, 6.

State of Tasmania v Lokendra Singh 11/11/16 file:///Volumes/KINGSTON/Supreme%20Court_%20SINGH%20L.

Szasz, T. (1961). *The Myth of Mental Illness.* Hoeber, New York.

Tsoi, W.F. (1973). *British Journal of Psychiatry, 123*, 567.

Tyndel, M. (1956). *Journal of Mental Science, 102*, 324.

Whitlock, F.A. (1967). *British Journal of Psychiatry, 113*, 19.

Weiner, H., Braiman, A. (1955). *American Journal of Psychiatry, 111*, 767.

Wirtz, G., Baas, U., Hofer, H., Nyffeler, T., Seifritz, E., Müri, R., Gutbrod, K. (2008). *Der Nervenarzt, 79*, 543.

Chapter 5

Couvade syndrome

> Hows'e'r the kind wife's belly comes to swell
> The husband breeds for her and first is ill.
> William Wycherley, *The Country Wife* (IV, iv)

Couvade syndrome is a disorder in which fathers-to-be suffer a variety of physical symptoms – the most striking of which resemble those with which pregnant women commonly suffer – during their partners' pregnancies or at the time of childbirth or both. It is also occasionally referred to as sympathetic pregnancy or expectant father syndrome (Kiselica and Scheckel, 1995; Markowska et al., 2018). It may, very rarely, affect other relatives and occasionally children.

Historical

"Couvade" as a term was first coined by Tylor (1865) within an anthropological context. The word is derived from the French Basque verb *couver*, to brood or hatch. The term defines an interesting ritual practised, subject to variations, by members of many pre-industrial cultures throughout the world. In essence the custom consists of the father-to-be retiring to bed during his wife's labour, fasting or abstaining from certain kinds of food, simulating labour pains and receiving attention usually shown to parturient women (Westmarck, 1921).

Although not given a name until relatively recently, reference to Couvade syndrome appears over several centuries in the historical literature. The ritual of Couvade is known to be of great antiquity. In 60 BC, Diodorus Siculus observed that "if a woman has borne a child in the Island of Crynos (Corsica) … the man lies down as if he were ill and remains for a definite number of days in child-bed."

One of the best historical references to Couvade occurs in the Provençal poem *Aucassin and Nicolette:*

The hero, Aucassin, comes to the palace of the King of Torelore, where he finds the king lying upon his bed. When he asks what is the matter with him, he is told that he is expecting a son at the end of the month. In this the king was only following the practice that has been reported by scientific investigators since the time of Strabo. Aucassin was no anthropologist, however, and instead of sympathising with the agonies of paternity, he belaboured the king with a cudgel. (Eden, 1958)

In 1627, Francis Bacon stated, "There is an Opinion abroad (whether Idle or no I cannot say) that loving and kinde Husbands have a Sense of their Wives Breeding Childe by some Accident in their Owne Body" (Hunter and Macalpine, 1963).

In 1677, Robert Plot, Fellow and Secretary of the Royal Society, wrote, "In the birth of man it is equally strange that the pangs of women in the exclusion of the child have sometimes affected the Abdomen of the husband" (Hunter and Macalpine, 1963).

It seems that Couvade syndrome also found a place in witchcraft beliefs, and it is on record that at least one witch, a certain Eufame Macalyane, was burned at the stake for, it was believed, having transferred labour pains from wife to husband (Frazer, 1910). According to Murray (1921), "It was a common thing for a witch to be accused of casting pain or illness from the patient on some other person or animal. When, as often happened, the pains were those of childbirth and were cast on the husband, he was most indignant, and his indignation was shared by the male judges to whom he related his woes." Midwives, too, were reputed to have this power (Pennant, 1772). It is also on record that when Mary Queen of Scots went into labour in June 1566, efforts were made by the Countess of Atholl to cast her pangs onto Lady Reres. The procedure does not appear to have been successful for although Lady Reres lay in bed "suffering likewise with her mistress" the Queen apparently obtained no relief (Fraser, 1969).

As with witchcraft so with folklore, there is one symptom in particular, toothache, which, when it afflicted husbands, was sometimes construed as a sign that their wives were pregnant: a belief which has been recorded in many parts of the British Isles (Rolleston, 1945). This was also referred to by the Elizabethan dramatists Dekker and Webster's *Westwood Ho,* a play written in 1607 (Flugel, 1921). During a scene in which three wives are discussing their husbands, one says to another, "The more happy she, would I could make such an ass of my husband too. I hear say he breeds thy children in his teeth every year."

It is also on record that toothache was regarded as a sign of unrequited love and was known in Norfolk as "the love pain." Shakespeare refers to it in this context in *Much Ado about Nothing* (III, ii) when Benedick, having fallen in love with Beatrice, complains of toothache and is teased about this by his companions. Apart from toothache, other Couvade symptoms are also mentioned in seventeenth-century drama and literature: for example, in the plays of Beaumont and Fletcher, Thomas Middleton and Wilkins (Lean, 1904), and, of course, Wycherley (1672 – see chapter heading), as well as in the poem written by Robert Heath in 1650 which comments on "reciprocity" between husband and wife (Lindsay, 1933).

Case reports

Case 1

A 38-year-old Englishman suffered from a variety of symptoms during each of his wife's six pregnancies. At other times he invariably enjoyed good health. Although somewhat shy as a child, he showed no overt neurotic traits. His sexual development seems to have been normal, though he had little contact with girls during adolescence. One younger brother was born when he was 16 years old.

He married three years after leaving the army, meeting his wife and becoming engaged to her during the time he was a baker's roundsman. His engagement was greeted by his parents with scorn, and they refused to attend his wedding. He was considerably hurt by this. His early married life was also somewhat marred by difficulties in accommodation. Then, following greater but not complete acceptance of his wife by his parents, both slept at night in his parents' home while she spent the daytime with hers. These difficulties persisted until after the start of her first pregnancy. The patient then obtained a caravan and later a house. His marital relationship was said to be good with a mutually satisfactory sexual relationship.

At interview he was assessed as reliable, easy-going and sensible in his judgements. He was affable in manner and a little circumstantial in speech.

During his wife's first pregnancy (11 years previously) he suffered from morning sickness. Curiously enough his wife never had this complaint. He also complained of severe toothache which lasted two weeks and led him to demand multiple extractions from a dentist, as a result of which all but eight molars were removed. During the day the child was born he was seized while at work by a severe stomach-ache which forced him to sit on the lavatory for an hour or so. This suddenly left him at 11.00 hours. He subsequently discovered that this was about the time that his son was born. (Coincidences such as these are not uncommonly described by sufferers from Couvade syndrome. Their significance is difficult to assess without invoking some kind of parapsychological explanation. It is more likely, however, that there is some retrospective falsification of memory in these cases.)

Early during his wife's second pregnancy (nine years previously) he suffered again from morning sickness. He then remained in good health until three weeks before the child's birth when for a week he suffered from severe cramps in his upper epigastrium which doubled him up.

During the months before the birth of his third child (now aged 8 years) he again suffered from chest and epigastric pain for one week. This disappeared spontaneously, and he remained well thereafter.

A year later when his wife was pregnant again he experienced the now familiar morning sickness. After this went he remained well until his wife's labour, during which he suffered severe, colicky, lower abdominal pain. Being in a state of some tension, he relieved himself by going into the garage and cutting up a large reel of wire into tiny pieces. He said that he did this to occupy his mind, admitting that he was very worried that something might happen to his wife.

During his wife's fifth pregnancy (three years previously) he had the easiest time of all. He suffered from only a few days' morning sickness and for a week or two from dermatitis on one thigh which he had never had before or since. He could recall no other symptoms during this pregnancy.

The birth of his sixth child took place two weeks before he was first interviewed. During this pregnancy he suffered from quite severe morning sickness starting in about the second month of pregnancy and again from toothache which disappeared spontaneously after about a fortnight. During the second trimester he suffered from low abdominal gripping pain also for about two weeks. This returned three weeks before the birth of the child and lasted for 10 days. Then came a new departure. Without being able to give any good reason for doing so he obtained an incubator and set some bantam's eggs. He gave these earnest attention, even to the point of assisting in the hatching of some of the chicks by easing the tough egg membrane open with tweezers. As soon as he did this his abdominal pain completely disappeared, and although he became extremely anxious and totally anorexic, on the day of the birth he suffered no pain.

During most of his wife's pregnancies he lost his appetite for three weeks early on, this together with morning sickness. During the third trimester, apart from periodic attacks of abdominal pain, he also tended to suffer from what he described as indigestion. He also complained of headaches which he associated with anxiety. During all his wife's pregnancies he confessed to much worrying in case anything should go wrong, especially when he was not present. This anxiety also tended to cause insomnia, frequency of micturition, restlessness and poor concentration. Despite having so many symptoms and being aware of their chronological relationship to his wife's pregnancies, he seemed to have very little if any insight into their likely cause. From the descriptive point of view, therefore, his symptoms must be regarded as a conversion reaction. An exact psychodynamic formulation of his case was hindered by the fact that he was seen on two occasions only, and then not at his own request but at the request of the investigator. (The authors wish to acknowledge the assistance of Dr W. Pryse-Phillips who provided details of this case.) This made deep probing somewhat difficult. However, enough was revealed to suggest that this patient had transferred some of the ambivalence he felt towards his mother to his wife. It was noteworthy how anxious he became during his wife's pregnancies, all of which were quite uncomplicated. This anxiety was associated with mild self-blame and guilt for putting her, as he felt, in jeopardy. What was even more obvious was a considerable degree of empathy and a need to protect and relieve his wife from danger and discomfort. Some degree of frustrated creativity was also apparent.

This first case illustrates many of the most essential aspects of the syndrome. The next case, however, is atypical in that the patient was overtly psychotic, despite his seemingly well-preserved personality.

Case 2

This was a 29-year-old man who earned his living as an itinerant house painter. He presented himself to the casualty department of the same general hospital immediately after his wife's admission there for her first confinement. He complained of "labour pains," which he said consisted of a sensation of pressure in his pelvis and tightness in his abdomen.

Retrospectively it was discovered that he had suffered from a variety of symptoms throughout his wife's pregnancy, including nausea, a feeling of abdominal distension and quickening sensations. As his wife's labour proceeded so did his own symptoms progress. When he learned that she had undergone an episiotomy he developed perineal soreness. During the early part of her lactation he complained of breast discomfort. Then, during her involution all his symptoms receded.

Despite the bizarre and prolonged nature of these symptoms and although no physical abnormality was evident, to him, his sufferings appeared to be real enough. Apart from these he was seen to have a well-preserved schizophrenic illness in that he showed fairly gross thought disorder, multiple delusions, or auditory and somatic hallucinations and other unequivocal symptoms of this condition. Although he did not appear to believe that he himself was pregnant, he was much preoccupied with ideas of thought transference, telepathy and extrasensory perception. His wife gave an interesting account of how, when she had a headache, he would place his hands on her head in the belief that he could transfer her headache to himself.

The only significant background factor uncovered was that when he was an infant of 8 months of age, his father suffered from a paranoid schizophrenic illness, leading to his admission to a mental hospital following which the patient's mother had refused to take him back.

After his wife's discharge from hospital, he too insisted on being discharged. Nothing further was heard from him until a letter arrived from a doctor in another part of the country asking for advice. It appeared that his wife was again pregnant, and his symptoms had begun to recur.

The following case represents a rare occurrence, the presentation with a physical sign, namely abdominal swelling.

Case 3

A 26-year-old Australian soldier was admitted while on active service to a military hospital with a swollen abdomen resembling that of fairly advanced pregnancy. While he suffered occasional "dry" vomiting, he had no pain or tenderness. Investigations showed no evidence of intra-abdominal disease. On being anaesthetised his abdomen became quite flat and no mass or abnormality could be felt on deep palpation. Once he had regained consciousness tumefaction returned.

He had married while on leave and had learned after returning to duty that his wife had become pregnant. She suffered greatly from morning sickness and importuned him by letter to return home. He worried greatly over this and at the irregularity of the mail. It was at this juncture that his abdominal swelling occurred and persisted for 22 months, until after his child was born, and he was able to return home, when it at once subsided. The military medical authorities made a diagnosis of "hysterical pseudocyesis."

While there is little doubt that this was a conversion reaction, to call it "pseudocyesis" was clearly incorrect. The patient himself did not believe he was pregnant; had he done so it would have been necessary to have diagnosed this as a delusion and to have regarded him as psychotic, which was certainly not the case.

It was curious to note that 12 years later his abdominal swelling recurred; on this occasion not in relation to his wife's pregnancy (there were no subsequent children) but following marital separation. Once again all physical investigations proved to be negative.

Variants of Couvade syndrome, in which a female relative of the pregnant woman is affected, have also been reported. Basil and Mathews (2006) described the case of a 36-year-old woman who went through the process and pain of delivery at the same time as her son's girlfriend was delivering the patient's first grandchild. Budur et al. (2005) reported "an unusual presentation in which the signs and symptoms described in Couvade syndrome occurred in a twin sister and not in the spouse."

Epidemiology

* Although gross examples are uncommon, if minor instances are included (for example where the expectant father experiences somatic accompaniments of anxiety), the condition is anything but rare with

widely reported incidences of anything from 11% to 65% and upwards.

- The highest incidence is during the third trimester of pregnancy (especially during the last month) with an earlier peak arising during the first trimester.
- Some association with certain social and emotional factors has been reported although the studies are contradictory in their results.

The results of the first controlled study published in Trethowan and Conlon, 1965 at first suggested that as many as one in nine men (11%) suffered some symptoms of psychogenic origin in relation to their wives' gestations, although a further consideration of their data indicated that this was an underestimate and that 19–20% might be nearer the correct figure. Other studies seem to have confirmed this. Lipkin and Lamb (1982) reported that 22% of the partners of 267 pregnant women sought medical attention for gastro intestinal complaints during their wives' pregnancies, these complaints being absent during the six months prior to conception and six months after delivery. Bogren (1983), who carried out the first prospective study of Couvade syndrome, again using husbands as their own controls and who randomly selected 112 primigravidae (later for various reasons reduced to 81) recorded that 20% of their husbands had symptoms which could be regarded as a reaction to their wives' pregnancies. Other studies in the United States have revealed a higher incidence than that reported by Lipkin and Lamb (1982), in some cases up to 79% (Munroe and Munroe, 1971; Clinton, 1987). Khanobdee et al. (1993) reported an incidence of 61% in a sample of Thai males.

Conner and Denson (1990) reported an increased incidence in anxious expectant fathers, individuals of black ethnicity and in those of lower socio-economic status. Other social and emotional associations include the absence of own father from home at an early age (Munroe and Munroe, 1971), unplanned pregnancy (Davis, 1978), a lower level of education (Wylie, 1976), lack of economic security (Wapner, 1975), ethno-religious background (Wapner, 1975; Davis, 1978) and marital disharmony (Reid, 1975). Bogren (1984) found a greater incidence amongst men whose father was aged over 30 and whose mother was aged over 25 years at the time of their birth, plus an increased incidence in those who were attached to their mother and who first experienced sexual intercourse after the age of 18 years; no association was found with the sufferers' financial situation or level of education.

Clinical features

Couvade symptoms may occur at any time from about the third month of pregnancy onwards. Very exceptionally they occur before the subject's spouse becomes aware that she is pregnant (Inman, 1941), although this becomes apparent fairly soon afterwards. A probable explanation for such premonitory symptoms is some kind of subliminal perception of the changes associated with very early pregnancy, which are sufficient to evoke Couvade symptoms in a susceptible subject. The incidence of symptoms tends to fall progressively after onset, with a secondary rise during the last trimester usually just before or at the time of labour.

In about a third of cases the symptoms disappear before labour begins, although they may recur at this time. Another third become symptom-free as soon as childbirth is over, while in the remainder symptoms may persist for a few days.

While there is an association between the occurrence of physical symptoms and anxiety, this is by no means invariable. Some subjects with marked physical symptoms exhibit little or no anxiety whatsoever. In the same way insight into the relationship between the occurrence of symptoms and pregnancy in the wife may be completely absent. In other cases insight is preserved or may develop but without necessarily bringing any relief.

Anxiety is apparent; this and the presence or absence of physical symptoms does not appear to be determined by whether the anxiety has a neurotic basis or whether there is a "genuine" obstetrical cause for it.

The symptoms of Couvade syndrome are variable and so widespread that almost any disorder without a well-defined organic basis which occurs only in chronological relationship to pregnancy and not at other times should be considered as possibly associated with this syndrome. The more common collections of symptoms are:

- Gastrointestinal disturbances including loss of appetite, toothache, nausea and vomiting (quite commonly morning sickness), indigestion, ill-defined abdominal pain or discomfort, constipation or diarrhoea
- Psychiatric symptoms such as depression, tension, insomnia, irritability, nervousness, weakness and headaches
- Pregnancy cravings may occur occasionally
- Abdominal swelling – as already described this is a rare phenomenon

This last symptom may also be a feature of pseudocyesis and was originally investigated by Sir James Simpson as long ago as 1860. Simpson observed that if a woman with pseudocyesis and a swollen abdomen was anaesthetised with chloroform, her distended abdomen flattens until it assumes its normal size and contour but, on recovering consciousness, "the muscles begin to arch and become as tense as before, so that by the time the patient is fully awake, her abdomen is as large and rounded as ever" (Simpson, 1872). Such swelling probably arises from a combination of depression of the diaphragm and lordosis of the spine.

Independent of abdominal swelling, some have suggested that weight gain may also be a relatively common symptom of Couvade syndrome (see Masoni et al., 1994). Indeed, in their recent study of psychosomatic symptoms in a total of 91 Finnish and Polish expectant fathers, Markowska et al. (2018) reported a progressive increase in the number of fathers experiencing weight gain during successive trimesters of their partners' pregnancies. The prevalence of potential Couvade symptoms in these expectant fathers is shown in Table 5.1 (Markowska et al., 2018). It can be seen that gastric symptoms (heartburn), mood swings and nervousness are common.

In respect of the occurrence of toothache, mentioned above, Steel (2017) has recently suggested that, "if a patient presents with unexplained toothache and has a pregnant partner, particularly if other unexplained symptoms are also present, perhaps the possibility of Couvade should be considered."

Aetiology and psychopathology

The aetiology of Couvade syndrome is obscure. Traditionally, it has been understood in the context of psychodynamic principles, with emphasis on factors such as parturition envy, identification with the expectant mother, ambivalence about fatherhood, latent homosexuality and the perception of the foetus as a rival. Such psychodynamic forces were also considered to form a common strand linking the Couvade ritual with Couvade syndrome.

Morse and Mitcham (1997) identify Couvade syndrome as a state of *compathy* or the contagion of physical distress. Compathy occurs when one person observes another person suffering a disease or injury and experiences in his own physical body a similar or related distress. Thus compathy is the physical equivalent of empathy.

More recently attention has focussed on biological mediators in the context of evidence provided by the discipline of ethology. All that can

Table 5.1 Prevalence of physical and emotional Couvade symptoms in a group of 91 Polish and Finnish expectant fathers. Based on data in Markowska et al. (2018)

Symptom	Polish fathers-to-be	Finnish fathers-to-be
Weight gain	78%	60%
Loss of appetite	2%	10%
Gastric symptoms (heartburn)	70%	10%
Nausea/vomiting	10%	Nil
Mood swings	60%	20%
Insomnia	51%	10%
Frustration	5%	20%
Nervousness	25%	50%

really be said, however, is that in the state of current knowledge the aetiology of Couvade syndrome is unproven and remains unknown. It is noteworthy that Piechowski-Jozwiak and Bogousslavsky (2018) point out that, "currently, there are several views on this phenomenon including medical, psychoanalytic, and psychological. Some explain this syndrome as part of men's preparation and participation in pregnancy and post-partum period." This syndrome may well help contemporary society with its gender problems to understand the complexity of male involvement in pregnancy and fatherhood.

The Couvade ritual

Many attempts have been made to explain the origin of this custom. It has been ascribed to feminine tyranny or henpecking or to a dim re-collection of the doctrine of original sin. It has been suggested that it is connected with androgyny, i.e. to the existence of imperfect but some-times functional mammary organs in man. It has even been ascribed to the "vanity of men and the submissiveness of women." The reason given by Marco Polo, who observed the custom in many Eastern countries, was that it was only fair that the husband should share in the pains of childbirth (Dawson, 1929).

Tylor (1865) saw Couvade as an act of simulation of childbirth carried out by the father in order to ensure the adoption of the child into his own family, thus marking the transition from matrilineal to patrilineal des-cent. Alternatively, and where polyandric marriage was permitted, Couvade may have been practised to establish paternity.

These views about Couvade rest on the assumption that the act does, in fact, consist of a pretence of paternity. However, according to Sir James Frazer (1910), this idea is unwarranted, it being unsupported by statements made by some of those who actually practised the ritual. Furthermore, the purpose of the custom cannot invariably be construed as an attempt to transfer parentage from the maternal to the paternal line of descent as it has also been observed amongst certain tribes who adhered to a system of maternal kinship.

An alternative explanation is that the ritual is one of many examples of sympathetic magic (Malinowsky, 1937), there being some other equally curious customs which, like Couvade, commonly express the notion of the vicarious suffering applied for the relief of women in labour at the expense of their husbands. In several countries it has been recorded as customary for the parturient woman's husband to dress himself in some of her clothes. In the west of Ireland, a woman in child-bed would secretly don her husband's vest; whereas in France and Germany it was said that de-livery could be greatly facilitated if she wore his trousers. These are obviously magical acts which Frazer classified as examples of the transference of evil based also on what Freud (1950) called "omnipotence of thought."

It was Reik (1931) who gave the first really comprehensive psychoanalytic interpretation of Couvade. Reik saw the practice as resting upon identification and ambivalence and suggested that because a man's hostility towards his wife is enhanced at the time of her labour, this tempts him to obtain pleasure from her suffering. The temptation is, however, strongly repressed and projected as a fear of demons (Flugel, 1921). Reik also thought that inhibition of sexual desire played an important part: "The participation of sexual wishes is certainly accessory to the high psychic tension of this period ... a man has no sexual intercourse with his wife when she is far advanced in pregnancy, and her increased helplessness through her condition is a constant temptation to him. On the other hand superstitious fear prohibits him from having sexual intercourse."

Phenomenology

From a phenomenological point of view, many cases can be seen as manifestations of relatively simple anxiety states accompanied by not so very unusual somatic symptoms and bearing in the time of their occurrence and direct chronological relationship to pregnancy or labour (Trethowan, 1972). In some cases the expectant father's anxiety of his wife's condition becomes completely somatised. In such cases, and in the presence of grosser physical symptoms, such as persistent vomiting and abdominal distension, the mechanism of conversion must be invoked.

It follows that in the majority of cases Couvade syndrome arises out of neurotic mechanisms. Cases arising through psychotic reactions, as in our Case 2, are rare with few case reports. Apart from this, delusions of pregnancy in men have occasionally been reported as symptoms in a wide variety of psychotic conditions, including schizophrenia, depressive psychosis and organic states.

Radhakrishnan et al. (1999) described a case of a male patient with schizophrenia who developed a delusion of pregnancy on two successive occasions when his wife became pregnant.

Psychodynamics

A number of psychodynamic interpretations of Couvade syndrome have been advanced:

- Parturition envy
- Ambivalence
- Identification

It has been suggested that the condition is an expression of frustrated creativity and a man's deep-rooted infantile envy of his wife's ability to bear a child (Jacobson, 1950; Jones, 1942). Certainly young boys, like their sisters, often indulge in mother-and-child play with dolls, but where psychological development follows the usual course, this is soon abandoned. It is claimed that if, during the Oedipal period, certain factors become operative, these may lead to the persistence of maternal trends in boys. Thus some adult patients with latent homosexual problems and strong creative trends are said to show, on analysis, intensely cathexed unconscious feminine reproductive fantasies (Macalpine and Hunter, 1955). In particular, persistent envy of female reproductive ability often concealed by an appearance of normal masculinity is said to occur in those men who at a certain stage of development are confronted by the birth of a younger sibling (Boehm, 1930).

It is probably unnecessary, however, to postulate that concealed or latent homosexuality is a factor in all such cases. Freeman (1951) came to the conclusion that the decisive factor must be the heightening of instinctual tension to an uncontrollable level. He observed that his patients were men dominated by childhood ideas and impressions about pregnancy which had become unconscious and that the occurrence of pregnancy in their wives stimulated their aggressive and sexual drives. However, as these could not find an adequate outlet and were repudiated by the adult ego, mental illness resulted and in some instances the conflict was somatised.

A somewhat although not altogether different explanation was advanced by Evans (1951), who reported in detail a case of simulated pregnancy in a male patient undergoing analysis. This patient had previously undergone a Couvade reaction during the first stage of his wife's labour. Evans saw in the patient's fantasy of pregnancy a dramatic expression of identification with his mother. For him a woman's supreme claim to womanhood was in her possession of a baby, which he too, in fantasy, sought to acquire.

It is difficult to judge to what extent concepts such as "parturition envy" or wish fulfilment in pregnancy fantasies in men contribute to the development of Couvade syndrome; in the majority of cases the evidence for this is slender.

An ambivalent relationship between man and his mother was apparent in two of our three cases. It appears in some instances that the subject can unconsciously identify with his wife as mother. He loves both, but doubting their love for him feels rejected and hates both. His wife's pregnancy may reinforce this because when he becomes aware of her loving contemplation of her unborn child, he may inescapably be reminded of how he once felt when his mother contemplated the birth of his younger brother or sister. Because his unborn child can hardly be regarded as a rival and it is his wife that contains the object which threatens his security, it is upon her that his feelings of hostility may be projected.

With regard to this hypothesis, Bogren (1985) observed a relationship between side preference in child holding, the occurrence of Couvade syndrome and the attachment of affected men to their mothers. Whereas about 80% of both women and men held their infants to the left of their body midline, men who were right-holders suffered more often from Couvade syndrome and were more closely identified with their mothers. In view of this finding, Bogren proposed that Couvade syndrome may be important, pointing to future difficulties in coping with fatherhood, and that right-holding in either sex is a sign of insecurity in the relationship with the infant.

The mechanism of identification has been postulated as an important aetiological factor (Trethowan, 1972). This may arise out of deep feelings of empathy between man and wife. Here the husband concerned about his wife's condition consciously or unconsciously takes upon himself her discomforts as a protective measure.

Tényi et al. (1996) reported two cases of psychotic Couvade and provided a psychodynamic interpretation of the cases. They emphasised the important role played by an ego defect and the phenomenon referred to as *double identification*. They postulated that identification with the foetus triggers an earlier ego deficit centred on a pathological relationship between subject and mother. The ego defect is characterised by poor ego boundaries and hence its manifestation in the form of clinical psychosis.

Biology

Mason and Elwood (1995) argue that there is a relationship between infanticidal behaviour and paternal behaviour in mammals including primates. A shift from the more (in biological terms) usual former behaviour to the latter occurs at certain times and may be related to a number of external factors including cohabitation with the pregnant female, the nature of the social interaction between female and male (including copulation) and the odours produced by the pregnant female. Such events are linked with internal physiological changes – particularly hormonal – within the male. The authors then postulate that Couvade symptoms are the result of an individual human male subject interpreting essentially normal internal physiological processes which are designed to bring about a state of parental responsiveness and are triggered by the partner's pregnancy. They further suggest that the Couvade ritual is simply a ritualisation of Couvade syndrome found in non-industrial societies.

Intriguingly, since Mason and Elwood (1995) put forward the above argument, evidence of a non-human primate analogue to the Couvade sign of weight gain has come from a study of the New World monkey

Saguinus oedipus (the cotton-top tamarin), which practises cooperative breeding. Sánchez Rodríguez et al. (2008) have found that during the cooperative pregnancy condition, "expectant" males gain weight during the final months of their partners' pregnancies. In contrast, after the infants' births, during the middle of the following cooperative breeding condition, both males and females lose weight – not just the fathers but also male helpers and female helpers.

It might be argued that a major weakness with the paradigm of Mason and Elwood (1995) is the difficulty in generalising the findings of studies conducted on lower animals to populations of human beings. However, humans do share many physiological and behavioural features with our mammalian cousins, and Mason and Elwood's postulates do at least provide the basis for a potentially testable hypothesis. Indeed, the hypothesis that hormonal changes take place within human expectant fathers has been tested by Storey et al. (2000). They measured serum prolactin levels in 20 expectant/new fathers who had two or more Couvade symptoms (using the criteria published by Masoni et al., 1994) and in 14 expectant/new fathers who had fewer than two such symptoms. The former group had significantly higher average prolactin levels (Storey et al., 2000). Interestingly, the partners of the first group also had higher prolactin and cortisol levels than the partners of the second (non-Couvade) group.

Management and treatment

Most sufferers from Couvade syndrome do not require treatment and indeed, in the majority of the cases, the condition may pass unrecognised so that few sufferers are referred to a psychiatrist. When a case is discovered, interpretation and relatively superficial psychotherapy aimed at reducing anxiety usually bring considerable relief. In the light of knowledge that the symptoms will resolve spontaneously as soon as childbirth is successfully concluded, it is not known whether better preparation for parenthood in fathers-to-be reduces the incidence of Couvade symptomatology.

Prognosis

The prognosis is benign. Although the condition may recur during future pregnancies, this is not an inevitable outcome.

References

Basil, B., Mathews, M. (2006). *Psychosomatics, 47*, 363.
Boehm, F. (1930). *International Journal of Psychoanalysis, 11*, 456.
Bogren, L.Y. (1983). *Acta Pschiatrica Scandinavica, 68*, 55.
Bogren, L.Y. (1984). *Acta Psychiatrica Scandinavica, 70*, 316.

Bogren, L.Y. (1985). *Linköping University Medical Dissertations No. 194*. Linköping University Press, Linköping.

Budur, K., Mathews, M., Mathews, M. (2005). *Psychosomatics*, 46, 71.

Clinton, J.F. (1987). *International Journal of Nursing Studies*, 24, 59.

Conner, G.K., Denson, V. (1990). *Journal of Perinatal and Neonatal Nursing*, 4, 33.

Davis, O.S. (1978). *Mood and Symptoms of Expectant Fathers During the Course of Pregnancy: A Study of the Crisis Perspective of Expectant Fatherhood.* Doctoral dissertation, University of North Carolina. Dissertation Abstracts International 38, 5841A.

Dawson, W.R. (1929). *The Custom of Couvade.* Manchester University Press, Manchester.

Eden, M. (1958). *The Philosophy of the Bed.* The Saturday Book. Hutchinson, London.

Evans, W.N. (1951). *Psychoanalytic Quarterly*, 20, 165.

Flugel, J.C. (1921). *The Psycho-analytic Study of the Family.* Hogarth Press, London.

Fraser, A. (1969). *Mary Queen of Scots.* Weidenfield and Nicholson, London.

Frazer, J.G. (1910). *Totemism and Exogamy*, Vol. 4. Macmillan, London.

Freeman, T. (1951). *British Journal of Medical Psychology*, 24, 49.

Freud, S. (1950). *Totem and Taboo.* Routledge and Kegan Paul, London.

Hunter, R., Macalpine, I. (1963). *Three Hundred Years of Psychiatry* Oxford University Press, London.

Inman, W.S. (1941). *British Journal of Medical Psychology*, 19, 37.

Jacobson, E. (1950). *Psychoanalytic Study of the Child*, 5, 139.

Jones, E. (1942). *Lancet*, 1, 695.

Khanobdee, C, Sukratanachaiyakul, V., Templeton Gay, J. (1993). *International Journal of Nursing Studies*, 30, 125.

Kiselica, M.S., Scheckel, S. (1995). *School Counsellor*, 43, 42.

Lean, V.S. (1904). *Collectanea, Simpkin.* Marshall Co., Bristol.

Lindsay, L. (1933). *A Short History of Dentistry.* Bole and Danielson, London.

Lipkin, M., Lamb, G. (1982). *Annals of Internal Medicine*, 96, 509.

Macalpine, I., Hunter, R. (1955). *Schreber; Memoirs of My Nervous Illness.* Dawson, London.

Malinowsky, B. (1937). *Sex and Repression in Savage Society.* Kegan Paul, London.

Markowska, U.S., Zyg, M., Kiełbratowska, B. (2018). *Ginekologia Polska*, 89, 35.

Mason, C., Elwood, R. (1995). *International Journal of Nursing Studies*, 32, 137.

Masoni, S., Maio, A., Trimarchi, G., de Punzio, C., Fioretti P. (1994). *Journal of Psychosomatic Obstetrics and Gynaecology*, 15, 125.

Morse, J.M., Mitcham, C. (1997). *Journal of Advanced Nursing*, 26, 649.

Munroe, R.L., Munroe, R.H. (1971). *Journal of Social Psychology*, 84, 11.

Murray, M. (1921). *The God of the Witches.* Sampson Low, London.

Pennant, T. (1772). *A Tour of Scotland and Voyage to the Hebrides*, quoted by Frazer, J.G. (1910).

Piechowski-Jozwiak, B., Bogousslavsky, J. (2018). *Frontiers of Neurology and Neuroscience*, 42, 51.

Radhakrishnan, R., Satheeshkumar, G., Chaturvedi, S.K. (1999). *Psychopathology*, 32, 1.

Reid, K.E. (1975). *Journal of Social Welfare*, 2, 13.

Reik, T. (1931). *Ritual.* Hogarth Press, London.

Rolleston, J.D. (1945). *British Dental Journal*, 78, 225.

Sánchez Rodríguez, S.M., Peláez del Hierro, F., Fidalgo de las Heras, A.M., Morcillo Pimentel, A., Caperos Montalbán, J.M. (2008). *Psicothema*, 20, 825.

Simpson, J. (1872). *Clinical Lectures on Diseases of Women*. Black, Edinburgh.

Steel, B. (2017). *British Dental Journal, 223*, 389.

Storey, A.E., Walsh, C.J., Quinton, R.L., Wynne-Edwards, K.E. (2000). *Evolution and Human Behavior, 21*, 79.

Tényi, T., Trixler, M., Jádi, F. (1996). *Psychopathology, 29*, 252.

Trethowan, W.H. (1972). *Sexual Behaviour, 2*, 23.

Trethowan, W.H., Conlon, M.F. (1965). *British Journal of Psychiatry, 111*, 57.

Tylor, E.B. (1865). *Researches into the Early History of Mankind and the Development of Civilisation, 2nd edn*. Murray, London.

Wapner, J.H. (1975). Quoted by Mason, C., Elwood, R. (1995).

Westmarck, E. (1921). *The History of Human Marriage, 3rd edn.*, Vol. 1. Macmillan, London.

Wycherley, W. (1672). *The Country Wife*. In *Famous Plays of the Restoration and Eighteenth Century*. The Modern Library, New York.

Wylie, M.L. (1976). Quoted by Mason C., Elwood, R. (1995).

Chapter 6

Munchausen's syndrome and related factitious disorders

> Disease has been simulated in every age, and by all classes of society. The monarch, the mendicant, the unhappy slave, the proud warrior, the lofty statesman, even the minister of religion, as well as the condemned malefactor, and boy "creeping like snail unwillingly to school," have sought to disguise their purposes, or to obtain their desires, by feigning mental or bodily infirmities.
>
> Hector Gavin, On Feigned and Factitious Diseases, Chiefly of Soldiers and Seamen, On the Means Used to Simulate or Produce Them, and on the Best Modes of Discovering Imposters (1843)

Munchausen's syndrome is a condition typically characterised by patients who are admitted to hospital with simulated acute illnesses supported by a plausible and often dramatic history which, at a later date is found to be false.

Historical

The term "Munchausen's syndrome" was first used in 1951 in the *Lancet* by Asher. Had Asher been less self-effacing, we might now talk of Asher syndrome (by proxy); one of his daughters, the famous actress Jane Asher, has commented that it was typical of her father not to name the condition after himself (Puri, 2006). The name was chosen because of the resemblance of the wanderings (peregrinations) and fabrications of these patients to the travels and fantastic anecdotes attributed to Karl Friedrich Hieronymus, Baron (Freiherr) von Münchhausen (1720–1797), as chronicled by the exiled German writer and geologist Rudolph Erich Raspe (1786).

Other suggested terms have included "peregrinating problem patients," "hospital hoboes," "kopenickiades (frauds)," "wandering Jew syndrome" "hospital addiction syndrome" and "polysurgical addiction." The multiplicity of synonyms reflects the multiple pathology and diagnostic complexity.

Cases had been reported in the medical literature before Asher's original description (Netherton, 1927; Grunert, 1932; Banzel, 1934; Chamoff and Sotina, 1935; Barrett and Hoyle, 1942; Ceiller, 1947; Gliebe and Goldman, 1949; Reinhard, 1950). Possibly the oldest is Chowne (1843), who cited an example of a male patient who underwent serial orchidectomies.

Case reports

The six cases summarised here are those originally investigated by the late Dr John Barker and reported both in his own writings on the subject and in the first edition of this book. Because of this and because they appear to be sufficiently characteristic of the disorder, it has not been felt necessary to add any fresh examples.

Case I

A 29-year-old lorry driver, a pathological liar, whose scarred abdominal wall bears the hallmark of having been a "veritable surgical battleground!" His first hospital admission took place when he was aged 13 years. Since then he has been admitted to several hundred hospitals over a 15-year period and has undergone some 15 unnecessary abdominal operations. Until recently he has had no mental hospital admissions and none for at least five years after the onset of his general hospital peregrinations.

In contrast to most of these cases, his home background appears to have been happy. His childhood development was reported to have been normal with no early neurotic traits. He was said, however, to be a poor mixer and to have few outside interests.

The conditions which he simulates vary widely, although he is mainly inclined to exhibit abdominal and neurological symptoms. The following conditions are some of those listed in his case records; post-traumatic anuria, pelvic abscess, peritonitis, intestinal obstruction, abdominal emergency, haematemesis, severe headaches (sometimes following an alleged head injury), meningitis, fractured skull, fractured spine, tetanus, disseminated sclerosis, subarachnoid and thalamic haemorrhage. All investigations and operative findings have been negative, except for some adhesions found during more recent laparotomies. He has made occasional histrionic suicidal attempts in hospital, has an affinity for pethidine and morphine and has requested to work as a nurse or orderly in some hospitals. Numerous psychiatric diagnoses have been suggested, but he is generally regarded as an aggressive, hysterical psychopath. This is supported perhaps by a non-specific EEG dysrhythmia. He has a long criminal record for motoring offences and larceny. Even a standard leucotomy performed in 1959 failed to prevent him from entering general hospitals afterwards, and he has since had at last one further laparotomy. Further details are available (Barker, 1958; 1960; 1962; Sanderson, 1957).

Case 2

A stout woman, aged 45 years with congenital ocular abnormalities (opaque nerve fibres and colobomata) and bifrontal burr-holes following a standard leucotomy performed in 1952 to relieve depression. Her condition began in 1935 when she underwent a chiasmal exploration for headaches, "blackouts," polyuria and increasing obesity with negative findings. She sometimes mentions tuberculous peritonitis and has undergone at least 13 laparotomies over 28 years, having had 126 known hospital admissions. Her hypogastrium is completely replaced by scar tissue. Many of her admissions have been for a presumed pituitary or cerebral neoplasm. She has a long criminal and psychopathic record. Her case has been widely reported (Barker and Grygier, 1957; Barker, 1958; 1962, Barker 1964a; Achte and Kaukp, 1964).

Case 3

An Irishman, aged 37 years with a "Beatle" hairstyle and the appearance of a mental defective. He is known as "The Baron." He has had hundreds of admissions since 1946 for haemorrhagic symptoms which are only occasionally observed to be factitious. He has a remarkable knowledge of blood diseases. Usually a severe dyscrasia such as haemophilia, Henoch-Schönlein purpura, polycythaemia, etc., is diagnosed, resulting in innumerable transfusions and frequently large quantities of steroids. He is addicted to pethidine but dislikes morphine. He has two abdominal scars, one of which, it is alleged, is the result of splenectomy. The records of his admissions are extraordinarily similar. Further details are available (Grant, 1952; Barker, 1960; Bagan, 1962).

Case 4

An educated plausible Cambridge graduate, aged 46 years, who is alleged to have fractured his skull at school. In 1953, he underwent bilateral craniotomy in Canada with negative findings, following his professed account of CSF rhinorrhoea after a flight over the Rockies. He often refers to a recent head injury occurring ostensibly while on important business and is usually admitted to hospital with headaches, epileptic fits, status epilepticus or epistaxes. Alternatively, he has sometimes been investigated for chest pain or haemoptyses caused by self-inflicted pharyngeal trauma (Wright, 1955; Barker, 1958; 1960; 1961; 1964a,b).

Case 5

A woman, aged 25 years, who had more than 45 admissions in three years during which she has undergone at least six laparotomies for abdominal pain, suspected salpingitis, tubal abortion, ovarian cysts and ingestion of safety-pins. Some nine pelvic examinations under anaesthesia have been performed at different hospitals for spurious pregnancies. Her hospital admissions followed marriage (Barker, 1960; 1962).

Case 6

An obese woman, aged 44 years, with some 60 admissions since 1946, for abdominal pain, self-inflicted stab wounds and safety-pin ingestion. Her abdominal wall is replaced by thin scar tissue following several laparotomies, and she has a large self-induced faecal fistula in the centre of her abdomen which she has kept open for six years (Barker, 1960; 1962).

These cases are reported in the present tense in order to illustrate the nature of communications which it was felt necessary to make to the casualty departments in order that the true nature of the condition of these patients should be recognised before further unnecessary investigations were undertaken.

Epidemiology

At the time of writing, the largest systematic review of Munchausen's syndrome is that of Yates and Feldman (2016), who identified and analysed 372 published studies, published between 1965 and 2015, containing 455 cases who fulfilled *DSM-5* and/or *DSM-IV* and/or *ICD-10* criteria for factitious disorder. Although the largest number were from the USA (249 reports) and the UK (94 reports), there were reports from all major continents and a wide variety of countries. Two-thirds of the patients were female. The average age at presentation was 34 years (median 32 years, minimum 18 years and maximum 79 years). The occupation was known in 214 of these patients; 122 (57%) had a healthcare/laboratory profession, with the commonest occupation being nursing (68/214 or 32%).

Clinical features

The clinical features are characterised by simulated disease, pathological lying and frequent wanderings:

- *Presentation* – often arrive at casualty departments "out of hours" or over weekends when less experienced doctors are on duty (Barker and Grygier, 1957); rarely possess a referring doctor's letter or attend ordinary outpatients; present a fairly constant history and demonstrate a remarkable knowledge of medical detail.

- *Symptoms and signs* – can involve the whole range of medical syndromes (see Table 6.1) that are sometimes given whimsical names. The large systematic review undertaken by Yates and Feldman (2016) referred to above confirmed the wide diversity of index medical presentations that have been recorded. The most numerous form of presentations of this sample were induced hypoglycaemia, reported retrosternal chest pain and induced generalised skin lesions.
- *Examination* – difficult to establish rapport; restless, evasive and attention seeking; intelligence ranges from learning disability range to superior; physical signs such as scars and fever; males often antisocial, females histrionic.
- *Associated features* – criminal records; pseudologia fantastica.
- *Demography* – tend to use a variety of aliases; extensive travelling and thus visit many hospitals; tendency towards chronicity.

Medical specialties

Munchausen's syndrome has an association with a large number of systems of the body so that a very large variety of medical specialties may be involved in its diagnosis. The large systematic study by Yates and Feldman (2016) referred to above revealed that most, if not all, major main-stream medical specialities are involved in the diagnosis of this syndrome, including for instance, allergy and immunology, dermatology, gastroenterology, HIV and sexual health, oncology, orthopaedics and trauma and rheumatology.

Finsterer and Stefan (2016) have reported that a mitochondrial disorder, caused by a complex I-IV defect, manifested in a female patient

Table 6.1 Common presentations in Munchausen's syndrome

acute abdomen (laparotomophilia migrans) – said to be the commonest variety
haemorrhagic type (haemorrhagica histrionica) – characterised by alarming episodes of bleeding with use of animal or human blood
neurological type (neurologica diabolica) – such as fits, faints, ataxias, sometimes even undergoing craniotomy or prefrontal leucotomy as a result
cutaneous type – (dermatitis autogenica) – self-inflicted skin lesions
cardiac type – presenting with angina, arrhythmias and even ECG abnormalities
respiratory type – infected sputum and traumatic pneumothorax
mixed and polysymptomatic types – miscellaneous false presentations including placenta praevia and even AIDS
psychiatric Munchausen type – presenting with apparent major mental illness such as depressive psychosis or schizophrenia

who had had 175 hospital admissions over 20 years. Her mitochondrial disorder had given rise to the following body system manifestations:

- Cerebral – Munchausen's syndrome (which dominated the clinical picture), rare epileptic seizures, frequent psychogenic seizures
- Myopathy – myalgia, fatigue, ptosis
- Endocrine – short stature, thyroid dysfunction
- Renal – mild Fanconi syndrome
- Bone marrow – iron-deficient chronic anaemia and elevated transferrin

Ophthalmological presentations can include recurrent corneal lesions, cataracts and uveitis (Valeina et al., 2016).

Reich et al. (2015) have suggested that Munchausen's syndrome appears to be poorly diagnosed by clinicians and surgeons working in oncology and that they need to bear this potential diagnosis in mind. Not unexpectedly, if the correct diagnosis is made, strong counter-transference feelings may ensue (Baig et al., 2016).

Brooks et al. (2015) have pointed out that the diagnoses of central line-associated bloodstream infection (CLABSI) and Munchausen's syndrome are not mutually exclusive (see also Kenneth et al., 2015). Indeed, as they point out, "the presence of a psychiatric disorder should be considered as a potential mechanism by which an infection may occur either intentionally [as in the case reported by Kenneth et al., 2015] or unintentionally. Rather than excluding psychiatric conditions from CLABSI prevention, we propose increased attention to the interplay between psychiatric conditions and CLABSIs in individual cases as well as systematically."

A series of cases of factitious angio-oedema, in which apparently refractory angio-oedema was mimicked by patients, was described by Feldman et al. (2014). In one case an 18-year-old woman presented with a several-year history of recurrent apparent swelling of the tongue and lips, which apparently occurred at least once each month. All investigations proved unremarkable. At the time of a subsequent apparent episode, she was found to have a clenched jaw with the tongue, which was not oedematous, protruding slightly. The authors explained that "palpation of her tongue revealed soft, pliable tissue without oedema or thickening. Her jaw was able to be loosened by gentle manipulation and her tongue retracted back into her mouth upon gagging." Feldman et al. (2014) described another similar case of an 18-year-old woman, this time with a two-year history of apparently "daily musculoskeletal pain and nausea associated with swelling of her lip, tongue, and lower back." These episodes would typically spontaneously resolve within 10 minutes. Again, investigations proved negative; "intra-attack laryngoscopy demonstrated vocal cord adduction and no oedema during a sensation of throat 'swelling.' All angioedema-specific therapies subsequently were stopped, and, along with hydration and rest, she was started on COX-2 inhibition for pain and antiemetics for nausea. She is currently seeing a psychologist for suspected factitious angioedema."

Cakmak et al. (2015) reported a case of a 27-year-old woman with psychogenic dystonia presenting with an acute onset of retrocollis, lower limb dystonia and bizarre gait. She was finally diagnosed with Munchausen's syndrome, which had started nine years earlier when she had been diagnosed with hemifacial spasm, which apparently only responded to treatment with botulinum neurotoxin. When Cakmak and colleagues injected her neck and facial area with a "placebo botulinum neurotoxin treatment" (namely, normal saline), there was a great improvement in all her symptoms, include hemifacial spasm, retrocollis and gait disturbance. Indeed, there were no abnormal neurological findings after this placebo treatment. Video recordings of the patient before and after the placebo treatment can be viewed via the hyperlink at https://www.ncbi.nlm.nih.gov/pmc/articles/PMC4462832/.

Feldman (2000) has used the term "Munchausen's by internet" to describe cases of Munchausen's syndrome in which patients feign illnesses in virtual support groups such as chat rooms and newsgroups. Feigned illnesses can also be ascribed to others (such as a child) in a form of virtual Munchausen's syndrome by proxy. These phenomena were previously described as *virtual factitious disorders* by Feldman et al. (1998).

It should be borne in mind that Munchausen's syndrome can be associated with death, for example as a result of direct self-injurious behaviour (e.g. as a result of thyroxine abuse leading to ventricular fibrillation), iatrogenic harm (e.g. anaphylactic reactions), invasive hospital procedures and suicide (Vaduganathan et al., 2014).

Kinns et al. (2013) have provided detailed advice regarding the role of laboratory investigations in the detection and diagnosis of Munchausen's syndrome. For example, mimicking of hypoglycaemia by the use of exogenous insulin or insulin secretagogues (e.g. sulphonylureas) may be suspected by simultaneously measuring levels of insulin, C-peptide, pro-insulin and insulin secretagogues from samples taken during hypoglycaemic episodes. Similarly, factitious Cushing syndrome by self-administration of exogenous glucocorticoids may be suspected by carrying out high-performance liquid chromatography analysis to distinguish between endogenous and exogenous steroids.

Reports of laboratory results may themselves be forged. Zittel et al. (2017) have described the first published case of *Munchausen's syndrome by genetics*, in which a 42-year-old nurse presented with apparent symptoms of dopa-responsive dystonia, fluctuating signs and, crucially, a three-year-old report from a certified genetics laboratory stating that she had heterozygous mutations in *CGH1* and *TH*, the respective genes encoding cadherin-1 (or CAM 120/80 or epithelial cadherin) and tyrosine hydroxylase (the enzyme catalysing the biosynthesis of L-3,4-dihydroxyphenylalanine from L-tyrosine). This document was in fact forged, and subsequent independent genetic testing did not show a mutation in either *CGH1* or *TH*. The nurse had used her apparent illness to obtain early retirement, and she had been prescribed daily levodopa and pramipexole. Commenting on this case, Oliveira (2017) has pointed out that "[this case] provided an instructive example of how to pay attention to details that we usually take for granted during the busy clinician routine. It would be crucial to check if the patient had a specific motivation, such as pension application or welfare."

Differential diagnosis

Conversion or dissociation hysteria – in which the individual cannot control the production of the symptoms.

Hypochondriasis – in which the patient believes that he or she is ill and has a disease and is worried about it, whereas in factitious disorder the worry is limited and not as pronounced.

Somatisation – sometimes it is difficult to differentiate between somatisation and factitious disorder in that both present with physical symptoms with underlying psychological distress. However, in somatoform disorders the patient does not produce the symptoms voluntarily and usually is not familiar with medical terminology or hospital procedures.

Malingering – especially when the gain is not readily apparent, for usually such gain is easily understandable in the context of the individual's personality.

Acute psychosocial crisis – presenting as an illness behaviour.

Substance abuse – although there is no history usually of multiple hospitalisations.

Psychopathic states – where self-mutilation is a gross and prominent feature often associated with multiple admissions.

Psychotic states – in which there is a hypochondriacal delusion.

Pseudologia fantastica – occurring in isolation.

Diagnostic criteria

The following factors must be taken into account to make as firm a diagnosis as possible (noting that an early diagnosis avoids unnecessary investigations and treatment and angry frustration on the part of the treating physician/surgeon).

Early factors

Be aware of this as a possible diagnosis
Evidence of falsified symptoms – physical and/or psychological

Evidence of lying regarding past, personal and medical history and use of aliases
Unexplained scars (post-operative and/or self-inflicted)
No fixed address

Suspicion can be reinforced with *later factors*

History of multiple presentations at casualty departments, admissions into hospital and surgery often with premature discharge
Paucity of family or friends or contact numbers or addresses
Disorders of personality, being aggressive and remote
History of criminal behaviour
History of alcohol/drug abuse
Disturbed sexual functioning
Often has much knowledge of medical symptoms and working of medical departments

Hyler and Sussman (1981) suggest that pseudologia fantastica, wandering and evidence of prior treatment, medical sophistication and disruptive hospitalisation, along with demands for medication and absence of visitors are key features.

In *ICD-10* (World Health Organisation, 1992), factitious disorder is included under the category of disorders of adult personality and behaviour in which the person, in the absence of confirmed physical or mental disorder, disease or disability, feigns symptoms *repeatedly* and *consistently*. Individuals with this pattern of behaviour also show other marked abnormalities of personality and relationships. At the time of writing, it also occurs in the beta draft of *ICD-11* under the category F68 "Other disorders of adult personality and behaviour" as F68.1 "Intentional production or feigning of symptoms or disabilities, either physical or psychological [factitious disorder]." The beta draft gives the following elaboration: "The patient feigns symptoms repeatedly for no obvious reason and may even inflict self-harm in order to produce symptoms or signs. The motivation is obscure and presumably internal with the aim of adopting the sick role. The disorder is often combined with marked disorders of personality and relationships." In the beta draft, both factitial dermatitis (included elsewhere under L98.1) and persons feigning illness (with obvious motivation) (included under Z76.5) are excluded from F68.1.

According to *DSM-IV* (American Psychiatric Association, 1994), the essential feature of factitious disorder is the *intentional* production of physical or psychological symptoms or signs. The presentation may include fabrication or subjective complaints (e.g. complaints of acute abdominal pain in the absence of any such pain), self-inflicted conditions (e.g. the production of abscesses by injecting saliva into the skin), exaggeration or exacerbation of pre-existing general medical conditions (e.g. feigning of grand mal seizures with previous history of epilepsy) or any combination or variations of these. In the more recent *DSM-5* (American Psychiatric Association, 2013), the diagnostic criteria include falsification of physical or psychological symptoms or signs, or induction of injury or disease, associated with identified deception; presentation to others as ill, impaired or injured; deceptive behaviour occurs even in the absence of obvious external rewards.

The motivation is to assume the sick role, and additional external incentives are absent. According to *DSM-IV* criteria, the disorder has three further subtypes – predominant psychological signs or symptoms, predominant physical signs or symptoms and a combination of both.

Aetiology and psychopathology

Munchausen's syndrome has been viewed as little more than malingering or a closely related variant. However, it is the authors' contention that although similar the two conditions are distinct, with Munchausen's syndrome representing a pathological state. This has important medical and legal implications.

The fundamental feature which separates the two concepts (Munchausen's and malingering) is the underlying *motivation*. In malingering the motivation is a conscious one of achieving some clear goal – laudable or otherwise; whereas in Munchausen's syndrome the motivation is pathological with the goal often obscure and ultimately self-destructive. The two conditions do share a final common pathway in that in both the subjects use a combination of lies and self-inflicted lesions to deceive others – usually doctors.

True malingering can be difficult to diagnose owing to the difficulty in establishing absolute proof, without which it is customary to give the subject the benefit of the doubt. It is thought that an element of malingering may often be present in compensation cases, although this may perhaps have been overstressed. Here, however, is a striking example.

Case 7

A labourer, aged 41 years, was first seen five years after having been injured at work. While using a power drill he sustained an electric shock which not only threw him to the ground but also resulted in burns to his hands, necessitating skin grafts. He also had some degree of residual stiffness of his right index finger. While these injuries were real enough, the final degree of his disability was only of a very minor kind. He had, however, not worked since his injury and complained of shaking continuously all over.

The way in which he presented this complaint was truly remarkable. During a one-and-a-half-hour examination, of both his physical and mental state, he shook all over, rather in the manner of a case of "shell-shock" as seen during World War I. While sitting in a chair, he showed a gross irregular tremor of his arms and head, while his legs and trunk remained stationary. While lying on the examination couch, his trunk and legs shook as well. All his muscles appeared tense, and he could not be made to relax. However, despite great difficulty in carrying out a physical examination, there appeared to be no other abnormal physical signs.

Before the examination the examiner (Professor W. H. Trethowan) was shown a film of the patient, taken without his knowledge and through a telescopic lens, by the insurance company's solicitors. This showed him walking down the street, entering and leaving a house and waiting at a bus stop, all the time without any evidence of shaking or tremor whatsoever. Further information about his behaviour was gleaned from a private investigator who had followed him into a public house and had observed him drink a full glass of beer without spilling any, roll a cigarette and play a game of bar billiards. None of these actions would have been possible had the shaking, which he exhibited during examination, been present. However, when specifically questioned he stated that this never stopped!

Because of the remarkable discrepancy in his account of himself as against that of others, it was decided, once the examination had been completed, to follow him and submit him to further observation unbeknown. Once again, while watching him through a car window, and at times as close as six or seven yards, and while he walked a quarter of a mile, there was no evidence of any abnormality. Subsequent to this he was twice observed, at even closer quarters, standing normally at a bus stop.

When the case came to court, evidence was produced for the plaintiff that he had been kept under continuous observation in a private hospital for a week, during which it was said that he had never once stopped shaking. However, on cross-examination, it appeared that this period of observation was by no means as continuous as had been at first made out.

As this subject could obviously turn his tremor on and off at will, controlling it completely when he thought himself unobserved and under circumstances when it might have caused him inconvenience, there can be no doubt of the entirely spurious nature of his disability. This was reinforced by the fact that his motivation for producing and at times sustaining it was fully conscious and known to be unethical, being directed to the purpose of monetary gain.

Other external motives for malingering include evading military conscription, avoiding criminal prosecution and attempting to obtain social and financial benefits.

What then is the *pathological* motivation in Munchausen's patients? This unfortunately remains unknown; indeed, it is probable that there is no one single uniform motivation common to all such patients. Motivation may even vary in the same patient at different times.

An inactive period following investigation in hospital may generate a state of growing tension which is only relieved when a fresh set of deceptions is practised on a fresh set of doctors at yet another hospital. Alternatively, a lack of sympathy or attention may cause the patient to discharge himself and seek solace elsewhere. Furthermore, all these patients are highly exhibitionistic, delighting apparently in displaying their abdominal scars to as many persons as possible and being presented at clinical meetings. In contrast to Walter Mitty, who craved the dramatic role of the surgeon, they appear to crave the drama of being submitted to surgery.

Physical association

The immediate motivation is more understandable in those who actually have some underlying organic disease. Some such condition, previously mishandled or misdiagnosed, may therefore tend to produce recurrent symptoms of a disabling or alarming nature, which may result in what has been called a *psychopathic accretion* (Small, 1955), also giving rise to the tendency to wander from one hospital to another. However, while this may be relevant in the case of those suffering from painful adhesions, it does not of course explain psychopathic behaviour which antedates the first operation, nor does it apply in the case of those without any disease of organic origin.

Attention seeking

The early environment of these patients may be unfavourable, leading in some way or another to their becoming conditioned, in a sense, to use symptoms as a means of seeking attention. This pattern may be reinforced both by repetition and possibly by the growth of a grudge against the medical profession, whereby the subjects begin to consider themselves to be victims of former mismanagement (MacKieth, 1957; Barker, 1962). Reinforcement may also be caused by, for example, a doctor who may have made an unfortunate remark in the patient's presence or aroused his curiosity by attending over-enthusiastically to some relatively unimportant physical sign such as dextrocardia (Davis, 1951) or some other essentially benign anomaly.

Drug addiction

While a desire to obtain drugs induces some admissions, these patients are, as a rule, not drug dependent. Some patients even discharge themselves from hospitals where liberal doses of pethidine may have been provided. Sometimes it seems as if those with a leaning towards medicine and nursing may attempt to resolve their personal problems through repeated hospital admissions (Hawkins et al., 1956). One patient used admission to hospital as a means of escaping her husband; others do to avoid the harsh realities of everyday life.

Psychopathology

At a deeper level, Menninger (1934; 1938), in a correlation of the psychopathology of self-destructiveness, enumerated such motives as avoidance of something more dreaded than surgery: the gratification of erotic needs and castration fantasies, possibly underlying a desire for a change of sex, the realisation of childbirth fantasies and the relief of deep-seated feelings of aggression and guilt through the self-induced suffering at the hands of surgeons.

Viewed in psychoanalytic terms, surgical operations may, therefore, be seen as symbolising castration, the implication being that successive parts of the body become genitalised, thus allowing some individuals almost literally to be cut in pieces. Menninger linked this tendency to invite operations (localised or focal self-destruction) with suicide, regarding them as different manifestations of the same morbid process. He observed how some patients were able to transfer responsibility for their actions onto the surgeon, thereby enabling "death of the whole organism to be averted by the sacrifice of a part of the whole," and also how "unconscious motives combine with conscious purposes to determine the surgeon's election to operate, no less than the patient's election to submit to a surgical operation."

Indeed, near-evisceration can result from the combination of a masochistic patient eager to be operated upon with a surgeon eager to perform operations (Weiss and English, 1957). Cases of this syndrome may also share a common background with those rare instances of patients who elect to carry out autosurgery (Menninger, 1938).

The psychologist Grygier (1954), who investigated a number of cases, produced the following formulation:

> Ambivalence is prominent everywhere. They are narcissistic and yet prepared to sustain injuries to their bodies and have attempted suicide. They crave attention, yet distrust their doctors as they are themselves distrusted. Their projective material reveals optimism that the next operation will cure them, but underlying pessimism is just beneath the surface. Although attention-seeking, they are self-effacing on tests, which suggests powerful unconscious exhibitionistic needs. Their dramatised symptoms contrast with their verbalisations, which show blandness, poverty of affect and *belle indifference*. A moralistic facade on projective tests contrasts with their proneness to criminal offences. Obsessive and paranoid features are apparent. There is evidence of homosexuality in the males, and in the females masochism has a pronounced sexual flavour, implying that operations may symbolise acts of rape, satisfying both aggressive and sexual needs.

Management and treatment

Although patients suffering from Munchausen's syndrome may pass through periods during which their behaviour becomes quiescent, there is a tendency towards chronicity, and the long-term outcome is probably intractable. Indeed only one case recorded in the literature has ever been treated successfully, and this patient was in hospital for three years and there is no detailed follow-up since then (Yassa, 1978).

Psychiatric treatment is difficult to carry out in this patient group and is rarely successful because (a) the condition does not respond to pharmacotherapy or other forms of biological treatment; (b) generally speaking, these patients do not wish to engage with psychiatrists, and they lack the motivation essential for a successful therapeutic alliance; (c) they have a tendency to wander from area to area and thus lose contact with healthcare professionals.

The following trends are emerging with regards to the treatment approach:

- Early recognition and accurate assessment. Many authors have advocated this since 1967, and this has been reinforced by Folks and Freeman (1985), thus avoiding unnecessary and dangerous interventions.
- The institution of central registers and periodic publication of so-called blacklists, though this is problematic (Wright et al., 1995).
- Inpatient treatment, usually compulsorily, owing to the tendency to abscond. The question of whether these patients are detainable under the current English and Welsh mental health legislation (Mental Health Act 1983, amended 2007) is controversial and must be left to each individual clinician's clinical judgement.
- Dynamic psychotherapy is usually unhelpful and indeed possibly harmful because the patients lack ego strength and have a tendency towards pathological lying.
- Supportive psychotherapy, however, is essential and best delivered by a clinician able to offer security and warmth, to tolerate aggression without returning it and to react phlegmatically to the attention-seeking behaviour exhibited (Ireland et al., 1967). To achieve this, attention to a physician's own counter-transference reaction is imperative (Scoggin, 1981; Scully et al., 1984; Snowden at al., 1978).
- Associated formal psychiatric disorders such as anxiety neurosis, depressive disorders, conversion symptoms and major psychosis must be distinguished and treated. Indeed some patients will accept such treatment while retaining their central disorder of personality and behaviour (Folks and Freeman, 1985).

These cases suffering from Munchausen's syndrome are complicated and demanding as well as often disruptive, but an early recognition, balanced handling and appropriate management can reduce the necessary dangerous interventions significantly. A team approach with psychiatrists meeting the referring physician or surgeon who confront the patient together with the facts can be most effective. Following this, however, it is essential that psychiatric help is offered immediately in such a manner that the psychiatrist can be seen by the patient thus, not as an adversary but as someone who is willing and prepared to help (Savard et al., 1988; Enoch, 1990).

Munchausen's syndrome by proxy

This is a variant of Munchausen's syndrome in which an adult, usually a parent or carer, deliberately simulates or fabricates symptoms or signs of illness in a dependent child, thus provoking unnecessary but potentially hazardous investigations and treatment.

Munchausen's by proxy is thus regarded as a variant of Munchausen's syndrome because the central essential lesion is within the perpetrator, the mother or carer, and the child is the victim. Cordess (1995), while accepting the term "Munchausen's syndrome by proxy" (MSBP), emphasises that there are two components to the aspect of "proxy": (a) the creation of illness in another and (b) the consequent distress caused by the doctor in investigations of the perplexing symptoms. He also refers to the similarities to Munchausen's syndrome, noting that in about a third of the cases there is a history of factitious illness behaviour in the perpetrator.

Schreier and Libow (1993), however, doubt whether there is a variant of Munchausen's syndrome, but their efforts to sub-classify the condition only lead to more confusion.

Meadow, a paediatrician, is regarded as having reported the first case in 1977, and he labelled it "Munchausen's by proxy." Initially, because paediatricians researched the condition, little attention was paid to the mothers involved and in whom the psychopathology lay. Although it was suggested initially that they did not exhibit any significant mental disturbance or disorder, it was when adult psychiatrists – the relevant experts – began to examine these mothers that it was increasingly shown that they did suffer from significant psychopathology. For example, they did exhibit personality disorder and often grafted onto this was a mental illness such as a depressive illness.

It may be that the fact that paediatricians had tended to make the diagnosis of Munchausen's by proxy without recourse to an adult psychiatrist examining the mother explains the increasing numbers who later made successful appeals against this diagnosis, albeit by then they certainly would have themselves suffered a great deal of stress in protesting and proving their innocence.

It must be emphasised that the diagnosis cannot be made without the mother undergoing an examination by a psychiatrist specialising in adult psychiatry, although it would be advisable for such an expert to co-operate closely with the paediatrician treating the child. This co-operation is essential in dealing adequately with a condition of such potential danger.

Epidemiology

The incidence and prevalence of MSBP have not been firmly established, although by 1987 over 100 cases had been reported (Rosenberg, 1987). By 1997, reported cases continued to escalate in number and gained national prominence through such cases as the nurse Beverley Allit. A report of the British Paediatric Association Surveillance Unit revealed a total of 128 cases of the following types of child abuse (victims under 16 years of age) in the UK and Republic of Ireland arising over a two-year period from September 1992 to August 1994: 55 cases of MSBP alone, 15 of non-accidental poisoning, 15 of non-accidental suffocation and 43 of more than one type of these three forms of child abuse (McClure et al., 1996). A total of 97 of these cases involved MSBP. However, it is obvious that for every published case there may be many more that are dealt with less publicly or which pass unrecognised. The reported age distribution of these victims of child abuse, at the time of diagnosis, revealed a range from infancy to 15 years with a median age of 20 months. The large majority of victims were aged less than two years.

At the time of writing, the largest systematic review of MSBP is that of Yates and Bass (2017), who identified and analysed studies relating to 796 perpetrators (487 in case series and 309 in the form of case reports), published between 1965 and 2016 (inclusive). Although the largest number were from the UK and Ireland (jointly accounting for 394 cases) and the USA (283 cases), there were reports from 30 other countries. Almost all (98%) of the perpetrators were female. The perpetrator was the mother of the victim in 96% of cases and the father in 2%; in the remaining cases the perpetrator had a different relationship with the victim, such as being his or her babysitter. The majority of perpetrators were married (76%). The average age of the perpetrators at presentation was 28 years (minimum 16 years and maximum 53 years). The occupation was mentioned in 292 cases; 133 (46%) claimed to belong to a healthcare or healthcare-related profession, although, as the authors point out, one must bear in mind the possibility of pathological lying when looking at this proportion. Psychopathological characteristics and psychosocial factors for the perpetrators were reported; a wide range of psychopathology was revealed, the most common disorders being factitious disorder imposed on self (31%), personality disorder (19%), depression (14%) and substance/alcohol abuse (14%). Perpetrators had a history of childhood maltreatment (30%), obstetric complications (24%)

and criminal behaviour (10%). In terms of the methods of abuse, fabrication by hands occurred in 79% of cases, and in 54% of the cases the fabrication continued during hospital admission. The outcome for victims was often poor or even catastrophic; 36% of victims were subjected to extensive healthcare use, and the perpetrator caused the death of the victim in 8% of cases. One particular clinical recommendation by Yates and Bass (2017), stemming from their results, is to "urge clinicians to consider mothers with a personal history of childhood maltreatment, obstetric complications, and/or factitious disorder at heightened risk" for perpetrating MSBP.

Clinical features

The whole range of childhood illnesses can be fabricated, and the syndrome can exist along a spectrum ranging from a slight exaggeration of real symptoms right through to deliberate actual physical harm. Rosenberg's (1987) authoritative review listed the following examples in a collection of 117 cases: epilepsy, otitis, bacteraemia, fever, poisoning, suffocation, apnoea, sudden infant death, developmental disability, impaired hearing, cystic fibrosis, airway obstruction, haemophilia, psychiatric disorder, cardiac disease, menorrhagia, haematuria and oesophageal perforation.

Wittkowski et al. (2017) reported an informative case report of a male child who presented with clinical signs from the age of 5 months onwards which were erroneously attributed, until the age of 3 years, to systemic autoinflammatory disease. A very large number of investigations were carried out, from blood tests and gene sequencing to bone marrow aspiration and skin biopsies; these all gave normal results. At the age of 3 years, the child was diagnosed as being a victim of MSBP, the perpetrator being his mother; the probable causes of some of the physical presenting signs were thought to be mechanical irritation (erythematous, bullous and necrotising skin lesions), addition of maternal blood (macrohaematuria) and the application of capsaicin (facial swelling).

MSBP may present with dental problems. A review of papers published between 1990 and 2015 (including their own case report) by Olczak-Kowalczyk et al. (2015) found six cases of MSBP presenting with oral lesions, including loss of teeth, oral mucosal ulceration, scars, haemorrhage, black tongue, polysialia and lip discolouration and swelling; in most cases, the mother was the perpetrator.

Victims

The victims are usually young children, the mean age at diagnosis being 39.8 months with a range of 1–252 months (Rosenberg, 1987). Males and females are involved in equal numbers. A high co-morbidity in siblings has been noted, including fabricated illness, non-accidental injury, failure to thrive, neglect and unexplained death (Bools et al., 1992).

Perpetrators and families

The perpetrators are usually mothers or female carers, e.g. grandmothers or babysitters. Father as perpetrator is unusual, but such cases do occur. A female perpetrator often has a detailed medical knowledge or sometimes a nursing background. Mental illness is uncommon, but personality disorder (especially histrionic and borderline types) is common. Factitious and somatoform disorders, Munchausen's syndrome and eating disorders are also common (Rosenberg, 1987; Bools et al., 1992; Samuels et al., 1992).

Non-perpetrating fathers are often described as passive or emotionally uninvolved in the family and even as passively colluding with the mother. High levels of family disturbance crossing generations also occur, including enmeshment, marital dysfunction, illness behaviour, and emotional, physical and sexual abuse (Griffith, 1988).

Case 8

Dee Dee Blanchard was the mother of Gypsy Rose, who for 17 years cared for her wheelchair-bound daughter, convinced that she suffered from a multiplicity of illnesses including muscular dystrophy, asthma, epilepsy, fatal sugar allergy and vision and hearing defects. Her growth was stunted and remained under 5 feet.

As a result she was given a great deal of public sympathy, special benefits and support from charities.

In spite of being examined by numerous physicians, only two suspected that this was a case of falsified illness, known as Munchausen's by proxy.

However, owing to the established condition and the widespread public sympathy, there was a reluctance to investigate her further.

However, Gypsy Rose, the daughter, was able to go online at night after her mother had gone to bed. In 2014, she contacted a man on an online dating agency, and they conspired to meet and also to consider killing Blanchard, though Gypsy Rose later denied that she had expected for her to be killed. However, they arranged together to meet in Blanchard's house, and while Gypsy Rose was in the bathroom her man friend fatally stabbed Blanchard while she was in bed asleep.

She pleaded to second degree murder in 2015 and was imprisoned for 10 years. Her man friend was found guilty of first degree murder in February 2019 and was sentenced to life imprisonment for murder. In 2018, when she was 26, Gypsy Rose said, "I feel like I'm freer in prison than living with my mom."

In our overview of the Munchausen's syndrome and Munchausen's by proxy over 50 years, this is first case where the victim instigated the murder of the perpetrator (Dean, 2016; Keegan, 2016; Herzog, 2017).

Management and treatment

Assessment and recognition

- Clinicians must be aware of the possibility of this diagnosis. Several warning signs have been proposed by many authors, including Meadow (1982). These include persistent or recurring illness which cannot be explained, investigations resulting in signs at variance with the child's health, symptoms and signs that make the specialists state that they have never seen such a case, symptoms and signs which do not occur in the absence of the parent; an overly attentive mother (who refuses to leave the hospital), treatments that are not tolerated, a very rare disorder, a mother who is not especially worried and clinical features that do not respond as expected to appropriate and careful administration of medication.
- Check the medical and background history in detail with a particular emphasis on the corroboration of information provided by the mother.
- Secure all medical records and charts, and retain samples for analysis.
- Laboratory investigations may help. For example, a clinical geneticist may be able to help distinguish rare mimics of abuse (e.g. osteogenesis imperfect) from genuine cases (Shur and Carey, 2015).
- Special surveillance which can include covert video camera surveillance, although this can be problematic.
- A multi-disciplinary approach involving psychiatrists, paediatricians and other clinical staff as well as social services and the police. Regular case conferences are essential.
- If deception is suspected and the child is in a potentially dangerous situation, it is essential that the child be removed from the scene and thus it may be necessary for recourse to legal proceedings to control the mother's access to the child. Given the difficulty of obtaining sufficient evidence to prove the mother's involvement, it may be necessary to undertake procedures which allow the child to be removed from the mother without proving the child has already suffered harm, provided the court is satisfied there is potential risk of harm.

Specific treatment

Although there is doubt about the efficacy of psychiatric treatment of the mother, she should have a full psychiatric examination, and the subsequent treatment would depend on the diagnosis. Although the management of these cases is often complicated because of the unwillingness of the mother to cooperate and because of continual denial on their part, if there is any form of psychiatric disorder present such as depression, then this should be treated intensively. Based on the findings of their systematic study, Yates and Bass (2017) recommend that caution be exercised in confronting perpetrators, given that some might have a history of suicide attempts or self-harm and also that it should not be assumed that the abuse will stop at the time of hospitalisation of the victim.

If the perpetrators are found to have damaged personalities or to be labouring under great social and family stress, then these features should be addressed. Family therapy can be especially helpful as long as the father, who has often proved to be remote if not absent, is included.

Prognosis

The available studies indicate that a significant proportion of children remain in the uncontrolled care of their mother and are thus at risk of emotional disturbance, ongoing mistreatment and even death. Eventually, Munchausen's syndrome develops in about a third of the children in adulthood. The approach most likely to succeed is a close working relationship between the paediatrician and the child and adult psychiatrists. The whole family, if at all possible, should be actively in-volved in the therapeutic process, including, and indeed especially, the "absent" father.

There is certainly a need for ongoing research in this important field where children are at risk of serious harm and even death, but it must be emphasised that the essential pathology is that of the perpetrator, usually the mother, and the child is simply the unsuspecting victim.

Munchausen's syndrome by adult proxy

Munchausen's syndrome by adult proxy (MSB-AP) is a variant of MSBP in which the victim is an adult. A review by Burton et al. (2015) of publications up to April 2014 (inclusive) found 13 published cases of MSB-AP. The victims (four male, nine female) ranged in age from 21 to 82 years. Presenting features included rashes, skin abscesses, coma, recurrent bacteraemia and fluid overload (with a false symptom history); in two cases there were no presenting signs. In two cases the outcome was death, while in another the victim be-came paraplegic. The majority of perpetrators (8 out of 13, or 62%) were female. In the vast majority of cases (85%) the perpetrator was a relative of the victim, such as the partner, mother, child or grandchild. Modes of abuse included poisoning (including by dermatological application), sometimes followed by subcutaneous injection of petrol or turpentine; injections of tranquillizers or insulin; and giving false medical histories, including a false history of memory loss.

Moreno-Ariño and Bayer (2017) have pointed out that the victim typically cannot speak for himself or herself with the result that, in response to a fabricated medical history or signs, "healthcare providers ... may unwittingly perpetuate the abuse by arranging unnecessary investigations and treatments that can themselves be potentially harmful." Moreno-Ariño and Bayer (2017) also caution that "a low index of suspicion of [MSB-AP] in older frail patients in whom atypical presentation and multiple morbidity are characteristics, together with their greater medical complexity and low physiological reserve, is likely to place them at ... significant risk of adverse outcome and death."

Pseudologia fantastica

Lying is a feature of everyday human existence and, as implied in the book of Genesis, has probably not only existed since the beginning of humanity but represents a core component of the human condition. A lie is a statement known by its speaker to be false and is intended to deceive in order to achieve a pre-conceived goal. Pathological lying or pseudologia fantastica is a morbid condition characterised by the production of gross falsifications disproportionate to any possible advantage, usually involving a web of fantastic untruths and sometimes amounting to a complex systematised deception. It therefore differs from ordinary lying in having its origins in pathological motives and psychopathological mechanisms.

Historical

*   In Delbrück, (1891 first described and used the term "pseudologia fantastica." The concept was introduced into the English medical literature by Healey and Healey, 1915).
*   Commentaries are found in some of the major contributions to the study of psychopathology (Jaspers, 1913; Kraepelin, 1921; Bleuler, 1924; Schneider, 1959; Fish, 1967). The "pseudologue swindler" is described and discussed in the criminological literature (Sparrow, 1962; Larsen, 1966).

Psychopathology

The basic mechanism is relatively simple: initially the deception of self and others is conscious and deliberate; however, after a time (depending upon the degree of pseudologia and the chronicity) the subjects themselves become convinced of the reality of their statements, at which point the process becomes an unconscious one and the statements may then become increasingly fantastic.

Traditionally, the progression from the first stage in the mechanism to the second has been thought to be aided by the absence of guilt and hence the observed association with personality disorders of a psychopathic nature (Kraepelin, 1921). Other personality traits have been described as being associated with the disorder, including borderline, narcissistic and histrionic.

This implies some relationship or similarity with the phenomenon of dissociation. Interestingly, Powell et al. (1983) reported a case in which the pathological lying was associated with psychological and physiological elements of guilt and thus suggested that the development of self-belief in the lies functioned as a guilt- or anxiety-reducing mechanism.

Psychodynamically the process has been viewed as a means of elevating low self-esteem, with the individual undertaking a flight from reality that is otherwise too uninteresting and painful to bear (Enoch, 1990). Strong reinforcement follows from the initial attention and powerful social rewards the stories may attract, at least in the short term.

Although the pathological liar is often intelligent and well educated (Enoch, 1990), cases are on record in which subjects have exhibited specific learning difficulties (Sharrock and Cresswell, 1989). This implies that, at least in some cases, there may be an underlying organically based deficit, which could account for some of the overlap seen in the clinical setting with the confabulation of gross organic states (Kerns, 1986).

Clinical presentation

The following list is by no means exhaustive but merely demonstrates some of the more commonly encountered clinical pictures:

- *The doctor impersonator* – unqualified individuals donning white coats and entering hospitals in order to adopt the role of a doctor, where they often proceed to minister to patients who are unaware as to their true status. Other roles, associated with high esteem in the eyes of the general public, may also be adopted, for example, priests, lawyers and police officers. Such actions, of course, frequently amount to a criminal offence.
- *The swindler* – the subject goes to great lengths to convey to others an image of wealth and great business acumen, often causing little harm other than disappointment and time wasting, as in the case of those unknown (as yet) people who hired expensive cars and suits and then proceeded to inspect large country properties throughout East Anglia, even putting in offers for purchase – only to vanish days later! On occasions, however, the activities of these individuals overlap with frank criminal deception and fraud.

- *Outraged females* – who allege fictitious sexual assault or inappropriate advances. Such examples comprised many of the original cases described in the literature (Healey and Healey, 1915).
- *False confessors* – who voluntarily and spontaneously claim to have committed a serious crime despite clear evidence to the contrary. This can occur in association with Munchausen's syndrome (Abed, 1997).

Treatment

There is no specific treatment for this disorder, and the general principles expressed in the section on Munchausen's syndrome probably apply. The findings of Powell et al. (1983) may prove to be of great importance in this area and suggest a differential behavioural therapy approach, depending on whether or not subjects show a psycho-physiological response to the process of lying.

The gaslight phenomenon

In December 1938, Patrick Hamilton's British play *Gas Light* (known as *Angel Street* in the USA) appeared, adapted twice for the big screen during the next six years (the British 1940 film *Gaslight* – but again appearing as *Angel Street* in the USA, and the American 1944 film also named *Gaslight*), in which a husband so manipulated a gaslight in order to make it seem that his wife's complaint about it was a sign of madness. His aim was to have her removed to an asylum so that he could have sole charge of their property.

From this plot Barton and Whitehead (1969) derived the term "gaslight phenomenon" to describe the unusual condition in which the presentation of apparent mental illness turns out on further enquiry to have been induced in a patient or to have been fabricated by another person for that person's gain. Initially, the intent was considered to be solely malicious (Barton and Whitehead, 1969; Smith and Sinanan, 1972; Tyndal, 1973; Lund and Gardiner, 1977), but further cases were subsequently reported where the motives to induce the apparent madness were based on psychoneurotic mechanisms rather than for any personal material gain (Cawthra and O'Brien, 1987; Calef and Weinshel, 1981).

This latter variant was referred to by Cawthra and O'Brien as "imposed psychosis" and, in the example they described, the *gaslightee* even became symptomatic. Such a process is obviously reminiscent of – and is very similar to – that which occurs in some cases of *folie à deux*. Both conditions involve the induction of symptoms in a weaker personality by a more dominant partner or relative; the symptoms, although genuine, soon subside when separation is effected.

There are few case reports in the literature, suggesting either a rare phenomenon or much undetected morbidity.

An awareness of this phenomenon is vital for all contemporary psychiatrists who practise in a complex, modern society. For example, if the accounts are accepted, then some elements of the state apparatus in the former Soviet Union engaged in large-scale gaslighting in presenting many political dissidents as being mentally ill, even going to the extent of releasing genuinely ill dissidents to the West in order to obfuscate the process (Fireside, 1979). Although the circumstances are very different, similar but perhaps more subtle pressures can be brought to bear upon psychiatrists working in Western liberal democracies, particularly in a forensic setting. All practising psychiatrists must remain constantly alert to their core role as physicians, whose primary obligation is to act for the welfare and best interests of their patients and not those of third parties.

References

Abed, R.T. (1997) *Irish Journal of Psychological Medicine, 14,* 144.

Achte, K.A., Kaukp, S.K. (1964) *Acta Psychiatrica Scandinavica, 40,* 121.

American Psychiatric Association (1994) *Diagnostic and Statistical Manual of Mental Disorders, Fourth Edition (DSM-IV).* American Psychiatric Association, Washington, DC.

American Psychiatric Association (2013) *Diagnostic and Statistical Manual of Mental Disorders, Fifth Edition (DSM-5).* American Psychiatric Association, Washington, DC.

Asher, R. (1951) *Lancet, 1,* 339.

Bagan, M. (1962) *Boston Medical Quarterly, 13,* 113.

Baig, M.R., Levin, T.T., Lichtenthal, W.G., Boland, P.J., Breitbart, W.S. (2016) *Psycho-oncology, 25,* 707.

Banzel, P. (1934) *Presse Medicae, 42,* 1731.

Barker, J.C. (1958) *British Medical Journal, 2,* 1274.

Barker, J.C. (1960) *The Nature and Features of the Munchausen Syndrome.* MD Thesis, University of Cambridge.

Barker, J.C. (1961) *British Medical Journal, 1,* 60.

Barker, J.C. (1962) *Journal of Mental Science, 108,* 167.

Barker, J.C. (1964a) *Journal of Mental Science, 1,* 1704.

Barker, J.C. (1964b) *Journal of Mental Science, 2,* 1136.

Barker, J.C., Grygier, T.G. (1957) *Lancet, 2,* 1069.

Barrett, N.R., Hoyle, C. (1942) *British Journal of Tuberculosis, 36,* 172.

Barton, R., Whitehead, J.A. (1969) *Lancet, 1,* 1258.

Bleuler, E. (1924) *Textbook of Psychiatry,* Trans. A.A. Brill. MacMillan, New York.

Bools, C.N., Neale, B.A., Meadow, R. (1992) *Archives of Disease in Childhood, 67,* 77.

Brooks, E., Christy, N.E., Mack, A.H., McFadden M. (2015) *Infection Control & Hospital Epidemiology, 36,* 996.

Burton, M.C., Warren, M.B., Lapid, M.I., Bostwick, J.M. (2015) *Journal of Hospital Medicine, 10,* 32.

Cakmak, M.A., Sahin, S., Cinar, N., Tiyekli, U., Karsidag, S. (2015) *Tremor and Other Hyperkinetic Movements, 5,* tre–5–297–6792–1.

Calef, V., Weinshel, E.M. (1981) *Psychoanalytic Quarterly*, *50*, 44.

Cawthra, R., O'Brien, G. (1987) *British Journal of Psychiatry*, *150*, 553.

Ceiller (1947) *Annales de Medecine Legale, Criminologie, Police Scientifique et Toxocologie*, *27*, 134.

Chamoff, V.N., Sotina, N.N. (1935) *Vrachebnoe Delo*, *18*, 9/5.

Chowne, M.D. (1843) *Lancet*, *1*, 131.

Cordess, C. (1995) In *Forensic Psychotherapy: Crime, Psychodynamics and the Offender Patient*, Eds. C. Cordess, M. Cox. Jessica Kingsley, London.

Davis, E. (1951) *Lancet*, *1*, 910.

Dean, M. (2016) *Dee Dee Wanted Her Daughter To Be Sick, Gypsy Wanted Her Mom to Be Murdered*. Buzz Feed, Buzz Feed Entertainment Group, New York.

Delbrück, A. (1891) *Die pathologische Luge und die psychischabnormen Schwindler. Ein Untersuchung über den allmahlichen Oberang eines normales psychologische Vorgans in ein pathologisches Symptom*. Enke, Stuttgart.

Enoch, M.D. (1990) In *Principles and Practices of Forensic Psychiatry*, Eds. R. Bluglass, P. Bowden. Churchill Livingstone, London.

Feldman, M.D. (2000) *Southern Medical Journal*, *93*, 669.

Feldman, M.D., Bibby, M., Crites, S.D. (1998) *Western Journal of Medicine*, *168*, 537.

Feldman, M.F., Khan, D.A., Brown, E.S., Bernstein, J.A. (2014) *Journal of Allergy and Clinical Immunology in Practice*, *2*, 795.

Finsterer, J., Stefan, L. (2016) *Indian Journal of Psychological Medicine*, *38*, 348.

Fireside, H. (1979) *Soviet Psychoprisons*. Norton, New York.

Fish, F. (1967) *Clinical Psychopathology*. Wright, Bristol.

Folks, D., Freeman, A. (1985) *Psychiatric Clinics of North America*, *2*, 263.

Gliebe, P.A., Goldman, L. (1949) *California Medicine*, *70*, 117.

Grant, A.P. (1952) *Journal of the Irish Medical Association*, *31*, 299.

Griffith, J.L. (1988) *Family Process*, *27*, 423.

Grunert, E. (1932) *Psychiatrisch-Neurologische Wochenschrift*, *34*, 611.

Grygier, T.G., Collie, I.F. (1954) *Lancet*, *2*, 1284.

Hamilton, P. (1939) *Gaslight*. London, Constable.

Hawkings, R.R., Jones, K.S., Sim, M., Tibbetts, R.W. (1956) *British Medical Journal*, *1*, 361.

Healey, W., Healey, M. (1915) *Pathological Lying, Accusation and Swindling. A Study in Forensic Psychology*. Heinemann, London.

Herzog, K, (2017) *"Mommy Dead and Dearest": How it Handles Munchausen Syndrome"*, New York: New York City Media, Retrieved June 3, 2017.

Hyler, S., Sussman, N. (1981) *Psychiatric Clinics of North America*, *4*, 365.

Ireland, P., Sapira, J., Templeton, B. (1967) *American Journal of Medicine*, *43*, 579.

Jaspers, K. (1913) *General Psychopathology*, Trans. J. Hoenig, M.W. Hamilton. Manchester University Press, London.

Keegan, H. (2016) *"Munchausen expert says Gypsy Blanchard case is unprecedented"*, *Springfield News- Leader, Springfield*, Missouri: Gannet Company, Retrieved June 2, 2017.

Kenneth, M., Zangwill, K.M., Marin, C., Vu, H. (2015) *Infection Control & Hospital Epidemiology*, *35*, 1550.

Kerns, L.L. (1986) *Psychiatry*, *49*, 13.

Kinns, H., Housley, D., Freedman, D.B. (2013) *Annals of Clinical Biochemistry*, *50*, 194.

Kraepelin, E. (1921) *Manic Depressive Insanity and Paranoia*, Trans. R.M. Barclay, G.M. Robertson. Livingstone, Edinburgh.

Larsen, E. (1966) *The Deceivers*. Baker, London.

Lund, C.A., Gardiner, A.Q. (1977) *British Journal of Psychiatry*, *131*, 533.

MacKieth, R. (1957) *Lancet*, *2*, 1069.

McClure, R.J., Davis, P.M., Meadow, S.R., Sibert, J.R. (1996) *Archives of Disease in Childhood*, *75*, 57.

Meadow, R. (1977) *Lancet 2*, 343.

Meadow, R. (1982) *Archives of Disease in Childhood*, *57*, 92.

Menninger, K.A. (1934) *Psychoanalytic Quarterly*, *3*, 173.

Menninger, K.A. (1938) *Man against Himself.* Hart-Davis, London.

Moreno-Ariño, M., Bayer, A. (2017) *Age and Ageing*, *46*, 166.

Netherton, E.W. (1927) *Ohio State Medical Journal*, *23*, 215.

Olczak-Kowalczyk, D., Wolska-Kusnierz, B., Bernatowska, E. (2015) *Central European Journal of Immunology*, *40*, 109.

Oliveira, J.R.M. (2017) *Neurology*, *89*, 307.

Powell, G.E., Gudjonsson, G.H., Miller, P. (1983) *Personal and Individual Differences*, *4*, 141.

Puri, B.K. (2006) *International Journal of Clinical Practice*, *60*, 1527.

Raspe, R.E. (1786) *Baron Munchausen's Narrative of his Marvellous Travels and Campaigns in Russia*. Oxford. In the British Library.

Reich, M., Clermont A., Amela, É., Kotecki, N. (2015) *Bulletin du Cancer*, *102*, 1036.

Reinhard, W.E. (1950) *Tuberkulosearzt*, *4*, 475.

Rosenberg, D.A. (1987) *Child Abuse & Neglect*, *11*, 547.

Samuels, M.P., McClaughlin, W., Jacobson, R.R., Poets, C.F., Southall, D.P. (1992) *Archives of Disease in Childhood*, *67*, 162.

Sanderson, P.H. (1957) *Lancet*, *1*, 483.

Savard, G., Andermann, F., Tettlebaum, P., Lehman, H. (1988) *Neurology*, *38*, 1628.

Schneider, K. (1959) *Clinical Psychopathology*, Trans. B.A. Hamilton. Grune and Stratton, New York.

Schreier, H., Libow, J. (1993) *Hurting for Love: Munchausen by Proxy*. Guildford, New York.

Scoggin, C. (1981) *Postgraduate Medicine*, *74*, 259.

Scully, R., Mark, E., McNeely, B. (1984) *New England Journal of Medicine*, *311*, 108.

Sharrock, R., Cresswell, M. (1989) *Medicine, Science and the Law*, *29*, 323.

Shur, N., Carey, J.C. (2015) *American Journal of Medical Genetics. Part C, Seminars in Medical Genetics*, *169*, 281.

Small, A. (1955) *British Medical Journal*, *2*, 1207.

Smith, C.G., Sinanan, K. (1972) *British Journal of Psychiatry*, *120*, 685.

Snowden, J., Solomans, R., Druce, H. (1978) *British Journal of Psychiatry*, *133*, 15.

Sparrow, G. (1962) *The Great Imposters*. Longman, London.

Tyndal, M. (1973) *British Journal of Psychiatry*, *122*, 367.

Vaduganathan, M., McCullough, S.A., Fraser, T.N., Stern, T.A. (2014) *Psychosomatics*, *55*, 668.

Valeina, S., Krumina, Z., Sepetiene, S., Andzane, G., Sture, E.A., Taylor, D. (2016) *Journal of Pediatric Ophthalmology and Strabismus*, *53*, e6.

Weiss, E., English, O.S. (1957) *Psychosomatic Medicine, 3rd edn.* Saunders, Philadelphia.

Wittkowski, H., Hinze, C., Häfner-Harms, S., Oji, V., Masjosthusmann, K., Monninger, M., Grenzebach, U., Foell, D. (2017) *Paediatric Rheumatology (Online)*, *15*, 19.
Wright, A.D. (1955) *Transactions of the Hunterian Society*, *14*, 13.
Wright, B., Bhugra, D., Booty, J. (1995) *Journal of Accident and Emergency Medicine*, *13*, 18.
Yassa, R. (1978) *Psychosomatics*, *19*, 242.
Yates, G., Bass, C. (2017) *Child Abuse & Neglect*, *72*, 45.
Yates, G.P., Feldman, M.D. (2016) *General Hospital Psychiatry*, *41*, 20.
Zittel, S., Lohmann, K., Bauer, P., Klein, C., Münchau, A. (2017) *Neurology*, *88*, 1000.

Chapter 7

Gilles de la Tourette's syndrome

"Whom do you want?" said the voice of Nikolay Levin, angrily.
"It's I," answered Konstantin Levin, coming forward into the light.
...
"Ah, Kostya!" he exclaimed suddenly, recognising his brother, and his eyes lit up with joy. But the same second he looked round at the young man, and gave the nervous jerk of his head and neck that Konstantin knew so well, as if his neckband hurt him; and a quite different expression, wild, suffering, and cruel, rested on his emaciated face.

Leo Tolstoy, *Anna Karenina* (1878)

Gilles de la Tourette's syndrome is a motor disorder classified within the realm of psychiatric disorders. A triad of components is necessary to make the diagnosis:

- Generalised tics
- Involuntary utterances which may be obscene or suggestively so
- Onset in childhood or adolescence

Historical

The evolution of the awareness and descriptions of the syndrome can be summarised as follows:

- Described by Gilles de la Tourette in 1885, who was the source of the eponymous syndrome, sometimes abbreviated to Tourette syndrome.
- The disorder was, however, described earlier in the nineteenth century.
- Many cases of the disorder have been described in the twentieth and twenty-first centuries.
- The disorder is acknowledged in the accepted major international classificatory systems, *ICD-10* and *DSM-5*, and is likely to appear in the forthcoming *ICD-11*.

- In recent years, much work has been undertaken focussing on the neurobiological and neurophysiological aspects of the condition.

The historical evolution of the syndrome of Gilles de la Tourette has been succinctly elucidated by Stevens (1964), who stated that when Beard's (1880) account of "The Jumping Frenchman of Maine" was translated by Gilles de la Tourette, this first generated his interest in such conditions. Charcot, whose staff he joined in 1884, encouraged him to continue the study in an attempt to classify the "chaos of the choreas." When Gilles de la Tourette isolated the condition which he called *maladie des tics compulsifs*, Charcot considered it to be an entity having sufficient characteristics to warrant a name of its own and suggested that it should be eponymous (Charcot, 1884; Tourette, 1884; 1885; 1889). Gilles de la Tourette described eight patients with persistent tics beginning in childhood, five of whom had verbal tics consisting of repeated expostulation of obscenities and swear-words (*coprolalia*):

About the age of 7 or 8, a child commonly with a wretched family history, begins to exhibit a series of tics. The attention of parents is soon drawn to the fact, but they seldom give much heed at first, since the twitches are limited preferably to facial musculature. At this stage, too, expiratory laryngeal noises are occasionally super-added. The movements may be confined for a long time to the face, but later they gradually invade the shoulders and arms... . The muscles of the larynx are also sometimes involved so that many sufferers from the tic give vent to quick expiratory "hems" and "ahs." The disease may be limited to this stage, but it is not uncommon to find, a few months or years after the beginning of the facial movements, that the inarticulate laryngeal sound becomes organised and develops in a particular direction: this being pathognomonic of the disorder. Under the influence of causes whose actions we are in the majority of cases powerless to appreciate, the patients give vent one day to a word or short phrase of quite special character, in so much as its meaning is always obscene. These words and phrases are explained in a loud voice, without any attempt at restraint... . Another physical stigma, echolalia, is occasionally, though less frequently observed.

A disorder comprising multiple tics accompanied by explosive utterances had been described previously, earlier in the nineteenth century by the French physician Itard (1825). He reported the case of the Marquise de Dampièrre, who, at the age of 7 years, began to tic and later to ejaculate bizarre cries and meaningless utterances, *"mais tout cela sans délière, sans aucun trouble des facultées mentales."* Following her marriage, there was an exacerbation of her symptoms so that her coprolalia, which contrasted with her otherwise refined manners, forced her to become a recluse for the last 70 years of her life. She died at over 90 years of age, still cursing.

In 1864, Hughlings Jackson described what could be regarded as an example of the syndrome, stating:

> I have a patient, the subject of chorea, who for several years has been in the habit of saying, quite involuntarily, the word "bloody." A few years ago, he was frightened by a man shouting the word after him. The fright produced Chorea, and if I may use such a term, Chorea of his mind, too; as, for three days, he said the word "bloody" and little else; and now he ejaculated it occasionally. The mental process for saying that word, is as little under his control as a few of the muscles of his face are, for the twitching of which he is now attending at the London Hospital.

Following Giles de la Tourette, Trousseau (1867) described other cases of the syndrome that had occurred earlier. Koester (1899) discovered two new cases among 2,500 patients admitted to the Leipzig University Polyclinic and found a total of 50 cases reported in the literature current at that time, including those described by Guinon (1886), Wille (1898) and Osler (1894). Prince (1906) described a further case of a male aged 35 years suffering from the condition.

No further cases were recorded for 30 years until the six reported cases of Creak and Guttman (1935): three males aged 10 to 15 years, another aged 22 years and two females aged 18 and 32 years, whom they found among cases in the Maudsley Hospital between 1932 and 1935. Then, Kinnier Wilson (1941) reported a case (posthumously) which he had encountered during the second decade of the twentieth century, and Kanner (1942) described another he had seen in 1929. A steady stream of new cases was then recorded, usually in the form of single case reports (Aberle, 1952; Balthasar, 1957; Rapoport, 1959; Schneck, 1960; Aimard and Kohler, 1961; Deshan, 1961; McDonald, 1963).

In *ICD-10*, the syndrome is classified as a disorder of childhood and adolescence, within the subgroup tic disorders, where it is referred to as "combined vocal and multiple motor tic disorder (de la Tourette syndrome)." The diagnostic criteria are the presence of multiple motor tics and one or more vocal tic (not necessarily concurrent) with an onset almost always in childhood or adolescence.

In *DSM-5*, the diagnostic criteria for Tourette disorder or Tourette syndrome include (American Psychiatric Association, 2013):

- The presence of at least two motor tics (e.g. blinking or shrugging the shoulders) and at least one vocal tic (e.g. humming, throat clearing or yelling out a word or phrase); these do not always have to occur at the same time

- Duration ≥ one year
- Onset before the age of 18 years
- Symptoms are not the result of medication, other drugs or another medical condition (e.g. seizures, Huntingtons' disease or post-viral encephalitis)

Other tic disorders in *DSM-5* include persistent (or chronic) motor or vocal tic disorder and provisional tic disorder. The diagnostic criteria are similar to those given above; for persistent (or chronic) motor or vocal tic disorder the criteria include:

- The presence of at least one motor tic or at least one vocal tic, but *not* both
- Tics occur many times daily or nearly daily or on and off for a period of more than one year
- Onset before the age of 18 years
- Symptoms are not the result of medication, other drugs or another medical condition which can cause tics (e.g. seizures, Huntingtons' disease or post-viral encephalitis)
- Not diagnosed with Tourette syndrome

Similarly, the diagnostic criteria for provisional tic disorder include:

- The presence of at least one motor tic or at least one vocal tic
- Present for no longer than 12 consecutive months
- Onset before the age of 18 years
- Symptoms are not the result of medication, other drugs or another medical condition which can cause tics (e.g. seizures, Huntingtons' disease or post-viral encephalitis)
- Not diagnosed with Tourette syndrome or persistent motor or vocal tic disorder

Case reports

Case 1

He was first admitted in 1959, aged 27 years. He complained of having had to utter monosyllabic noises to interject short obscenities and to make compulsive gestures and movements in his arms, tongue and neck continuously for the past 21 years. This had followed tonsillectomy at the age of 6 years. Shortly afterwards there began flicking of his head backwards, spontaneous movement of his hands and tongue and the use of foul language. Noises and movements abated during sleep. He had a convulsion at 2 years and was enuretic until 12 years of age. He received little understanding from his father, who locked him up when his movements were excessive. He missed much schooling and was frequently caned for his complaint. He worked as a hod-carrier on building sites and often lived rough. He drank heavily and frequently became depressed about his condition.

Physical examination was normal, apart from his movements and utterances. He put his tongue in and out repeatedly in rapid succession. This was frequently accompanied by grimacing and contracting of the platysma, producing a rather leonine expression. The grimacing occasionally occurred alone. Movements and gestures of the arms were more pronounced on the right side, and one gesture of the right arm appeared to have sexual significance. The movements and utterings, "Phtt, phtt," appeared aggressive in character. Echophenomena were absent. He maintained he wished to die if he could not be cured.

There were no psychotic features. His intelligence was average. His EEG showed a generalised dysrhythmia. Hypnotherapy, with posthypnotic suggestion that his symptoms would shortly abate, was unsuccessful as was the suggestion when made with intravenous thiopentone. Carbon dioxide therapy (Meduna, 1943) exacerbated his symptoms. Chlorpromazine and myanesin (a muscle relaxant) produced limited improvement during a subsequent admission. In 1965, his condition was reported to be in remission.

Case 2

Her illness began in 1954, at the age of 11 years before the 11-plus examination, and when her sister, to whom she was very attached, left home. It was preceded by an attack of croup. She rebelled against her authoritarian father with frequent screaming attacks. A nail-biter, she was an immature, nervous and awkward child with retarded speech who became enuretic between the ages of 11 and 12 years. In 1956, she became maladjusted and had to leave school because of swearing, screaming, grimacing and outrageous behaviour. On admission in 1956, physical examination revealed early mitral stenosis and some equivocal neurological signs (an eccentric left pupil, limb hypertonia and Rombergism). She exhibited repetitive, quasi-purposeful multiple tics, involving her face, neck, trunk and limbs, which had progressively increased but which were abolished by concentration. Her coprolalia, which seemed compulsive, occurred incidentally, "Bloody old things," "Buggers," etc. If corrected, she shouted and stamped and seemed compelled to restart the sentence if interrupted. Her intelligence was average and her EEG normal. She wanted to become an authoress but not to write anything by hand.

Later, in an adolescent unit, her multiple tics, shouting, screaming, swearing, scribbling on walls, obscenities and climbing everywhere did not respond either to a sympathetic environment or to tranquillisers.

Three years later she still had a number of minor tics and admitted to using foul language, but she believed she could control this. Her improvement was ascribed to the fact that she recently left home. In 1965, her condition was reported to be in a state of remission while she herself was working regularly.

Case 3

She was first admitted in 1953, aged 60 years. She was a recluse giving a history of almost continuous shouting for several months. The noise was of a crowing, barking or screaming character which she could not prevent, especially when excited. She had always been nervous since having chorea at the age of 7 years and had had much strife in her family. At the age of 21 years, she had been advised to sit in front of a mirror to cure her facial tic.

On examination, her nervous system was normal. She had an obsessional personality, and there was no evidence of psychosis. She had a "soul-destroying" compulsive tic when she turned her head up and barked in a staccato fashion, concluding with an explosive "Shut up" as if to mitigate her display. She exhibited twisting and twitching movements and was constantly grimacing. She frequently ejaculated "Hey, hey," followed by "Shut up," and her cries could be heard in the corridor outside the ward. Ordinary sedation was ineffective. She had been blind in her right eye for two years, and a large retinal detachment was discovered, caused by, it was thought, all her excessive head shaking and shouting.

Her last admission occurred in 1963 following a prolonged admission during which she had received chlorpromazine as an outpatient. She had drug-induced Parkinsonism which responded to orphenadrine. Her copro-lalic interjections were largely in abeyance, although she was occasionally noticed talking to herself. Her whereabouts then became unknown.

Case 4

She was admitted in 1964, aged 47 years. She had had an unhappy childhood and resented her mother's lack of interest in her, which started with the birth of her younger brother. She did not love her father, and her early life was marred by quarrels. She is now happily married with two sons. She has little social life, being interested only in her home and family.

At the age of 10 years, following the death of her grandmother, to whom she was particularly attached, there began peculiar "bleeping" noises, twitching movements of the face, grinding of her teeth, involuntary movements of her arms and legs and later the utterance of obscenities. She had some voluntary control over these, but this was incomplete. Her husband alleged that her "noises" had increased since marriage and have even occurred during childbirth. They were exacerbated by stress and by mention of the patient's mother.

Inhibition of the "bleeping" could occur when she was alone and when writing a letter. They recurred with renewed vigour when she had to inhibit them in public. Physical examination was normal, and she was of average intelligence.

Methedrine abreactions revealed material which suggested that she had been rejected in childhood and had tended to interpret all interpersonal relationships in terms of early parental rejection. Lysergic acid was tried, but she could not tolerate its somatic affects. Her noises and twitching were unaffected by a variety of tranquillising drugs, and at times she became depressed and hysterical.

She terminated treatment while undergoing behaviour therapy. This therapy caused no overall improvement at the time, although it demonstrated that she could voluntarily produce noises which were identical to the involuntary ones, and it showed her that in contrast to her usual complaint of needing to keep the noises in, a stage could be reached when no noises could be made in spite of intensive voluntary efforts to do so. She was not improved when she left hospital. Nine months later she was scarcely making any noises but was definitely more tense.

Epidemiology

Gilles de la Tourette's syndrome, once thought to be a rarity, is found in all cultures, ethnic and religious groups, presenting with similar characteristics. The exact prevalence of the condition is unknown, depending, at least in part, on the method of assessment and the operational criteria used in making the diagnosis.

Mahler et al. (1945) found that 18 of 541 children admitted to a children's ward in a New York hospital had tics. However, only 11 of them suffered from the "tic syndrome," the synonym he used for Gilles de la Tourette's disorder. Ascher (1948) found only four cases among 9,000 inpatients and 50,000 outpatients of the Henry Phipps Psychiatric Clinic, Baltimore, between 1918 and 1947. Salmi (1961) detected only one case among 5,300 children attending an education guidance centre in Turku, Finland. Kelman 1965, surveying reports of Gilles de la Tourette's syndrome in children, found 44 reported cases over the period 1906 to 1964.

In 1967, Fernando, while noting its rarity, emphasised the necessity to review all published cases as this was the only feasible method of surveying the condition in its broader aspects. He considered that only 69 cases then reported in the English-language journals were sufficiently detailed to allow him to agree with the diagnosis as being correct. In 1976, he accounted for an additional 69 published cases, again reported in the English-language journals between 1964 and 1974.

Abuzzahab and Ehnlen (undated) have taken a special interest in Gilles de la Tourette's syndrome. This led them to establish an international register at the University of Minnesota for the purpose of studying the subject, following which they were able to collect 500 documented cases of the disorder.

Scahill et al. (2013) have reviewed the prevalence of childhood Tourette syndrome in studies carried out between 2000 and 2012. The 10 studies in question revealed a prevalence rate ranging from 2.6–38 per 1,000 population.

Hansen et al. (2018) interviewed the parents of 407 consecutively referred children, aged 7 to 13 years, at the time of admittance to child and adolescent mental health services outpatient clinics in the Akershus county/Oslo area of Norway, using the semi-structured Schedule for Affective Disorders and Schizophrenia for School-Age Children, Present and Lifetime Version (Kaufman et al., 1997); 72 (18%) of the children had a tic disorder (chronic tics, transient tics, Tourette syndrome).

Although most of the case reports are from the USA and Europe, it should be noted that the disorder is found in all parts of the world, and cases have been reported from Germany, Switzerland, Poland, France, Spain, Canada, Ireland, Sweden, Norway, Australia, New Zealand, India, China, Taiwan, South Africa, Israel and Saudi Arabia.

Clinical features

The clinical features of the syndrome are:

- Generalised tics
- Coprolalia
- Occasionally, echo phenomena
- Onset in childhood or adolescence
- Associated psychological symptoms – poor concentration, restlessness, depression and obsessional features
- In some cases, behavioural and personality disorder

The disorder usually starts in childhood, in 85% of cases before the age of 11 years. In those patients whose symptoms are of later onset, unusual circumstances are usually present, and the syndrome follows an atypical pattern. Males are affected three times as commonly as females. Thus, in the large Norwegian study mentioned above, the mean age of the children presenting with a tic disorder was 10.3 years (standard deviation 2.1 years), and 78% of them were boys (Hansen et al., 2018). The authors also studied the course of tic severity during the first two decades of life, based on the earlier work of Leckman et al. (1998; 2002). There was a sharp rise in severity from the age of 5 years onwards, reaching a peak at around 10 years of age, with a steady decline thereafter.

The abnormal movements usually begin in the muscles of the face, especially around the eyes or the mouth. The tics, unlike those of 20% of the population, persist and gradually extend to involve other muscles in the neck, collar, arms, legs and trunk. The muscular contractions affect synergistic muscles in an apparently systematic fashion in any one patient, but the particular combination of muscles and types of contractions vary from one patient to another. The intensity of the tics can also vary greatly from patient to patient and also in the same patient at different times. They can be very severe and manifest themselves as violent spasmodic jerking which may also catapult a patient from his chair (Stevens, 1964). In general, motor and vocal tics take place in bouts with relatively stable time intervals between bouts, as demonstrated by the work of Lin et al. (2002) and Leckman (2002). Also, there is a fractal nature to the temporal character of these bouts, such that over different time-scales the pattern of motor and vocal tics looks similar (Lin et al., 2002).

The repeated shouting and head shaking of our Case 3 probably provoked unilateral blindness following retinal detachment. Another patient dealt himself such violent blows to his eyes that he induced vitreous haemorrhages and lost his sight (Seignot, 1961). The movements usually cease during sleep, and, unlike coprolalia, which may occur only in the presence of others, usually persist unaltered whether other people are present or not. They are usually intensified, however, by emotional factors such as fear and embarrassment and by fatigue. They have been reported to be diminished during febrile illnesses (Ascher, 1948; Walsh et al., 1986) and relieved by alcohol (Bockner, 1959), and it is generally accepted that they can be modified or completely suppressed by voluntary control.

Abnormal movements may be the only symptom present for a very long time, ranging from a few days to several years, but the next manifestation of the syndrome is almost invariably the utterance of inarticulate sounds: vocal tics. These sounds are usually emitted at the point of climax of the motor tic and may resemble grunting and barking. They may then develop into articulate sounds and into fully formed ejaculation and fully formed sentences, progressing typically to the compulsive shouting of obscenities (*coprolalia*), which was considered by Giles de la Tourette to be a distinctive feature of the illness, although one occurring less frequently than other symptoms, being present in only about half the cases. Thus many patients do not progress to the point of explosive obscene utterances, whilst others may succeed in concealing these by modifying their speech slightly or by coughing. On the other hand, a number of coprolalic interjections are sufficiently severe to compel the patient to retreat from public life, living virtually as a recluse. Mental coprolalia – that is a compulsion to *think* obscenities – is probably commoner than vocal coprolalia, although the former can transform itself into the latter. Very rarely do vocal tics precede motor tics, although sometimes they commence simultaneously.

The explosive and stereotyped tics and abrupt repetitive utterances already described, together with echophenomena, constitute the characteristic symptom-triad for the syndrome. Echophenomena consist of compulsive repetition of words spoken by others (*echolalia*) or even of a repetition of the patient's own words (*pallilalia*), also compulsive imitation of the experiences, movements and actions of others (*echomimesia, echokinesis* and *echopraxia*). Although Giles de la Tourette included echolalia in his original description of the syndrome, even he noted that it only occurred in half his cases. Since then, it has become progressively apparent that the many patients with generalised tics and coprolalia do not exhibit echophenomena; and even when these are present they may seem insignificant.

Sometimes the noise made by these patients may be extremely loud and distressing to others; for example, the cries of our Case 3 could be heard outside her ward. Mazur (1953) examined the speech abnormality of his patient and concluded that the patient could not adjust the volume of his voice except by trial and error, and he described this disability as a form of dysmetria or dysnergia affecting the muscles of phonation. Although the handwriting of the sufferers may be reduced to a mere scrawl, it is never interrupted by automatic written words in the same manner as is their speech.

A number of quantitative studies have suggested that it might not be appropriate to consider Gilles de la Tourette's syndrome as a unitary condition. One of the largest such studies was the factor analysis by Cavanna et al. (2011) of data from 639 patients. The following three factors were delineated in their study.

* Complex motor tics (i.e. tics involving more than one muscle group) and echo-paliphenomena (echolalia, echopraxia, palilalia)
* Attention-deficit hyperactivity symptoms plus aggressive behaviours
* Complex vocal tics and coprophenomena

Obsessive-compulsive behaviours were loaded on the first two factors, and together all three factors accounted for almost 49% of total symptom variance (Cavanna et al., 2011).

Associated psychological symptoms are often present, although these vary considerably and are non-specific. They include absent-mindedness and an inability to concentrate, together with restlessness and depression of various degrees. Controlled studies have shown increased rates of depression. Depression is more severe among those with a longer history of the syndrome, possibly suggesting that it is a reactive phenomenon to a chronic, disabling and stigmatising disorder.

There are increased rates of obsessive-compulsive disorder and behaviours among sufferers of Tourette syndrome. Studies have also revealed raised rates of such disorders in first-degree relatives. The phenomenology observed in Tourette syndrome sufferers differs slightly from the obsessions and compulsions found in those without the disorder. For example, obsessions in Tourette syndrome are more often sexual, violent and symmetrical, while touching, counting and self-damaging compulsions are more frequent in the others (Eapen 1993).

In the large Norwegian study of Hansen et al. (2018), the co-morbidity figures for tic disorders were 10% no co-morbidity, 50% attention-deficit hyperactive disorder, 15% ASD, 35% anxiety disorder, 11% depressive disorder, 26% disruptive behaviour disorder, and 7% obsessive-compulsive disorder. The median number of diagnoses was two (including a tic disorder). Leckman (2002) demonstrated that in cases of co-morbidity ADHD manifestations emerge at a slightly earlier age than tic disorder, whereas obsessive-compulsive features manifest at a slightly later age.

An affected child often exhibits abnormal behaviour patterns, in many cases before the tics or vocal manifestations begin. Other abnormal movements or behaviour patterns commonly occur, along with the tics and vocalisations. These may include stuttering, repeated protrusion of the tongue, pounding of the chest or abdomen with the fist, hissing and temper tantrums. High rates of discipline problems and other antisocial behaviours are found.

In a large North American (USA and Canada) study of 811 patients with Tourette syndrome (mean age at interview 19 years, mean age of onset 6 years), Greenberg et al. (2018) found that 4% met the DSM-5 criteria for trichotillomania (hair-pulling disorder), while 13% met the criteria for excoriation (skin-picking disorder). Predictors of hair-pulling disorder and/or skin-picking disorder in the Tourette syndrome patients included female sex, obsessive-compulsive disorder, tic severity and severity of obsessive-compulsive symptoms.

Physical antecedents appear prominently in many of the cases reported in the literature. Examples include head injury, encephalitis lethargica and chorea. It is not known whether this is a significant observation or simply represents reporting bias.

Clinical examination of the nervous system is often normal, and although there has been an increasing number of neurological abnormalities reported, these are always of a minor nature and difficult to assess clearly in an objective fashion. Examples include mild motor asymmetries, decreased muscle tone, impaired arm swinging and a Babinski sign. Sweet et al. (1973) from the Cornell Medical Institute, New York, after carrying out a careful clinical examination of 22 patients with Gilles de la Tourette's syndrome, found 11 with such neurological abnormalities.

Intelligence would appear to be normally distributed, although it can range widely from the learning disability range to superior, and there is sometimes a verbal-performance discrepancy (performance being the lower). Psychological test results have indicated a marked preponderance of obsessional personalities among those suffering from the syndrome (Morphew and Sim, 1969).

The differential diagnosis includes:

- Organic movement disorders such as Sydenham chorea and Huntingtons' disease (chorea)
- Post-encephalitic states
- Hysterical disorders
- Simple tic disorders
- Schizophrenic mannerisms and catatonic states
- Autism and other pervasive developmental disorders
- Other movement disorders including *latah*, *myriachit* and "*The Jumping Frenchman of Maine*"

Coprolalia is not only a symptom of psychiatric disorders but is also a very common social "grace," found in a proportion of the normal population. Prince (1906) distinguished the swearing of normal individuals from the automatic obscene ejaculations found in this syndrome on the grounds that the former would cease when attention was drawn to it and a conscious effort made to stop, whereas the latter were not only involuntary but persisted even when the patient made a deliberate attempt at suppression. Hughlings Jackson (1884), with his inimitable powers of observation, was of the opinion that swearing is, strictly speaking, not a part of language. He regarded it as a habit that has grown up from the impulse to add the force of passing emotions to the expression of ideas, and it belongs, therefore, to the same general category as loudness of tone and violence of gesticulation. The distinction of such utterances from language as an intellectual act may be illustrated best by the remark Dr Johnson once made to a boisterous antagonist: "Sir, you raise your voice when you should enforce your arguments."

Some authors see a close resemblance between Gilles de la Tourette's syndrome and stammering, both being conditions with compulsive movements, the connection being even closer if we accept the contention of Fenichel (1945) and others that stammering itself means the utterance of obscene, especially *anal words* and is an aggressive act directed against the listener.

Latah is a condition that was first observed to occur in Malayans by O'Brien, 1883 and was described by Yap (1952) as "a curious behavioural quirk or aberration, normal but not quite so." The Latah reaction, comprising a severe startle response, imitative behaviour, automatic obedience and coprolalia, is alleged to occur in cultures with a limited control over their environment. The victim is compelled against his will to imitate the commands and actions of others, although this may be detrimental to him. There are, however, fundamental differences between Latah and Gilles de la Tourette's syndrome. Tics never occur in Latah, and imitative phenomena are often absent in Gilles de la Tourette's syndrome.

Coprolalia in Gilles de la Tourette's syndrome is spontaneous, whereas it is always provoked in Latah. Another essential feature of Gilles de la Tourette's syndrome is its onset in childhood, while Latah is never seen before late adolescence and occurs most commonly in middle and old age.

Myriachit is the transliteration of a Russian word which is used to describe a syndrome identical to Latah and reported by Hammond (1884) as occurring in Siberia and known also as "Arctic hysteria." The "Jumpers" or "Jumping Frenchman of Maine," also known as "Shakers" or "Barkers," were a peculiar religious sect who emigrated to North America, and exhibited violent jumping and twitching movements when startled, accompanied by echolalia and echokinesis. Strangely enough this syndrome disappeared completely so that no further reference was made to it until 1964, when Stevens described two new cases.

Aetiology and psychopathology

Gilles de la Tourette's syndrome along the years has bestridden the frontier between neurology and psychiatry. But increasingly it has perhaps tended to cross the porous boundary separating these two disciplines as have other movement disorders, albeit not to the extent of some.

Genetics

Gilles de la Tourette's syndrome undoubtedly has a genetic component. The genetic basis, however, comprises a vulnerability to developing the condition along with other related tic disorders. Indeed it is likely that it is the vulnerability to a tic disorder that is inherited, which may, in any individual case, be manifested as Tourette syndrome.

Price et al. (1985) conducted a twin study involving 43 same-sex twins in which at least one twin suffered with Tourette syndrome. Concordance rates of 53% for monozygotic twins and 8% for dizygotic twins were reported. This demonstrated good evidence for the genetic basis. Furthermore, if the diagnostic criteria were broadened to include the presence of minor tics, then the concordance rate of monozygotic twins increased to 77%. Leckman et al. (1987) re-examined the studies' original data and found that in the case of discordant dizygotic twins, the unaffected twin was often of a higher birth-weight than the affected co-twin. It was therefore suggested that prenatal factors may influence the development and expression of the disorder in an individual with the genetic propensity towards Tourette syndrome.

The vulnerability inherited was thought to be transmitted in an autosomal-dominant pattern with a variable penetrance which is greater in males than females (Curtiss et al., 1992); the existence of an X-linked mechanism had previously been postulated to account for the increased prevalence in males (Comings and Comings, 1986). However, in their review of genetic studies of Tourette syndrome, Qi et al. (2017) point out that:

> Both family and twin studies have shown that the etiology of [Tourette syndrome] is at least partially of genetic origin; however, the inheritance is more likely to be complex than [following a] simple [Mendelian pattern]. In general, [Tourette syndrome] and associated comorbidities have much lower heritability compared to other neuropsychiatric disorders, ... indicating other factors during development and from the environment also play some roles in [the] pathogenesis of [Tourette syndrome] and its comorbidities.

Reviewing the main findings of linkage and association studies of neurotransmitter-related genes and Tourette syndrome, Qi et al. (2017) found no evidence of an association with $DRD1$ (the dopamine D1 receptor gene), $DRD3$, $DRD5$, TH (tyrosine hydroxylase), $COMT$, $5\text{-}HT3A$, $5\text{-}HT3B$, $5\text{-}TH7$, $HRH3$, $ADRA1C$ or $ADRA2A$.

The A1 allele of the $Taq1$ polymorphism of $DRD2$, at chromosomal location 11q22–23, has been reported to be significantly increased in Tourette syndrome (44.9%, $n = 147$) compared with controls (24.5%, $n = 314$) (Comings et al., 1991); it was also increased in patients with attention-deficit hyperactivity disorder, autism and alcoholism and might act as a modifier rather than a primary aetiological factor. Lee et al. (2005) have reported that this polymorphism is also associated with Tourette syndrome in Taiwanese children. An association with the seven-repeat $DRD4*7R$ allele of the exon 3 VNTR (variable number of tandem repeats) polymorphism, at 11p15.5, was reported by Grice et al. (1996) and also more recently by McGill University and the Montreal Tourette Syndrome Study Group (Diaz-Anzaldúa et al., 2004).

The dopamine transporter gene $DAT1$ (or $SLC6A3$) has chromosomal location 5p15. Its genotype (a 40-base-pair VNTR) has been found to account for variations in tic severity in Tourette syndrome (Tarnok et al., 2007). The $DAT1$ Ddel polymorphism has also been found to be associated with Tourette syndrome (Yoon et al., 2007). Comings et al. (1996) have reported evidence of polygenic inheritance in Tourette syndrome involving polymorphisms of the three dopaminergic neurotransmission-related genes $DRD2$, $DAT1$ and DBH (dopamine beta-hydroxylase, located at 9q34.2); the degree of loading for markers of these genes was found to be linearly related to behaviour scores for attention-deficit hyperactivity disorder, stuttering, oppositional defiant, tics, conduct, obsessive-compulsive, mania, alcohol abuse and general anxiety (in that order).

So far as genes relating to the serotonergic system are concerned, there is weak evidence of an association between Tourette syndrome and the following two missense mutations in the $HTR1A$ receptor gene (at 5q11.2–13): Arg219Leu; and Asn417Lys (in the carboxyl tail) (Lam et al., 1996). Stronger evidence has been reported by Huang et al. (2001) of an association between the T102C polymorphism in *HTR2A* (13q14–21), on the one hand, and Tourette syndrome co-morbid with obsessive-compulsive disorder in a Chinese cohort, on the other hand. A weak association has been reported between Gilles de la Tourette's syndrome, particularly for male patients, and the following *HTR2C* polymorphisms: C759T and G697C (Dehning et al., 2010). A large European study of alleles of the serotonin transporter gene *SERT* (or *SLC6A4*), at 17q11.2, in 151 Tourette syndrome patients compared with 858 controls found that the former group were more likely to express the 5-HTTLPR/rs25531 L_A (the long allele) than were the controls, while the 5-HTTLPR/rs25531/rs25532 L_{AC} haplotype was also more common in Tourette syndrome (Moya et al., 2013); in both cases, these alleles were more common in patients with Tourette syndrome alone compared with those patients who also suffered from co-morbid obsessive-compulsive disorder.

Turning to the biosynthesis of serotonin, Mössner et al. (2007) have studied *TPH2* in Tourette syndrome; this gene encodes the enzyme tryptophan hydroxylase 2, which is associated with serotonin biosynthesis in the brain and has chromosomal location 12q21. In this German study, 98 Tourette syndrome patients were compared with 178 controls. The single-nucleotide polymorphism (SNP) rs4565946 showed an association with Tourette syndrome; no such association was found for the other SNP studied, namely rs4570625 (which the authors may have chosen because of previous functional neuroimaging study findings).

There is also some evidence of an association with glutamatergic-related neurotransmission genes. The E219D allele, a missense variant, of the glial high affinity glutamate transporter gene *EAAT1* (or *SLC1A3*), located at 5p13.2, has been reported to be 2.4 times higher (though not conventionally statistically significantly higher; $p = 0.09$) in a Tourette syndrome cohort compared with controls (Adamczyk et al., 2011). Non-significant (after correcting for multiple testing) associations with Tourette syndrome were also reported in the same year in respect of *SAPAP3/DLGAP3* (SAP90/PSD95-associated protein 3; a post-synaptic scaffolding protein which is highly expressed in striatal glutamatergic synapses), located at 1p34.3, for the SNP rs11264126 and two haplotypes containing rs11264126 and rs12141243 (Crane et al., 2011).

Histamine is biosynthesised by decarboxylation of L-histidine; this reaction is catalysed by L-histidine decarboxylase, encoded by *HDC*, located at 15q21–22. Tagging SNPs in this gene were interrogated in a large study totalling 520 Tourette syndrome nuclear families, of Polish, Italian, Hungarian, Greek, Albanian, German and Spanish ancestry, and including 150 families from Canada (Karagiannidis et al., 2013). A strong association was reported between Tourette syndrome and the SNPs rs854150 and rs1894236 as well as with a five-SNP haplotype and two-SNP haplotypes. These results point to an important potential role of the histaminergic system in Tourette syndrome.

In their large study of 162 Polish Gilles de la Tourette's syndrome patients and 270 controls, Janik et al. (2015) found evidence of an association of the disorder with polymorphisms of two SNPs of the adenosine A1 and A2 receptor genes, namely rs2228079 in *ADORA1* at 1q32.1 (GG + GT genotypes were underrepresented in the patient group) and rs5751876 in *ADORA2A* at 22q11.2 (overrepresentation in the patient group of the T allele). There were also associations with the co-morbid disorders depression, obsessive-compulsive disorder, attention-deficit hyperactivity disorder and anxiety disorder. The GG genotype of rs2228079 was also found to be associated with an earlier age of onset of tics.

In the Tourette syndrome study mentioned above by McGill University and the Montreal Tourette Syndrome Study Group (Diaz-Anzaldúa et al., 2004), an association was also found between the disorder and "high activity" alleles (defined in terms of the number of 30-base-pair repeat sequences of five alleles) of the promoter VNTR polymorphism of the X-linked (Xp11.3) *MAO-A* gene. Interestingly, six years earlier Gade et al. (1998) reported a correlation between the length of VNTR alleles of the same gene and both behavioural phenotypes and drug dependence in Tourette syndrome patients.

Currently, two genome-wide association studies (GWASs) have been carried out of Tourette syndrome as well as one replication GWAS; just one marginally significant result has been found (Qi et al., 2017). Qi et al. (2017) have also reviewed genomic structural abnormalities in Tourette syndrome; patients have been reported to have variations (translocations, deletions, [micro]duplications, insertions and inversions) affecting the following candidate genes: *GPR63*, *NDUFA4* and *KLHL32* (6q16); *IMMP2L* (7q22-q31); *CNTNAP2* (7q35-q36); *CBFA2T1* (8q); *OLFM1* (9p); *SLITRK1*, *ERCC5* and *SLC10A2* (13q); *CDH7* and *CDH19* (18q); and *NLGN4* (Xp22.3).

Neuroimmunology

It has been suggested that childhood tic disorder and/or obsessive-compulsive disorder may be associated with a history of a group A β-haemolytic streptococcal (GABHS) infection, as part of paediatric autoimmune neuropsychiatric disorders associated with streptococcal infections (PANDAS; previously known as paediatric autoimmune neuropsychiatric disorders, with the same acronym), which were originally diagnosed on the basis of the following five criteria (Allen et al., 1995; Swedo et al., 1998):

The presence of obsessive-compulsive disorder and/or a tic disorder
Prepubertal symptom onset
Episodic course of symptom severity
History of GABHS infection
Association with neurological abnormalities

Martino et al. (2011) compared 168 children with Tourette syndrome
and 177 children suffering from epileptic or sleep disorders. The Tourette
syndrome children were more likely to have experienced a group A
streptococcal infection (8% versus 2%) and had a higher mean anti-
streptolysin O titre and a higher anti-basal ganglia antibody frequency
(25% versus 8%). It could therefore be speculated that the infection
might have led to molecular mimicry, with the corresponding antibodies
cross-reacting with cerebral targets such as the basal ganglia. Furthermore,
Frick and Pittenger (2016) have suggested that Tourette syndrome, as
well as PANDAS and obsessive-compulsive disorder, may be related to
neuroinflammation associated with microglial dysregulation.

However, although there are other studies favouring an association of
Tourette syndrome with streptococcal infection (e.g. Müller et al., 2000),
some studies have been less clear or indeed have given a negative result
(Loiselle et al., 2003; Singer et al., 2000).

Morbid anatomy

There is still little neuroanatomical information about the syndrome
available, and this may be related to the fact that the illness is not fatal. A
few post-mortem studies have been performed, and these have not revealed any specific cerebral pathology (Wulf and Boggart, 1914; Clauss
and Balthasar, 1954).

Neuroimaging

Greene 2017 carried out a large voxel-based morphometry MRI study
of 103 children and adolescents with Tourette syndrome compared with
103 matched controls who did not suffer from tics. The white matter
volume was lower bilaterally in the orbital and medial prefrontal cortex in
the Tourette syndrome patients. The grey matter volume of the patients
was higher in the posterior thalamus, hypothalamus and mesencephalon.
The authors commented on the possible significance of their findings: "as
orbital cortex is reciprocally connected with hypothalamus, structural
abnormalities in these regions may relate to abnormal decision making,
reinforcement learning or somatic processing in [Tourette syndrome]."

Electrophysiology

Direct electrical recordings from eight awake Tourette syndrome patients, aged 19 to 55 years, during bilateral implantation of deep brain stimulation (DBS) electrode placement into the anteromedial globus pallidus internus under local anaesthesia, showed that the basal neuronal firing rate was low in both the globus pallidus internus and the globus pallidus externus (Israelashvili et al., 2017). Furthermore, the rate of firing was state-dependent, varying according to whether or not tics were present. These findings mirror those of Zhuang et al. (2009), also from eight Tourette syndrome patients, who were undergoing pallidotomy for severe tics. The anterior globus pallidus externus/internus represent associative/limbic domains and appear, according to these findings, to point to a functional interaction between the motor and associative/limbic circuits of the cortico-basal ganglia loop in Tourette syndrome (Israelashvili et al., 2017).

Biochemistry

Recently attention has focussed on neurochemical processes that may mediate the disorder's symptomatology at the cerebral level. Essentially it is postulated that the clinical features arise as a result of an imbalance in cerebral neurotransmitters, particularly dopamine (Chase et al., 1986). The basis for this hypothesis lies in the fact that haloperidol, a dopamine antagonist, suppresses the various symptoms, whereas an agent such as methylphenidate, a dopamine agonist, tends to exacerbate the symptoms. Further support comes from the finding of abnormal levels of homovanillic acid (a metabolite of dopamine) in the CSF of some patients.

More recent post-mortem studies have implicated other transmitter systems including endogenous opioids (Chappell, 1994), glutamate and serotonin, in addition to monoamines such as dopamine (Robertson, 1994). The abnormal activity of these various transmitter agents tends to be located in the basal ganglia and related structures.

An *in vivo* proton magnetic resonance spectroscopy study of 32 children with Tourette syndrome and 43 age-matched healthy controls, carried out at the relatively high magnetic field strength of 7 T, reported an elevated glutamate concentration in the patient group across a combination of the regions of interest studied (namely, the dorsolateral prefrontal cortex, the ventromedial prefrontal cortex, the premotor cortex and the striatum) and also in the premotor cortex alone (Mahone et al., 2018). Furthermore, in the Tourette syndrome group, the left premotor cortical glutamate concentration was negatively correlated with the motor overflow total on the Revised Physical and Neurological Assessment of Subtle Signs.

Neuropsychology

Baron-Cohen et al. (1994) have suggested that a neuropsychological function referred to as the *intention editor* is dysfunctional in Tourette syndrome. Channon et al. (1992) reported specific deficits in attention. The intention editor is described as a key mechanism underlying the concept of *the will* and is said to start to function during early childhood. Further, it is said to be activated whenever there are several intentions all competing in parallel with each other. This function forms a sub-component of the *supervisory attentional system* (Shallice, 1988) and is mediated by the frontal lobes (Robertson, 1994).

Morand-Beaulieu et al. (2017) have reviewed the neuropsychological dimensions of Tourette syndrome. Only slight impairments in intellectual abilities, memory functions and attentional abilities are found in Tourette patients. This also appears to be the case for language and motor skills. Executive function deficits appear to be limited to inhibition and cognitive flexibility; planning and decision-making abilities seem to be intact.

Social decision-making

O'Connell and Hofmann (2011) have suggested that two neural circuits, the social behaviour network and the mesolimbic reward system, form a larger social decision-making network which regulates adaptive behaviour. Given that the corpus striatum is part of the mesolimbic reward system, and given also that a major role of facial and head movements is social signalling, Albin (2018) has suggested that "Tourette syndrome may be a disorder of social communication resulting from developmental abnormalities at several levels of the social decision-making network." Morand-Beaulieu et al. (2017) make the point that few data are available in respect of social cognition.

Psychodynamics

Mahler and Rangell (1943) alleged that tics are manifestations of emotional conflicts arising from attempts at gratification of repressed instinctive urges and their control. They regarded the involuntary interjections and animal-like noises of their patients as both aggressive and neurotic in character and considered that they were equivalents to coprolalia which could not be expressed because of powerful reaction formation against obscene ideas.

Coprolalia has, indeed, been regarded as a hostile reaction towards authority figures, especially within the family, usually towards one or both parents (Hammond, 1892; Tobin et al., 1961). Children with coprolalia often exhibit very rigid behaviour and do not have sufficient outlets for their hostility, being afraid of punishment. Their pent-up feelings of hostility towards their parents build up to the point where they are released in a crescendo of explosive tics and utterances. This view is supported by the fact that an unusually high proportion of one or both parents are very strict or rigid, demanding exceptionally good behaviour, tidiness, obedience and educational excellence. In this setting the birth of a younger sibling appears to be particularly stressful, increasing the demand of the child to a point which weakens his control and induces illness. Such children may be so aggressive as to have homicidal fantasies towards their parents, who are starving them of affection. It is possible that the sexual and faecal content of such utterances are culturally determined, i.e. equated with something repulsive and dirty.

The aggressive component of tics and coprolalia tends to lessen with repetition and, thereby, becomes more acceptable to the patient and those around him (Ascher, 1948). Also, a number of patients seem to become more comfortable when their vocal tics assume a scatological quality. Similarly, the change from *mental tic* to vocal coprolalia implies that the hostile feelings have been transferred from a particular person onto society in general, in the form of vulgar language.

Other psychodynamic models have been described in the literature. For example Menninger (1938) investigated the psychopathology of a case where violent, involuntary movements were directed against the patient's own body and postulated that this was a form of neurotic self-mutilation. Ferenozi (1921) believed that tics of all types are narcissistic in nature and inferred that they are "stereotyped masturbatory equivalents."

Management and treatment

The management of Gilles de la Tourette's syndrome requires an eclectic approach involving a combination of drug therapy and psychological intervention. The following regime is recommended:

- Initially a trial of butyrophenones (or other antipsychotics or possibly SSRI antidepressants) in conjunction with supportive psychotherapy.
- The treatment of any associated disorders, e.g. depression or obsessive-compulsive features.
- If the above fails to achieve adequate symptom relief, consider the addition of a course of behavioural therapy.

The European Society for the Study of Tourette Syndrome have published a decision tree for the treatment of Gilles de la Tourette's syndrome and other tic disorders (Roessner et al., 2011), and a modified version of this was published by Robertson et al. (2017). The decision tree covers a range of interventions: psychoeducation, monitoring, treatment of co-morbid conditions, behavioural therapy, pharmacotherapy and alternative therapies provided in specialist centres such as DBS, cannabinoids and botulinum toxin.

Drug therapy

Ever since their introduction for the treatment of this condition in 1961, the *butyrophenones* have been the mainstay of the drug treatment approach. They have been demonstrated to be effective, so that in a large number of patients symptoms disappeared, in both recent and long-standing cases (Connell et al., 1967; Boris, 1968; Fernando, 1976). Children seem to tolerate the drug well (Connell et al., 1967). The period of time necessary for haloperidol to work varies from 24 hours to 30 days or more, and the necessary dose varies from patient to patient. The drug needs to be taken regularly, and at least two years of symptom-free existence is advised before any dosage reduction is undertaken. If there is a recurrence of symptoms, then the drug should be recommenced and the dose adjusted according to the severity of the symptoms. Sometimes tolerance to the drug develops, a phenomenon that can be counteracted by alternating haloperidol with another antipsychotic (see below). Yet another hazard is the possible development of subtle changes in personality coincidental with the relief of symptoms. For example, one patient lost her creative ability, while another was so frightened of her subjective feelings as to prefer her symptoms to the overall effect of the drug.

Other antipsychotic drugs have also been shown to be effective in relieving the disorder's symptoms. Examples include the *phenothiazines* (Hunter, 1969) and *pimozide* (Ross and Moldofsky, 1977), while, of the more recently introduced antipsychotics, aripiprazole may be better tolerated than, say, risperidone (Robertson et al., 2017).

Antidepressant drugs of the *SSRI* category have been increasingly used following favourable reports in the late 1980s (Wetering et al., 1988). Cipriano et al. (1999) reported the successful treatment of a possible organically induced Tourette syndrome with a combination of clomipramine, fluvoxamine and pimozide. Antidepressants should certainly be considered if depressive symptoms are present. Successful treatments with other drug groups have also been reported, including calcium antagonists (Berg, 1985; Vieregge, 1987), lithium carbonate (Messiha, 1979), naloxone and tetrabenazine (Sandyk, 1985). In the United States, the α_2-adrenergic agonists clonidine and guanfacine tend to be used as first-line drug treatments (Robertson et al., 2017). Other drugs treatments which may be helpful for Tourette syndrome and which may have a more tolerable side-effect profile than antipsychotic medication include baclofen, topiramate, botulinum toxin A, tetrabenazine and deutetrabenazine (Quezada and Coffman, 2018). These authors also have developed a treatment algorithm for Tourette syndrome; after behavioural intervention as the proposed first-line therapy, it includes three levels of pharmacotherapy, and it also mentions drugs which are currently under investigation.

Psychotherapy

There are conflicting reports of the efficacy of behaviour therapy in this condition. Various types of behaviour therapy have been used since the early 1960s (Polites et al., 1965; Cohen and Marks, 1977). Yates (1958), Walton (1961) and Clark (1966) have used a form of treatment based on Hullian learning theory, which involves the *massed practice* of tics. They account for a reduction of tics following massed practice by the rapid build-up in reactive inhibition. Subsequent dissipation of inhibition during rest serves, they suggest, as a reinforcing state for responses occurring during the rest period. Yates examined experimentally the effects of varying the duration of the massed practice on the tic rate. Walton reported a reduction in tic movement following massed practice with improvement maintained at two-monthly and yearly follow-up. Clark successfully treated two cases by this method and claimed that massed practice may be a treatment of choice in this condition. Each of Clark's patients was asked to repeat his currently most frequent obscenity as often and as loudly as possible during two 30-minute treatment sessions daily. When the patient substituted other words, an electric shock just below the pain threshold was delivered. During the latter treatment sessions, patients showed progressively fewer responses and could no longer emit the agreed-upon obscenity. The massed practice of tics, however, was ineffective in one case and only partially successful in another.

Reinforcement techniques based on operant conditioning have been attempted. Jeste et al. (1973), however, reported that behaviour therapy in the form of negative practice was ineffective in a 13-year-old with the disorder. Conditioning, attempted with a device that automatically followed shouts with an electric shock, was ineffective in another patient (Challas and Braver, 1963). Reciprocal inhibition modified the symptoms of one of our own cases, but unfortunately she failed to complete the course of treatment. Hutzel et al. (1974) described a case whose control of symptoms by self-monitoring resulted in remission. A randomised trial in 122 adult Tourette syndrome patients, aged 16 to 69 years, by Wilhelm et al. (2012) has demonstrated the efficacy and safety of behavioural therapy for tics. A similar finding has been reported from a trial in 126 children, aged 9 to 17 years, with Tourette syndrome or chronic tic disorder (Piacentini et al., 2010).

Other physical therapies

ECT is usually ineffective, although it has proved successful in isolated cases of bizarre psychogenic movements (Edwards, 1972). The disorder has also been treated with psychosurgery, the first prefrontal leucotomy for this condition taking place in 1955 was reported as having beneficial effects lasting for nearly 10 years (Stevens, 1964). Another case remitted for nearly a year following bimedial frontal leucotomy (Baker, 1962). This type of psychosurgery, however, seems unusually drastic for most patients, who mostly exist on reasonable terms with their tics. On the other hand, DBS appears to be both effective and safe in treatment-refractory obsessive-compulsive disorder and may also have a role in Tourette syndrome (Figee et al., 2018). Indeed, a 10-country study of the outcome of DBS in 185 patients with medically refractory Tourette syndrome, using the International Deep Brain Stimulation Database and Registry, found an improvement of just over 45% in tic severity after one year; the most common adverse events were dysarthria (6%), paraesthesia (8%), infection (3%) and haemorrhage (1%) (Martinez-Ramirez et al., 2018).

Family therapy

The quality of life for patients suffering from Tourette syndrome is very much determined by their relationships with other people, especially members of their own family. It must be accepted that the very symptoms of the disorder can be extremely irritating and tension-producing, hence tolerance and understanding, although difficult to give, are absolutely necessary in order for the family to live in peace. Sometimes the tension is so great and the conflicts between patient and family so intense that family counselling is indicated.

Parents should be encouraged to allow their child as much freedom as possible to express himself or herself, to have outside interests and to make relationships with other people outside of the family. Rigid restrictions should be kept to an absolute minimum. Certainly a child should not be made to feel compelled to stop the tics or vocalisations.

Prognosis

It remains difficult to determine the long-term prognosis of the syndrome – the natural history of the disorder with its spontaneous remissions and exacerbations makes evaluation of treatment regimens difficult, especially when based on small numbers of cases. It is certainly not, however, as poor as Gilles de la Tourette himself predicted. Little was known about the risk of suicide in this patient group until the study of de la Cruz et al. (2017), who compared 7,736 patients with Tourette syndrome and chronic tic disorders from the Swedish National Patient Register over the period 1969 to 2013 with general population controls; the patient group were found to have an increased risk of dying by suicide (odds ratio 4.39) and of attempting suicide (odds ratio 3.86); the increased risk remained even after adjustment for psychiatric co-morbidity. In general, however, complete mental deterioration does not usually occur in this patient group, and very rarely does psychosis develop (Jankovic et al., 1984). Nevertheless, there may well be some truth in Gilles de la Tourette's dictum: *Une fois tiqueur, toujours tiqueur.*

As the life of Tourette patients is not threatened, they often live to an old age, and several celebrated cases have had a lifelong history of the disorder (Itard, 1825; Bockner, 1959). Famous sufferers may have included the British lexicographer Samuel Johnson (Monaco et al., 2009). It has often been suggested that the composer Wolfgang Amadeus Mozart may have suffered from Tourette syndrome (Monaco et al., 2009), but this is disputed by others (e.g. Ashoori and Jankovic, 2007). In any case, although Mozart tragically died at the age of just 35 years, there is no reason to suspect that his death was related to Tourette syndrome.

References

Abule, D.F. (1952) *Transactions of the New York Academy of Sciences, 14,* 291.

Abuzzahab, F.S., Ehnlen, J K. (undated) *Tourette's Syndrome. A Guide for Parents.* USA: University of Minnesota.

Adamczyk, A., Gause, C.D., Sattler, R., Vidensky, S., Rothstein, J.D., Singer, H., et al. (2011) *Psychiatric Genetics, 21,* 90.

Aimard, P., Kohler, C. (1961) *Rev. Neuro. Psychiatr. Infant., 9,* 110.

Albin, R.L. (2018) *Brain, 141,* 332.

Allen, A.J., Leonard, H.L., Swedo, S.E. (1995) *Journal of the American Academy of Child Adolescent Psychiatry, 34,* 307.

American Psychiatric Association (2013) *Diagnostic and Statistical Manual of Mental Disorders, Fifth Edition (DSM-5).* American Psychiatric Association, Washington, DC.

Ascher, E. (1948) *American Journal of Psychiatry, 105,* 267.

Ashoori, A., Jankovic, J. (2007) *J Neurol Neurosurg Psychiatry, 78,* 1171.

Baker, E.F.W. (1962) *Canadian Medical Association Journal, 86,* 746.

Balthasar, K. (1957) *Arch. Psychiatr. Nervenkr., 195,* 36.

Baron-Cohen, S., Cross, P., Crowson, M. (1994) *Psychological Medicine, 24,* 29.

Beard, J.M. (1880) *Journal of Nervous and Mental Diseases, 7,* 487.

Berg, R. (1985) *Acta Psychiatrica Scandinavica, 72,* 400.

Bockner, S. (1959) *Journal of Mental Science, 105,* 1078.

Boris, M. (1968) *Journal of the American Medical Association, 205,* 648.

Cavanna, A.E., Critchley, H.D., Orth, M., Stern, J.S., Young, M.B., Robertson, M.M. (2011) *J Neurol Neurosurg Psychiatry, 82,* 1320.

Challas, G., Braver, W. (1963) *American Journal of Psychiatry, 120,* 283.

Channon, S., Flynn, D., Robertson, M.M. (1992) *Neuropsychiatry, Neuropsychology and Behavioural Neurology, 5,* 170.

Chappell, P.B. (1994) *Lancet, 343,* 556.

Charcot, J.M. (1884) *Ritorma Med, 1,* 184.

Chase, T.N., Geoffrey, V., Gillespie, M. (1986) *Revue Neurologiques, 142,* 851.

Cipriano, P., Silvestrini, C., Peronti, M. (1999) *Rivista di Psichiatria, 34,* 145.

Clark, D.F. (1966) *British Journal of Psychiatry, 112,* 771.

Clauss, J.L., Balthasar, K. (1954) *Arch. Psychiatr. Nervenkr.*, *191*, 398.

Cohen, D., Marks, F.M. (1977) *British Journal of Psychiatry*, *130*, 315.

Comings, D.E., Comings, B.G. (1986) *Proceedings of the National Academy of Sciences (USA)*, *83*, 2551.

Comings, D.E., Comings, B.G., Muhleman, D., Dietz, G., Shahbahrami, B., Tast, D., et al. (1991) *JAMA*, *266*, 1793.

Comings, D.E., Wu, S., Chiu, C., Ring, R.H., Gade, R., Ahn, C., et al. (1996) *Am J Med Genet*, *67*, 264.

Connell, P.M., Corbett, J.A., Horne, D.J., Matthews, A.M. (1967) *British Journal of Psychiatry*, *113*, 375.

Crane, J., Fagerness, J., Osiecki, L., Gunnell, B., Stewart, S.E., Pauls, D.L., et al. (2011) *Am J Med Genet B Neuropsychiatr Genet*, *156b*, 108.

Creak, M., Guttman, E. (1935) *Journal of Mental Science*, *81*, 834.

Cubo, E., Gabriel Y., Galan, J.M., Villaverde, V.A., Velasco, S.S., Benito, V.D., Macarron, J.V., et al. (2011) *Pediatr Neurol*, *45*, 100

Curtiss, D., Robertson, M.M., Gurling, H.M. (1992) *Br J Psychiatry*, *160*, 845.

Dehning, S., Muller, N., Matz, J., Bender, A., Kerle, I., Benninghoff, J., et al. (2010) *Psychiatr Genet*, *20*, 35.

Deshan, P.W. (1961) *Journal of Oklahoma State Medical Association*, *54*, 636.

Diaz-Anzaldua, A., Joober, R., Riviere, J.B., Dion, Y., Lesperance, P., Richer, F., et al. (2004) *Mol Psychiatry*, *9*, 272.

Eapen, V., Pauls, D.L., & Robertson, M.M., (1993), *British Journal of Psychiatry*, *162*, 593.

Edwards, J.G. (1972) *British Journal of Clinical Practice*, *26*, 387.

Fenichel, O. (1945) *The Psychoanalytical Theory of Neurosis*. Norton, New York.

Ferenozi, S. (1921) *International Journal of Psychoanalysis*, *2*, 1.

Fernandez de la Cruz, L., Rydell, M., Runeson, B., Brander, G., Ruck, C., D'Onofrio, B.M., et al. (2017) *Biol Psychiatry*, *82*, 111.

Fernando, S.J.M. (1976) *British Journal of Psychiatry*, *128*, 436.

Figee, M., Schuurman, P.R., Denys, D. (2018) *Ned Tijdschr Geneeskd*, *162*, D2333.

Frick, L., Pittenger, C. (2016) *J Immunol Res*, *2016*, 8606057.

Gade, R., Muhleman, D., Blake, H., MacMurray, J., Johnson, P., Verde, R., et al. (1998) *Mol Psychiatry*, *3*, 50.

Greenberg, E., Tung, E.S., Gauvin, C., Osiecki, L., Yang, K.G., Curley, E., et al. (2018) *Eur Child Adolesc Psychiatry*, *27*, 569.

Grice, D.E., Leckman, J.F., Pauls, D.L., Kurlan, R., Kidd, K.K., Pakstis, A.J., et al. (1996) *Am J Hum Genet*, *59*, 644.

Greene, D.J., Williams, A.C., Koller, J.M., Schlaggar, B.L., & Black, K.J. (2017). Brain structure in pediatric Tourette syndrome. *Molecular Psychiatry*, *22*, 972.

Guinon, H. (1886) *Revue Medicale*, *6*, 50.

Hammond, W.A. (1884) *New York Medical Journal*, *39*, 191.

Hammond, W.A. (1892) *Medical Record*, *41*, 236.

Hansen, B.H., Oerbeck, B., Skirbekk, B., Petrovski, B.É., Kristensen, H. (2018) *Nord J Psychiatry*, *72*, 285.

Hornsey, H., Banerjee, S., Zeitlin, H., Robertson, M. (2001) *J Child Psychol Psychiatry*, *42*, 1035.

Huang, Y., Liu, X., Li, T., Guo, L., Sun, X., Xiao, X., et al. (2001) *Zhonghua Yi Xue Yi Chuan Xue Za Zhi*, *18*, 11.

Hughlings Jackson, J. (1884) *Clinical Lectures and Reports to the London Hospital*, *1*, 452.

Hunter, H. (1969) *British Journal of Psychiatry*, *115*, 443.

Hutzel, R.R., Platzek, D., Logue, P.B. (1974) *Journal of Behaviour Therapy and Experimental Psychiatry*, *5*, 1.

Israelashvili, M., Smeets, A., Bronfeld, M., Zeef, D.H., Leentjens, A.F.G., van Kranen-Mastenbroek, V., et al. (2017) *Mov Disord*, *32*, 1091.

Itard, J.M.G. (1825) *Archives of General Medicine*, *8*, 404.

Janik, P., Berdynski, M., Safranow, K., Zekanowski, C. (2015) *PLoS One*, *10*, e0136754.

Jankovic, J., Glaze, D.G., Frost, J.D. (1984) *Neurology*, *34*, 688.

Jeste, D.V., Sule, S.M., Ate, J.S., Vamain, S. (1973) *Indian Journal of Paediatrics*, *41*, 435.

Jin, R., Zheng, R.Y., Huang, W.W., Xu, H.Q., Shao, B., Chen, H., et al. (2005) *Eur J Epidemiol*, *20*, 925.

Kadesjo, B., Gillberg, C. (2000) *J Am Acad Child Adolesc Psychiatry*, *39*, 548.

Kanner, L. (1942) *Child Psychiatry*. Thomas, Springfield, Illinois.

Karagiannidis, I., Dehning, S., Sandor, P., Tarnok, Z., Rizzo, R., Wolanczyk, T., et al. (2013) *J Med Genet*, *50*, 760.

Kaufman, J., Birmaher, B., Brent, D., Rao, U.M.A., Flynn, C., Moreci, P., et al. (1997) *Journal of the American Academy of Child & Adolescent Psychiatry*, *36*, 980.

Kelman, D.H. (1965) *Journal of Child Psychology and Psychiatry*, *6*, 219.

Khalifa, N., von Knorring, A.L. (2003) *Dev Med Child Neurol*, *45*, 315.

Kinnier Wilson, S.A. (1941) *Neurology*. Williams and Wilkins, Baltimore.

Koester, G. (1899) *Deutsche Zeitschrift Nervheith.*, *15*, 147.

Kraft, J.T., Dalsgaard, S., Obel, C., Thomsen, P.H., Henriksen, T.B., Scahill, L. (2012) *Eur Child Adolesc Psychiatry*, *21*, 5.

Kurlan, R., McDermott, M.P., Deeley, C., Como, P.G., Brower, C., Eapen, S., et al. (2001) *Neurology*, *57*, 1383.

Lam, S., Shen, Y., Nguyen, T., Messier, T.L., Brann, M., Comings, D., et al. (1996) *Biochem Biophys Res Commun*, *219*, 853.

Leckman, J.F. (2002) *Lancet*, *360*, 1577.

Leckman, J.F., King, R.A., Bloch, M.H. (2014) *Journal of Obsessive-Compulsive and Related Disorders*, *3*, 372.

Leckman, J.F., Zhang, H., Vitale, A., Lahnin, F., Lynch, K., Bondi, C., et al. (1998) *Pediatrics*, *102*, 14.

Leckman, J.F., Price, R.A., Walkup, J.T. (1987) *Archives of General Psychiatry*, *44*, 100.

Lee, C.C., Chou, I.C., Tsai, C.H., Wang, T.R., Li, T.C., Tsai, F.J. (2005) *Pediatr Neurol*, *33*, 272.

Lin, H., Yeh, C.B., Peterson, B.S., Scahill, L., Grantz, H., Findley, D.B., et al. (2002) *J Am Acad Child Adolesc Psychiatry*, *41*, 1070.

Loiselle, C.R., Wendlandt, J.T., Rohde, C.A., Singer, H.S. (2003) *Pediatr Neurol*, *28*, 119.

Mahler, M.S., Rangell, L. (1943) *Psychiatry Journal*, *17*, 579.

Mahler, M.S., Luke, J.A., Daltroff, W. (1945) *American Journal of Orthopsychiatry*, *15*, 631.

Mahone, E.M., Puts, N.A., Edden, R.A.E., Ryan, M., Singer, H.S. (2018) *Psychiatry Res Neuroimaging*, *273*, 46.

Martinez-Ramirez, D., Jimenez-Shahed, J., Leckman, J.F., Porta, M., Servello, D., Meng, F.G., et al. (2018) *JAMA Neurol*, *75*, 353.

Martino, D., Chiarotti, F., Buttiglione, M., Cardona, F., Creti, R., Nardocci, N., et al. (2011) *Dev Med Child Neurol,* *53,* 951.

Mazur, W.P. (1953) *Edinburgh Medical Journal,* *60,* 427.

McDonald, J. (1963) *British Journal of Psychiatry,* *109,* 206.

Meduna, L.J. (1943) *Journal of Nervous and mental Disease,* *117,* 39.

Menninger, K. (1938) *Man Against Himself.* Hart-Davis, London.

Merskey, H. (1974) *British Journal of Psychiatry,* *125,* 593.

Messiha, F.A. (1979) *Proceedings of the Western Pharmacology Society (Seattle),* *22,* 22.

Monaco, F., Servo, S., Cavanna, A.E. (2009) *J Psychosom Res,* *67,* 485.

Morand-Beaulieu, S., Leclerc, J.B., Valois, P., Lavoie, M.E., O'Connor, K.P., Gauthier, B. (2017) *Brain Sciences,* *7,* 106.

Morphew, J.A., Sim, M. (1969) *British Journal of Medical Psychology,* *42,* 293.

Mössner, R., Muller-Vahl, K.R., Doring, N., Stuhrmann, M. (2007) *Mol Psychiatry,* *12,* 617.

Moya, P.R., Wendland, J.R., Rubenstein, L.M., Timpano, K.R., Heiman, G.A., Tischfield, J.A., et al. (2013) *Mov Disord,* *28,* 1263.

Müller, N., Riedel, M., Straube, A., Gunther, W., Wilske, B. (2000) *Psychiatry Res,* *94,* 43.

O'Brien, H.A. (1883) *J. Straits Branch R. Asiat. Soc.,* *11,* 143.

O'Connell, L.A., Hofmann, H.A. (2011) *J Comp Neurol,* *519,* 3599.

Osler, W. (1894) *On Chorea and Choreiform Affections.* London: H.K. Lewis.

Peterson, B.S., Pine, D.S., Cohen, P., Brook, J.S. (2001) *J Am Acad Child Adolesc Psychiatry,* *40,* 685.

Piacentini, J., Woods, D.W., Scahill, L., Wilhelm, S., Peterson, A.L., Chang, S., et al. (2010) *JAMA,* *303,* 1929.

Polites, D.J., Kruger, D., Stevenson, I. (1965) *British Journal of Medical Psychology,* *38,* 43.

Price, R.A., Kidd, K.K., Cohen, D.J. (1985) *Archives of General Psychiatry,* *42,* 815.

Prince, M. (1906) *Journal of Nervous and Mental Disease,* *33,* 29.

Qi, Y., Zheng, Y., Li, Z., Xiong, L. (2017) *Brain Sciences,* *7,* 134.

Quezada, J., Coffman, K.A. (2018) *CNS Drugs,* *32,* 33.

Rapoport, J. (1959) *American Journal of Psychiatry,* *116,* 177.

Robertson, M.M. (1994) *Journal of Child Psychology and Psychiatry,* *35,* 597.

Robertson, M.M., Eapen, V., Singer, H.S., Martino, D., Scharf, J.M., Paschou, P., et al. (2017) *Nat Rev Dis Primers,* *3,* 16097.

Roessner, V., Plessen, K.J., Rothenberger, A., Ludolph, A.G., Rizzo, R., Skov, L., et al. (2011) *Eur Child Adolesc Psychiatry,* *20,* 173.

Ross, S.R., Moldofsky, H. (1977) *Lancet,* *1,* 103.

Salmi, K. (1961) *Acta Psychiatrica Scandinavica,* *36,* 157.

Sandyk, R. (1985) *Annals of Neurology,* *18,* 367.

Scahill, L., Williams, S., Schwab-Stone, M., Applegate, J., Leckman, J.F. (2006) *Adv Neurol,* *99,* 184.

Schneck, J.M. (1960) *American Journal of Psychiatry,* *117,* 78.

Scahill, L., Dalsgaard, S., & Bradbury, K. (2013). In Martino, D. & Leckman, J.F. (Ed.), *Tourette Syndrome.* Oxford: Oxford University Press.

Seignot, J.M. (1961) *Annales Medico-Psychologiques,* *119,* 578.

Shallice, T. (1988) *From Neuropsychology to Neural Structure*. Cambridge University Press, Cambridge, UK.

Singer, H.S., Giuliano, J.D., Zimmerman, A.M., Walkup, J.T. (2000) *Pediatr Neurol*, *22*, 380.

Stevens, H. (1964) *Med. An. D.C.*, *33*, 277.

Swedo, S.E., Leonard, H.L., Garvey, M., Mittleman, B., Allen, A.J., Perlmutter, S., et al. (1998) *Am J Psychiatry*, *155*, 264.

Tarnok, Z., Ronai, Z., Gervai, J., Kereszturi, E., Gadoros, J., Sasvari-Szekely, M., et al. (2007) *Am J Med Genet B Neuropsychiatr Genet*, *144b*, 900.

Sweet, R.D., Solomon, S.E., Wane, H., Shapiro, E., & Shapiro, A.K. (1973). *Journal of Neurology, Neurosurgery and Psychiatry*, *36*, 1.

Tobin, W.G., Reinhart, J.B. (1961) *American Journal of Diseases of Children*, *101*, 778.

Tourette, G. Gilles de la (1884) *Archives of Neurology*, *8*, 68.

Tourette, G. Gilles de la (1885) *Archives of Neurology*, *9*, 17, 158.

Tourette, G. Gilles de la (1889) *Seminars in Medicine*, *19*, 153.

Trousseau, A. (1867) *Lectures on Clinical Medicine, delivered at the Hotel Dieu*, Paris. Trans. and ed. P.V. Bazire, Hardwicke, London.

Vierogge, P. (1987) *Journal of Neurology, Neurosurgery and Psychiatry*, *50*, 1554.

Walsh, T.L., Lavenstein, B., Licamele, W.I. (1986) *American Journal of Psychiatry*, *143*, 1467.

Walton, D. (1961) *Journal of Child Psychology and Psychiatry*, *2*, 148.

Wang, H.S., Kuo, M.F. (2003) *Brain Dev*, *25*(Suppl 1), S29.

Wetering, B.J.M. van de Cohen, A.P., Minderaa, R.B. (1988) *Nederlands Tijdschrifte Voor Geneeskunde*, *132*, 21.

Wilhelm, S., Peterson, A.L., Piacentini, J., Woods, D.W., Deckersbach, T., Sukhodolsky, D.G., et al. (2012) *Arch Gen Psychiatry*, *69*, 795.

Wille, H. (1898) *Monatsschrift Psychiatrie Neurologie*, *4*, 210.

Wulf, A., Boggart, L. van (1914) *Monatsschrift Psychiatrie Neurologie*, *104*, 53.

Yap, P.M. (1952) *Journal of Mental Science*, *98*, 33.

Yates, A.J. (1958) *Journal of Abnormal Psychology*, *56*, 175.

Yoon, D.Y., Rippel, C.A., Kobets, A.J., Morris, C.M., Lee, J.E., Williams, P.N., et al. (2007) *Am J Med Genet B Neuropsychiatr Genet*, *144b*, 605.

Zhuang, P., Hallett, M., Zhang, X., Li, J., Zhang, Y., Li, Y. (2009) *J Neurol Neurosurg Psychiatry*, *80*, 1075.

Chapter 8

Cotard's syndrome
(le délire de négation)

To be or not to be ...

William Shakespeare, *Hamlet* (III, i)

This is an uncommon condition in which the central feature is a nihilistic delusion, which, in its complete form leads a patient to deny his or her own existence and that of the external world.

Historical

The Parisian neurologist Jules Cotard, in 1880 at a meeting of the Société Médico-Psychologique, described this condition in a report entitled *Du délire hypochondriaque dans une forme grave de la mélancolie anxieuse*. He reported a case of a 43-year-old woman who believed that she had "no brain, nerves, chest, or entrails and was just skin and bone," that "neither God nor the Devil existed," that "she was eternal and would live forever" and had tried to commit suicide more than once, asking to be burned alive (Cotard's, 1880; Berrios and Luque, 1995a; Pearn and Gardner-Thorpe, 2002). He believed that he had identified a new type of depression. Later, in 1882, he used the term *délire des négations* to describe the condition and gave a further account of it in his book *Maladies Cérébrales et Mentales* published in 1891.

In 1788, Charles Bonnet, the French physician, had reported a person believing she was dead; she was an elderly lady who insisted on being dressed in her shroud and placed in a coffin. She stayed in it for weeks until the feeling (though not the lady herself) passed away (Förstl and Beats, 1992).

The disorder was commented upon by many other authors during the last years of the nineteenth century: in 1893, Régis coined the eponym *delire de Cotard* and Séglas in 1897 greatly consolidated the use of the phrase "Cotard's syndrome." In the first half of the twentieth century, the condition was discussed periodically and new cases were reported in the French literature (Capgras and Daumezon, 1936).

The Second World War was followed by a renewed interest in the condition. In 1956, de Martis described a case occurring in a 38-year-old woman who, following surgery, probably for an ovarian neoplasm, became hostile, irritable and withdrawn with a tendency to depressive episodes.

In previous editions of *Uncommon Psychiatric Syndromes*, this and several of the other cases which follow were given in some detail, since they were being reproduced in English for the first time. This pattern is replicated here:

> She had been overtly ill for three years, the onset of her illness occurring four months following the death of her father from heart disease. His death was untimely in that it occurred when there was considerable conflict between them, although they had always been very close. She suffered for years from extreme guilt and from accusatory hallucinations which would tell her, "It was you who made your father ill." She was given ECT in a private clinic on nine occasions, but her condition worsened and she began to have feelings of derealisation and depersonalisation in addition to auditory hallucinations. She also believed that she had been transformed both inwardly and outwardly.

> After her discharge and an initial period of improvement there was a recrudescence of her illness. She became extremely withdrawn and was admitted to another clinic where she protested that "all is dead within and outside me." She was preoccupied in contemplating what de Martis vividly described as "her own abyss of dejection." On rare occasions she would respond to questioning and revert to making spontaneous remarks. Once she pointed to the surrounding countryside and said that all that encircled her "the sun, earth and the very stars do not exist." She believed that she alone survived the initial explosion that created the world, and that she wandered in an empty world as a "carbonized star." She believed that even time had been consumed and that she was thus condemned to wander eternally in this form.

The case exhibits the major features of Cotard's syndrome – namely, an initial period of anxiety leading to the ideas of objective negation, with a patient denying the existence of the outside world, together with ideas of subjective negation whereby she denied the existence of parts of her own body and, finally, ideas of immortality associated with the state of despondency, depersonalisation and mental pain. She also exhibited a rarer manifestation of the syndrome – namely, the ideas of enormity of her body.

In 1968, Ahlheid described three cases with an emphasis on organic components:

The first patient suffered from poliomyelitis in childhood. A heavy drinker for most of his life, he was admitted to hospital at the age of 61 years with a depressive illness, complaining of "feeling like death." He improved with ECT but had to be readmitted aged 65 years when he was again described as depressed and as having "alcoholic agitation" when treated with anti-depressants. His next admission occurred at the age of 67 years when he suffered from a severe depressive state with evidence of organic deterioration. He stated "I am already dead," "I am finished," "I am poisoned." He was preoccupied with his bowels. After 25 days in hospital he asked to be buried because he said he was a "corpse which already stinks." A month later he said that he had no flesh and no legs or trunk. These ideas were unshakeable, so that the clinical picture remained unchanged for months.

The second patient developed syphilis at the age of 37 years and paranoid ideas at the age of 39 years which then cleared completely. At 62 years his paranoid ideas recurred and gradually worsened. He was in poor physical health and was extremely despondent, "because people are dead and corpses are on the wall." He was convinced that he too was dead, that his bowels did not work and that they were calcified. He insisted that his toes were dead. He was extremely depressed and although when treated with anti-depressants he initially improved, after a few days he relapsed and again stated that he was "a living corpse with no stomach and bowels; which do not exist." ECT was felt to be contraindicated because of his poor physical state. He remained inaccessible for three months, and although he developed other delusions as well, his nihilistic delusions persisted throughout.

The third patient suffered from typhoid at 10 years of age and suspected syphilis at 20 years. Since childhood he had complained of various psychosomatic disorders but was not admitted to a psychiatric hospital until aged 38 years, when he was possibly deluded. At 60 years of age he complained of vague physical disturbances and stayed in bed for most of the time "waiting for death." ECT did not alter his condition at all and he protested that he had "no blood and no veins" and repeatedly said, "I am dying," while refusing to eat. At 65 years he showed early signs of arteriosclerosis. He was prescribed imipramine for his depressive symptoms with some improvement, but two months later he again deteriorated, became agitated, stating that his body was already dead. He explained that he was still able to speak because "his spirit was waiting to die." He demanded to be buried as he was very depressed. At 67 years he improved for a short period but then developed delusions of grandeur, stating that he had become a saint. He added that he did not bother about a body "because a saint is immortal and does not need a body." At 68 years he was obviously euphoric and his nihilistic delusion was completely encapsulated.

In 1971, Dietrich described a fascinating case of a nihilistic delusion in a neurologist. There have since been other case reports, discussion and passing reference to Cotard's syndrome in various journals and textbooks, particularly in the French and Italian psychiatric literature (Leroy, 1920; Nardi, 1935; Zilboorg and Henry, 1941; Poli, 1942; Cremieux and Cain, 1948; Kretschmer, 1952; Perris, 1955). In recent years interest in the clinical, neurobiological and nosological aspects of the disorder has been resurrected within the English-speaking world.

The condition's nosological status has attracted considerable discussion and, currently, remains uncertain. In the authors' view, it is justifiable to regard it as a distinct clinical entity not only because it can exist in the pure and complete form but, even when symptomatic of another mental illness, such as depressive psychosis or schizophrenia, the nihilistic delusions tend to dominate the clinical picture. Furthermore, it has a complex psychopathology of its own which must occupy a central position in the study of mental disorder because it brings us face to face with the very meaning of existence itself.

Case reports

Case I

A widow, aged 65 years, presented with a severe depressive illness precipitated by the death of her husband and that of a close friend, both within six weeks of one another. Her own father had died in 1930, and following this she had suffered from a depressive illness resulting in her admission to hospital where she remained for over three years. She had been a timid, shy child who later became more outgoing. After remaining at school until the age of 15 years, she learned shorthand and typing and after six months in her first job moved to her second job where she remained for 39 years, eventually becoming a personal secretary and remaining so until she retired. Her physical health was good. She was also quite strong-willed and took up driving at the age of 64 years in order to be able to transport her invalid husband around. She had met him, a widower, when she was 59, having known him in her younger days. He was a retired printer, and they had one adopted daughter. It was six weeks after his death that she began to be depressed with a considerable exacerbation occurring as a result of the second death, that of the close friend with whom she had stayed shortly after her husband's death.

On admission, she was extremely depressed, looked physically ill and was dehydrated and agitated. Her speech was coherent and relevant, although she was preoccupied with her own condition. She said that she was affecting all the other patients in the ward and was responsible for their illnesses. She stated that she had strange unreal feelings and felt also that she was going to live forever. Yet at other times she would say, "I am no longer alive; I am dead." She felt that she had done great wrong, although she could give no details, but believed that as a result of her wrongdoings her family were going to be harmed. She thus presented with a severe depressive illness with nihilistic delusions and paradoxical feelings of immortality occurring in the late involutional period. She was treated with imipramine together with ECT (a total of eight treatments), and she recovered; all her depressive symptoms cleared, including the nihilistic delusions and other features of Cotard's syndrome.

Case 2

A married woman of 69 years of age was first admitted following a domiciliary visit in 1971, when she was found to be suffering from a severe endogenous depression, worse in the mornings and with considerable feelings of guilt, unworthiness and hopelessness. In addition, she complained of persistent early-morning wakening, loss of libido and loss of interest in everything, and was very agitated. She was perturbed by the fact that she had strange feelings about her own body and believed that she was turning into an animal, such as a dog. At times she stated, "I have no body. I am dead."

The patient had had a happy childhood. After marriage she went to live with her in-laws in Shropshire and had lived in their house for 39 years. Although she had a sister living nearby, she began to feel increasingly lonely and isolated. She had never really liked the place, and during the year after she had become ill, she began to detest it. For years she had tried to persuade her husband to move, but this he would not countenance. As she became more and more depressed, her hatred for the house grew, and she became less effective in looking after it, herself and her husband. His health was also causing her some concern.

The patient herself had no history of any previous psychiatric disorder, although three months before entering hospital, she had had an attack of influenza and was advised to stay in bed for a month. It was on getting up that she immediately felt stranger and confused as well as depressed. It was at this juncture that she began to have the symptoms found on her admission.

After a month in hospital, during which she was given clomipramine and amitriptyline, she began to improve. The delusions of her existence and body lessened in intensity, although she still insisted that she had strange feelings and that she did not feel like other people. Within another month she was markedly improved and was eating and sleeping well for the first time in many months. Her previous delusions had cleared completely; she was rational and sensible in her speech but still complained about lack of concentration and of an apparent inability to memorise. She also lacked interest and still suffered from extreme lethargy. Weekends spent at home only tended to aggravate her condition, and on return to hospital she would feel more depressed because of the amount of work that she realised she would have to do on returning home. However, she eventually did leave hospital, although reluctantly, much improved, and was seen regularly as an outpatient being maintained on antidepressant therapy.

A year after her discharge she was seen again at home. There had been a slight worsening in her condition, resulting mainly from the fact that she had become even more worried about her husband, whose physical state had deteriorated very markedly. On this occasion she again improved with increased doses of antidepressants. While being seen regularly as an outpatient for a further year, there was no recurrence of her nihilistic delusions or of the strange ideas and feelings which she had had about her body, but she never regained her customary drive, energy and interest. No doubt her surroundings, her house and her husband's physical ill health, all of which were a constant source of worry to her, were a barrier to further improvement.

Case 3

A 61-year-old housewife was referred by her family doctor on account of loss of weight, thought originally to be from an oesophageal stricture or carcinomatosis, but for which no physical cause had been found. On admission she weighed only 39.3 kg.

Her presenting complaint was of inability to swallow and of a choking sensation in her throat. She stated, "It is ridiculous, I know, but there is a force stronger than me, against me. I can't think clearly, it just goes blank. I'm pulsating a lot; it sounds ridiculous but I can't swallow. I don't go to the toilet; my bladder and bowels are not working at all; my front passage has shrivelled away completely; my muscles and nerves are not co-operating."

It appeared that these symptoms had first started about a year previously when, following a throat infection, she had begun to feel "rather nervy" and to experience a bad taste in her mouth. She then developed dysphagia and was admitted on this account to a general hospital where a diagnosis of hiatus hernia and reflux oesophagitis was made. Oesophagoscopy was carried out, whereupon it was reported that she had a stricture. This was said to have been dilated, but in view of subsequent events, it seems likely that this diagnosis was incorrect, although some oesophageal spasm may have been present at the time. Other investigations revealed nothing abnormal, apart from a barium enema which showed a minor degree of diverticulosis.

Her previous history seems to have been relatively unremarkable. Her somewhat dominating mother had died when aged 82 years from gastric carcinoma, and her father at aged 69 years from cardiac failure. She had one brother. She married when aged 30 years but remained childless and continued her work as a domestic science teacher. Her sexual relationship with her husband, which had probably never been keen, seems to have dwindled further over their later years. Whereas her physical health appeared to have been satisfactory until the start of her mental illness, it became clear that she had always been somewhat hypochondriacal. Five years before admission, she was treated by a psychiatrist who regarded her as suffering from a state of depression, noting at the time that she was a woman of anxious, rigid and somewhat obsessional personality. She was first treated psychotherapeutically but was later given amitriptyline tablets, which, however, she claimed to be unable to swallow.

On admission she was clearly deluded about her bowels, particularly her rectum, from which she maintained something offensive was emanating, her bladder, which she said did not work, and indeed about most parts of her body, except for her heart which she knew must be functioning because she was aware of its thumping. She again insisted that she could not swallow, but when given a glass of water to drink she swallowed it successfully. When asked where the liquid had gone, she replied, "Into the tissues of my neck." Despite these numerous bodily delusions, she did not seem to be particularly depressed but, if anything, gave the impression of being somewhat affectively flattened, an appearance which seemed, nevertheless, to conceal a not inconsiderable degree of anxiety. She also had some difficulty in sleeping.

Apart from her hypochondriacal ideas, she expressed some rather vague notion about her husband trying to poison her, maintaining also that some eggs in her refrigerator had been giving off some sort of gas, possibly hydrogen sulphide, which was "making her inside go funny." She stated that she had thrown these away with the utmost care so as to avoid breaking them.

On mental state examination, there was no evidence of any organic condition nor anything to suggest a schizophrenic illness. In view of her previous psychiatric history and her present complaints, a diagnosis of depression accompanied by marked hypochondriasis and nihilistic delusions was made. Although hesitant in view of her anxiety about what might happen to any food she might attempt to swallow, because she was convinced that she had no digestive tract which could absorb it, she was fairly readily coaxed to eat. Despite this, she adamantly refused any oral medication and accordingly was treated with ECT. After eight treatments her condition improved considerably so that when discharged she had lost her delusional ideas altogether, although remaining vaguely hypochondriacal. Her weight on discharge was 45 kg, which was considered satisfactory in view of her somewhat slight build.

The above cases are fairly typical examples of the syndrome. All were females in their late middle years. Note (Cases 1 and 2) the prominent feelings of unreality as well as nihilistic delusions. The following patient was of a younger age and was particularly interesting in that she exhibited both Capgras' and Cotard's syndromes, although at different times.

Case 4

In 1949, when aged 21 years and while serving in the Women's Royal Naval Service, she was admitted to hospital with a vague history of gastric symptoms of one month's duration. She was also found to be euphoric and to have an inappropriate affect, with ideas of reference and thought disorder. Her condition was diagnosed as schizophrenic. Within a week as an inpatient, she became restless, difficult to manage and actively hallucinated. She responded well to ECT in that the acute symptoms cleared, but she remained detached and preoccupied. She was not tranquil but rather facile, having no insight. A course of deep insulin coma therapy produced a gradual but definite improvement; she attended a rehabilitation course to relearn shorthand and typing and then returned to work, where she remained until 1959. It was then that she was admitted again into a mental hospital now aged 31 years. She was apathetic with poverty of speech and movement, and she appeared perplexed; she ate little and had no insight. She had also lost a considerable amount of weight. Once again her condition was diagnosed as schizophrenic. This second illness began during the puerperium; two and a half months before being admitted, she had given birth to a son following which she began hearing voices. She had also begun to have strange ideas about herself. She believed that her hometown was full of people she had known in her childhood and her earlier life in London, and it seemed odd to hear that they did not acknowledge her. She recognised strangers as old acquaintances (a phenomenon which appears to be the reverse of Capgras' syndrome). She felt very depressed, believing that "things were going on in the house;" for example, she believed that the Bible belonging to her sister-in-law with the words "To Margaret" written on it had been replaced by a black one with "To Margaret" written in italics. On admission, she believed that she recognised many of the patients in the ward as having been with her in the hospital to which she had been admitted 10 years earlier. She was also generally suspicious and grimaced frequently and inappropriately. Her speech, although generally coherent, appeared to be under pressure and revealed flights of ideas. She was giggly and fatuous, and her affect was incongruous at times.

She was treated with chlorpromazine but continued to misidentify people on the ward and began to doubt that her husband was really her husband, thinking that he was somebody else and might have been replaced. Within 10 days, however, she no longer misidentified him but explained her previous mistake, saying that he had had "his teeth scraped and therefore looked different."

In July 1959, she became very depressed, with little spontaneous speech. She asked, "Can I go to some institution where there are people like me? I have no intellect, I can learn nothing; I am not capable of running a home. I don't want to do anything." She protested that she had let down both her husband and her sister and that she was useless. She had feelings of hopelessness regarding her future, believing that she would never be fit to return home. She wished to be locked away forever so that her husband would forget about her. At this point a diagnosis of severe depression was made, there being no evidence of schizophrenia. She looked a picture of abject misery, expressing feelings of despondency and despair. However, on being asked if she felt depressed, she answered, "I have no feelings," thus expressing nihilistic delusions. Her condition improved markedly following ECT, and she was discharged; she was soon readmitted, however, in a very apathetic and withdrawn state, so that on this occasion her condition was diagnosed as catatonic schizophrenia, although the possibility of atypical manic-depressive psychosis was considered. In October 1959, she received two ECT treatments and was stated to be "alive again." She was now cheerful and showed some insight, although following discharge she still had episodes of depression.

In 1960, her EEG was considered to be unequivocally abnormal for a 32-year-old woman who had been off drugs for 10 days, and while being unspecifically *organic* was thought to be consistent with a diagnosis of a toxic confusional state or a reversible metabolic condition. Detailed psychological testing, while reinforcing the diagnosis of schizophrenia, showed some degree of intellectual deficit. However, the variability of her performance on various tests at different times suggested that this deficit had a functional rather than an organic basis.

Each of the four cases we have so far described involved females which, unlike most of those reported by the European authors who have been quoted, appear nonetheless to suggest a higher incidence of the condition among women.

A further case is described in detail in the chapter on *folie à deux*. While the central figure of the case was the father of the family, his delusion that he was deceased appears to have been shared by the majority of other family members of both sexes.

There follows a further case of Cotard's syndrome involving a single man.

Case 5

When first seen in 1973, the patient, aged 59 years, had been continuously resident in a mental hospital for 31 years. During this period he exhibited a variety of symptoms which were thought to be of schizophrenic origin but which, with the passage of time, became increasingly more characteristic of depression of endogenous type. He was a man of limited intelligence, having an IQ within the dull normal range, and was unable to read, apparently because anxiety while at school had interfered with his ability to study. His history of nihilistic delusions extended back over 32 years, tending to become more prominent during his phases of severe depression. He often said, "I am a ghost" or "I am dead" and sometimes denied the existence of certain parts of his body, saying, for example, "I have no blood." He admitted to having suicidal thoughts and over 21 years was given to attacks of window smashing, which he explained were the result of uncontrollable destructive urges. He also insisted that he was being controlled by outside forces and by God, who, he believed, commanded him to kill children, although he had never attempted to do so. During periods of severe agitation occurring in association with his depressive symptoms, he believed that the nurses were trying to poison him. Despite a considerable amount of treatment with ECT and various antidepressants, together with a variety of other tranquillisers (except chlorpromazine to which he proved sensitive), no such measures alleviated his condition other than offering him transient and limited relief.

The next case is a good example of Cotard's symptomatology occurring in the setting of an acute schizophrenic episode.

Case 6

A 26-year-old male patient of Arabic origin who had resided in the UK since the age of 12 years. In early 1995, he was transferred to hospital from prison, where he was on remand facing a serious charge of violence. There was a history of two previous admissions to an acute psychiatric unit with acute psychosis.

On admission he was extremely disturbed and greatly distressed by bizarre somatic hallucinations comprising twisting sensations within his body and the feeling that parts of his anatomy were disappearing. In addition, he held the delusional beliefs that he was about to die imminently and that several of his organ systems had ceased to function.

The florid features of psychosis resolved within weeks of the commencement of antipsychotic drugs and, although mildly disabled by negative deficits, the patient was successfully returned to the community.

Epidemiology

The various contexts in which the term "Cotard's syndrome" has been used clinically have been explored by Berrios and Luque (1995b). These authors analysed more than 200 scientific articles containing reports of the disorder published between 1880 and 1993 (inclusive) and took the view that in their sample 100 complete cases of the syndrome were on record. Using the same methodology, in collaboration with Berrios and Luque, a further 26 reports in English or French, containing sufficient details of 38 patients, were identified by Cohen's group between 1994 and 2005 (inclusive) (Consoli et al., 2007).

Although the disorder has been described in all age groups between 10 to 82 years, most examples occur in late middle life. The condition seems to be rare in adolescence, and only a few cases are reported in the medical literature (Halfon et al., 1985; Dugas, 1985; Degiovanni et al., 1987). Of the 138 patients reported between 1880 to 2005 (Consoli et al., 2007), 21 (15%) were aged less than 26 years; the mean age of all 138 patients was 47.7 years (standard deviation 17.8 years), with the youngest patient being 10 years of age and the oldest 82 years. The sex ratio in this cohort, of female to male of 94 (68%) to 44 (32%), is consistent with the clinical impression of the present authors that the syndrome is more frequently encountered in women than in men. This sex ratio remained almost the same for those aged below 26 years: 15 (71%) female to 6 (29%) male (Consoli et al., 2007).

Chiu (1995) carried out a retrospective study of the case-notes of all outpatients and inpatients treated over a two-year period, between 1991 and 1993, by the psychogeriatric unit of the Chinese University of Hong Kong. The catchment area served 750,000 people, of whom 8.7% were aged 65 years or older. Of 349 patients (262 female and 87 male, all ethnically Chinese), two female patients, both widows suffering from major depression, were diagnosed as suffering from Cotard's syndrome. This gave a prevalence of Cotard's syndrome of 0.57% in psychogeriatric patients. 18.1% of the cohort were diagnosed as suffering from major depression, yielding a prevalence of Cotard's syndrome in elderly patients with major depression of 3.2%.

The disorder has been described in a moderately mentally handicapped man (see also Case 5) (Kearns, 1987). Another case, also in a man with moderate intellectual disability, which developed following an important episode of fear in which he witnessed an attempted theft, was described by Sottile et al. (2018). However, such occurrences must be considered exceptional.

Clinical features

The clinical features of the condition vary greatly in terms of the extent and number of nihilistic delusions. The concept of a spectrum of completeness/incompleteness of syndrome has long been recognised by authors who have written on the disorder.

The essential symptom of Cotard's syndrome is a delusion of negation. This can vary in severity along a continuum from a belief held by a patient that she is losing her powers of intellect and feeling to the severest form when she believes that she no longer exists, leading her to deny both her own existence and that of the cosmos. This nihilistic delusion is often associated with a depressive illness and sometimes with a schizophrenic or a psycho-organic syndrome.

Of the 138 patients reported between 1880 to 2005 (Consoli et al., 2007), almost all were retrospectively diagnosed as suffering from a primary psychiatric diagnosis, using *DSM-III-R* criteria for the cases reported up to 1993, and *DSM-IV* criteria reported after 1994, as follows:

* Depression 79 cases (57%)
* Bipolar disorder 27 (20%)
* Schizophrenia 14 (10%)
* Organic 17 (12%)

Of note, 22 (81%) of the 27 patients with bipolar disorder (depressive phase) were female. Interestingly, the observed age of onset in all 27 of these patients with Cotard's syndrome associated with bipolar disorder was better described as existing in two distinct distributions, an early onset with median age of onset of 18.7 years and a late age of onset with median age of 50.5 years, rather than by one overall normal distribution.

The onset of Cotard's syndrome in general is often sudden with no previous history of any psychiatric disorder. Typically, however, there is a phase of initial anxiety which can vary in length from a few weeks to several years. The anxiety is vague and diffuse and often associated with irritability.

In milder cases the patient may well complain of becoming depressed and of beginning to believe that she is losing her powers of reasoning and feeling. She feels that things are different inside and outside her, which in turn leads her to become even more anxious than before. The condition progresses to a more severe form when the anxiety gives way to despair having a frankly nihilistic colouring. The patient may then state that she is ruined and that she has lost all of her material wealth as well as her intellectual capacity, this often leading to her self-loathing.

In the presence of a completely nihilistic delusional state, ideas of negation occur, leading the patient to deny any link with reality or the surrounding world, the existence of which she may also deny.

Simultaneously, ideas of subjective negation lead the patient to deny the existence of parts of her own body. This usually begins with the denial of one specific part of the body. As one patient stated, "I used to have a heart. I have something which beats in its place." From then on she went to say, "I have no stomach, I never feel hungry. When I eat I get the taste of food but once past my gullet, I feel nothing. It seems that food falls into a hole." Subsequently, the subject may proceed to deny her very existence, even dispensing altogether with the personal pronoun "I." One patient even called herself "Madam Zero" in order to emphasise her non-existence. One of Anderson's (1964) patients said, referring to herself, "It's no use. Wrap it up and throw 'it' in the dustbin."

The patient reaching such a state of utter despair may profess an overriding desire "not to exist," yet paradoxically the possibility of death may be seen as impossible, leading to ideas of immortality. This, then, becomes the greatest despair of all, wishing to die but condemned to live forever in the state of nihilism, reminiscent of Kierkergaard's (1941) living hell.

Such ideas of immortality may be associated with other megalomanic ideas, such as ideas of enormity (*délire d'énormité*) and other similar bodily delusions. Such patients may be convinced of the massive increase in the size of their bodies, believing that they may even extend to merge with the universe. Thus they may claim that their heads touch the stars. The paradox becomes even more pronounced when those patients at one time protesting that they did not exist start to claim to be all pervading the earth. This development constitutes the *manic* Cotard's syndrome. There is also an obvious parallel to be drawn here between such patients and those who, after suffering from persecutory delusions for many years, become grandiose, believing that their supposed persecutors have been finally defeated and they themselves have become omnipotent.

Cotard's syndrome may occur in the context of pregnancy and childbirth. Kuppili et al. (2017) described the case of a 24-year-old patient with schizophrenia who, from the second month of pregnancy, denied the existence of her pregnancy, stating that her uterus and foetus were dead; at two weeks post-partum, she denied the existence of her baby. Similarly, Walloch et al. (2007) described a 28-year-old primigravida with first onset of a depressive episode who, in spite of clear abdominal enlargement consistent with the start of the third trimester, was convinced that she was not pregnant; the authors considered this to be a special form of Cotard's syndrome.

Accessory symptoms of Cotard's syndrome may include analgesia, mutism, self-mutilating urges, suicidal ideas, illusions and, in some cases, hallucinations. The latter may be visual but are much more commonly auditory. Their content always reflects a preoccupation with guilt, despair and death. Thus, one patient "sees the walls tremble" and believes the house to be mined. He fears the preparations for his execution, "the guillotine being erected." Such experiences are more likely to be illusions based on strong effect rather than hallucinations. Others may have hallucinations of taste and smell, believing that they are rotting away, that their food is completely changed or that they are being offered filth, faecal matter or human flesh. Such patients have a tendency to self-mutilation and suicide.

Herein is another paradox, for although they believe that they are dead, or that they can never die, they still try to destroy themselves. This is not altogether surprising, however, especially in those who believe themselves to be damned and who are in utter despair; as their lives are already a veritable hell, suicide is the only way of escape. Those who believe they are immortal are in the greatest hell of all because they believe that their state of despair must continue forever.

Based on the staging of depression put forward by Fava and Kellner (1993), Yarnada et al. (1999) have proposed that the clinical course of Cotard's syndrome may be considered to fall into the following three consecutive stages:

i   The germination stage – a prodromal period in which hypochondriasis and cenesthopathy may, for example, occur.
ii The blooming stage – a period characterised by the full development of symptoms of Cotard's syndrome.
iii The chronic stage – according to Yarnada et al. (1999), "Cotard's syndrome shows two chronic courses, one of which involves persistent emotional impairment with chronic change of depression (depressive type), while the other involves systematization of delusions with depression receding to its 'background,' chronic change to paranoia (paranoid type)."

Negativistic attitudes and behaviour are not uncommon. Self-starvation because of negation of existence or of self may occur (Silva et al., 2000; Grover et al., 2014). Others less severely disordered who have, nevertheless, ideas of guilt and self-reproach may only pick at their food, fasting being a penance. Refusal to take food may be absolute, as in our Case 3, who believed she had no stomach. Nejad (2002) described a 65-year-old male patient who refused to eat and drink, showing evidence of panic reactions when offered a glass of water; hydrophobia is a rare presentation of Cotard's syndrome.

As Cotard's syndrome often occurs in association with other psychotic states, the symptoms of these disorders are also likely to be present. For example, when nihilistic delusions are grafted onto a depressive illness, other symptoms often characteristic of depression will be found. Similarly, within the psycho-organic syndrome, there will also be symptoms and signs of an impairment of the sensorium such as disorientation, defects of grasp, attention and concentration, together with memory loss. More rarely, the syndrome may occur in acute schizophrenic states, when of course other schizophrenic symptoms will be present. Saavedra (1968) referred to this particular state as "coenaesthetic schizophrenia."

Psychopathology and aetiology

The great debate concerning Cotard's syndrome, which is rare and remains poorly understood (Dieguez, 2018), is whether the condition only exists as a syndrome and, therefore, is always symptomatic of another mental illness or, in some cases, can be viewed as a specific disease entity in its own right. This question has not been completely resolved but, for a considerable period of time now, the syndromal hypothesis has occupied the orthodox position. This is reflected in the fact that the term "Cotard's syndrome" does not find itself defined as a category, in either of the major internationally accepted classificatory systems, *DSM-5* or *ICD-10*.

The picture is further clouded by the total absence of any operational definition and, hence, a lack of uniformity as to how the concept has been applied by both clinicians and researchers alike. This must be borne in mind when one attempts to interpret published studies of Cotard's patients. The historical development of the term "Cotard's syndrome" is usefully explored by Berrios and Luque (1995a).

Nosology

Whatever the nosological significance, as mentioned above numerous authors have reported patients diagnosed as suffering from a wide range of mental illnesses (affective, schizophrenic and organic) and who also exhibit delusions of negation and other related nihilistic features. Cotard himself, in 1882, described a series of 11 patients and divided them into three categories: those with simple nihilistic delusions (eight cases), associated with GPI (one case) and a third group with a more complex clinical picture who also demonstrated persecutory delusions (two cases). A modern interpretation of this work would suggest that the first group represent depressive psychosis, whereas the third category probably displayed schizophrenic components.

A similar picture was produced by Saavedra (1968), who described 10 cases, classifying them into three types: depressive (four cases), mixed (three cases) and schizophrenic (three cases). Furthermore, two out of the eight patients in the organically based study of Joseph and O'Leary (1986) were said to have an underlying schizophrenic illness.

Applying factor analysis to their cohort of 100 cases (from 1880 to 1993), Berrios and Luque (1995b) extracted three factors: a depressed group (psychotic depression), a mixed group (Cotard II) and a group with no loadings for depression (Cotard I) which, the authors postulated, could constitute a "pure" syndrome whose nosology may be more closely aligned to delusional than affective disorders. In the light of this suggestion, it may be significant to recall that, at least until relatively recently, the condition in the USA was viewed as a paranoid type of involutional psychosis (Arieti, 1974).

In recent years some attention has focussed on organic and neurobiological factors which, it has been postulated, form the aetiological basis of the syndrome. Such evidence is examined in this section, along with an exploration of other factors – psychological, psychodynamic, existential – which, in the authors' view, is essential for a more complete understanding of the psychopathology of nihilistic delusions.

Biology

An hereditary component has long been postulated in the pathogenesis of Cotard's syndrome; in fact this was mooted way back in 1892 by Arnaud and has since been supported by other authors (Coen-Bonifante, 1926; Mignot and Lacassagne, 1937; Fattovich and Niccolani, 1938; Saavedra, 1968). These views, however, amount to little more than clinical and anecdotal impressions, and there is no hard, systematic evidence to suggest that Cotard's syndrome has a specific genetic aetiology.

It has long been suspected that Cotard's syndrome has an underlying organic substrate. Case reports abound in the literature revealing an association with such frank organic states such as general paralysis and senile dementia; indeed, such a relationship is evident from a study of Cotard's (1891) original work. This theme has been maintained in recent years with descriptions of the syndrome – or partial syndrome – in typhoid fever, following head injury and in association with temporal lobe seizures (Campbell et al., 1981; Greenberg et al., 1984). Helldén et al. (2007) described two cases of Cotard's syndrome, one in a 35-year-old female patient with a failing renal transplant and the other in a 36-year-old male bone marrow transplant recipient, which occurred as an adverse drug reaction to the antiviral aciclovir and its prodrug valaciclovir. Furthermore, the tendency for Cotard's patients to be of late middle age also hints at some aetiological role for organicity.

If such an association between the disorder and organic factors is accepted, then this immediately begs the question, what is the nature of this relationship? Is it an indirect one, whereby diffuse organic impairment operates as a background factor "releasing" the Cotard's phenomenology, or are the clinical features a direct manifestation of some specific, focal brain lesion? Recent studies have shed light on this, as is now discussed.

Many authors have postulated the presence of a focal cerebral pathology. The view of Saavedra (1968) that the condition involved atrophy of the basal ganglia has not been confirmed by more recent neurobiological studies.

Given the central delusion of Cotard's syndrome, i.e. the denial of one's own existence, and its immediate (although probably superficial) resemblance to such neurological features as disordered body image and denial syndrome, it is only logical that suspicion for the site of the presumed lesion should fall upon the parietal lobes. Such speculation, however, has not been subsequently confirmed by organic studies on Cotard's patients. Joseph and O'Leary (1986) reported an experimental study involving CT brain scanning of eight patients with Cotard's syndrome along with eight controls matched for age, sex and psychiatric disorder. The Cotard's group had greater diffuse cerebral atrophy and inter-hemispheric fissure enlargement than the controls, but no specific parietal lobe pathology was evident. The inter-hemispheric fissure enlargement was thought to be a manifestation of medial frontal lobe atrophy and may yet prove to be an important finding. Other case reports involving the investigation of organic variables have similarly failed to reveal any specific, or even predominant, parietal lobe pathology and often unveil evidence of disturbed structure and function in other brain regions – such as the frontal and temporal regions (Joseph, 1986; Young et al., 1994). Sahoo and Josephs (2018) reviewed the records of all patients over the age of 18 years who had been diagnosed as suffering from Cotard's syndrome at the Mayo Clinic between 1996 and 2016; the 12 patients identified had a median age of 52 years (ranging from 30 to 85 years) and showed the following neuroimaging changes:

- Frontal lobe changes – four (33%) patients
- Generalised volume loss – four (33%) patients
- Ischaemic changes – five (42%) patients
- Right-sided or bilateral hemisphere lesions – seven (58%) patients

It must be emphasised that all these reports share the frustration of not having available a universally acceptable clinical definition of what constitutes the disorder and, therefore, sample validity is open to question.

The first [18F]-fluorodeoxyglucose (FDG)-PET study of a patient with Cotard's syndrome, by Charland-Verville et al. (2013), showed extensive cortical hypometabolism compared with a cohort of 39 age-matched healthy controls. The patient was a 48-year-old male with a previous short depressive illness and no other obvious reason for this hypometabolism. Indeed, this finding led the authors to entitle their publication "Brain dead yet mind alive."

More recently, the results of cerebral FDG-PET neuroimaging on another 48-year-old male patient who had developed Cotard's syndrome were reported by Ozkan and Caliyurt (2016). This time the patient was suffering from schizophrenia, for which he had been treated with antipsychotic medication; he had developed upper limb cogwheel rigidity. Again, widespread hypometabolism was found, along with hypermetabolism in the basal ganglia, presumably related to his extrapyramidal side-effects.

Greenberg et al. (1984) described four cases, all exhibiting cerebral manifestations of serious physical disease who, whilst having prolonged complex partial seizures, experienced death-related phenomena such as the sensation of being dead and alive at the same time and a morbid fear of impending death. Cotard's syndrome has, in addition, been described in cases of temporal lobe disease. Greenberg's cases did not, however, share any typical features of Cotard's phenomenology, and their significance for the latter syndrome is debatable. Parks et al. (2014) described the case of a 59-year-old woman with a long history of migraine with aura who developed dysmetropsia and Cotard's syndrome as a result of a migrainous infarction associated with right temporal-parietal-occipital changes and apparent cortical laminar necrosis.

It is well known that tumours of the brain may be associated with neuropsychiatric symptomology. Reich et al. (2012) described the case of the development of Cotard's syndrome in a 60-year-old male patient suffering from inoperable glioblastoma multiforme on the splenium of the corpus callosum. They make the important point that, in such cases, there needs to be close collaboration between psychiatrists, neuro-oncologists and radiation oncologists.

Matsukura et al. (1981) investigated ß-endorphin activity in a patient with schizophrenia, delusions of negation and immortality, associated with pain insensitivity, but found this to be normal.

Neuropsychology

Recently, focus has softly shifted away from the study of stark biological lesions to more subtle functional neuropsychiatric aspects. Indeed, harbingers of such a theme can be found in the literature from the 1960s; authors such as Anderson (1964) and Ahlheid (1968), while emphasising the importance of organic factors, nevertheless accepted that the syndrome does occur in functional psychosis. Anderson also indicated that these cases are often the cumulation of a lifelong anankastic personality disorder which under the influence of the ageing process, with or without cerebral arteriopathy, has "crystalised out" into a rigid, monotonous clinical picture, with a grotesque exaggeration of pre-psychotic personality traits, notably hypochondriasis (see also Case 3 in this chapter).

These states form fertile ground for the formation of both *délire de négation* and *délire d'énormité*.

Cases have been reported in which Cotard's and Capgras' symptomatology is seen in the same patient, often sequentially (see also Case 4 in this chapter). Young et al. (1994) reported the neuropsychological investigation of both Capgras' (three examples) and Cotard's (two examples) cases. Such detailed examinations revealed a largely specific impairment in facial recognition. Those authors argued that in both syndromes the underlying psychopathological processes may be similar in that they represent the patient's attempts to make sense of a shared fundamental morbid experience. In other words, Cotard's syndrome amounts to a delusional interpretation (a psychological mechanism) of an organically determined cognitive/perceptual disturbance. Important superimposed factors, such as an affective element and/or depersonalisation, would then determine the final outcome, manifesting as delusions of negation (Young and Leafhead, 1996). Interestingly, such a conceptual framework may well have its roots in the early medical literature as the relationship between delusions of persecution and delusions of nihilism was discussed by Cotard himself. In addition, Séglas (1897) believed that there was a failure in the mechanism of mental synthesis, and in particular mental vision (i.e. visual memory), which led on to depersonalisation and which in turn resulted in the formation of ideas of negation.

The patient suffering from Cotard's syndrome certainly experiences deep feelings of change within and without, and the fundamental aetiological importance of this sensation is commented upon by many authors and is sometimes described as a "fundamental disturbance of coenaesthesia" (Bianchi, 1924; Poli, 1942). Anderson (1964) has shown how extreme depersonalisation can give rise to bizarre delusional ideas such as the non-existence of the body, the rotting away of the bowels and at times the belief by the subject that she is dead. Ahlheid (1968), in discussing the concept of *leib* (body for me) and *korper* (body in itself), stated that when *korper* takes prevalent place, ideas or feelings of depersonalisation emerge.

Psychodynamics

Psychodynamic concepts favour the explanation that the delusion of negation arises from the death wish inherent in the collective unconscious, as reflected sometimes in self-punishment and at other times in the total denial of self. Thus feelings of guilt which arise from the depressed mood distort the relationship between *I* and *them* and immobilise the activity of the super-ego. As a result of the possibility of *being*, a feeling of alienation arises, so deep and ineffable as to identify *I* with nothingness. The *I* therefore no longer exists (Vitetta, 1962).

Bolzani (1958) points out that the denying of the existence of an organ is a morphobiological way of believing in its death. In the psychopathology of the condition, the denial of recognition, observed by Fuster (1955), and the "existential transposition" are emphasised. It has been suggested by Saavedra (1968) that the fundamental disturbance is an "abnormal intuition of subjective time." It is also suggested that such patients usually have conflicts in the narcissistic, oedipal or homosexual sphere and may freely resort to fatalistic symbolism to describe their experiences. A persistent deep sense of guilt may engender self-punishment, with a desire to sever contact from all human relations in a world in which the existence of space and time is completely denied.

When the patient comes to believe that she is not only dead but also immortal, it means that she will remain in her "I am dead" state forever, with no possibility of release through death; in effect, a state of "everlasting death" and hence everlasting despair. This, as has already been suggested, is the greatest despair of all. As Kierkegaard (1941) stated:

> When death is the greatest danger, one hopes for life, but when one becomes acquainted with an even more dreadful danger, one hopes for death. So when the danger is so great that death has become one's hope, despair is the disconsolateness of not being able to die.

Sociology

The suggestion that many of the more overt features of Cotard's syndrome are artefacts, the products of chronic institutionalisation, has been made by certain continental observers (Lafand, 1973; Bourgeois, 1980; Trémine, 1982). This would, on the face of it, appear to be unlikely but, if true, should be associated with the decline in the frequency of case reporting in forthcoming years.

In the context of the case of a 42-year-old woman who believed that she had been killed by a ghost, consistent with her Persian background and belief system, Nejad et al. (2013) have pointed out that "cultural and superstitious beliefs could affect the forming of the complex constellation of the patient's symptoms including Cotard's syndrome symptoms."

Existential aspects

Cotard's symptomatology essentially amounts to the most extreme degree of denial of self. This is a vital point to emphasise because of what it illustrates about the human condition. Before one can deny self, one must firstly be aware of self. By this is meant the totality of self – somatic sensations, emotions, cognitions, mental imagery, continuity with one's past, one's anticipated future and, therefore, the relationship one has with time. This phenomenon is perhaps, at least in phylogenetic terms, the highest mental experience and probably most distinguishes man from other known life forms. It is first and foremost an introspective experience, and in the words of Eccles (1989): "It implies knowing that one knows."

This theme is further developed by Dobzhansky (1967): "Self-awareness is, then, one of the fundamental, possibly the most fundamental, characteristic of the human species ... Self-awareness has, however, brought in its train sober companions – fear, anxiety and death awareness."

This unique possession of man may help, therefore, perhaps to explain some aspects of Cotard's syndrome, such as the rarity of the symptomatology in adolescence and in those of low IQ. It can be postulated that both of these groups are characterised by an immaturity not conducive to the development of such a sophisticated condition. Furthermore, if the seat of self-awareness is accepted as residing in (at least some) areas of brain activity, then the potential full significance of Joseph and O'Leary's (1986) findings of inter-hemispheric atrophy becomes apparent and may well resurrect an idea proposed by Flechsig, who in 1920 regarded the frontal lobes to be the anatomical substrate for consciousness.

Management and treatment

The *specific treatment* of Cotard's syndrome is essentially that of the underlying condition of which it is part. As it seems to be more frequently observed in patients with affective psychosis, antidepressants may be effective. These are usually administered orally, but Lopes et al. (2013) described the successful use of intravenous clomipramine in a 50-year-old female patient whose symptoms had not responded to oral treatment with paroxetine and olanzapine.

Augmentation with the dopamine agonist bromocriptine has been reported to be effective in a 72-year-old female patient in whom Cotard's syndrome and depressive symptoms had failed to respond to treatment with a combination of clomipramine and lithium (Kondo et al., 2003), while the dopamine agonist pramipexole has been similarly used to avoid fibrotic cardiac valvopathy (Takahashi et al., 2010). Maruo et al. (2016) have described a case in which the use of pramipexole as augmentation therapy in the case of a 62-year-old female patient with Cotard's syndrome whose symptoms were resistant to quetiapine, olanzapine, aripiprazole and duloxetine (in this order), given in addition to mirtazapine and lorazepam, was associated with improvement in nihilistic delusions and depressive symptoms within about two months. However, after a further two months the patient developed abnormal behaviours, such as eating the food of other patients; these behaviours gradually disappeared during the two months following discontinuation of pramipexole treatment.

Owing to the presence of delusions, ECT may be more strongly indicated, and indeed it is advocated by some authors as the treatment of choice (e.g. Mughal and Menezes, 2013; Mamaeva et al., 2016). It is noteworthy how our Cases 1-3, and to a lesser extent Case 4, responded to treatment by these means (Majeron and Finavera, 1975).

When the syndrome is linked to a chronic schizophrenic illness, as in Case 5, who suffered with nihilistic delusions for over 30 years, the prognosis is clearly much worse. However, in other schizophrenic patients where the onset is more acute, although the symptoms are bizarre and severe, there may well be a rapid improvement with the administration of neuroleptic drugs, as was the situation in our Case 6. Sulpiride has been successfully used to treat Cotard's syndrome in schizophrenia (Shiraishi et al., 2004), while amongst third generation antipsychotics, aripiprazole monotherapy has been reported to be successful (De Berardis et al., 2010). In some cases, therapeutic success may follow the combined use of an antidepressant and an antipsychotic drug; reported cases include the successful use of imipramine with risperidone (Machado et al., 2016) and escitalopram with aripiprazole (De Berardis et al., 2015).

One implication of Berrios and Luque's (1995a) findings, regarding the possible existence of a pure Cotard's syndrome, is that it would suggest that neuroleptics are the treatment of choice in this group rather than antidepressants. This, however, is an hypothesis that remains to be tested.

If the syndrome occurs in association with some organic state, the treatment will be that of the underlying condition, if this is possible. If it is part of a pre-senile or a senile dementia, then there is little likelihood of improvement. If, however, it is part of a toxic confusional state, then it may clear completely with adequate treatment, and examples of this are reported in the literature, including a case of typhoid fever manifested as an acute Cotard's syndrome (Campbell et al., 1981). Ahlheid's (1968) three patients with mixed pathology give us an indication of the prognosis in such cases.

Apart from those forms of treatment, which may be considered as more or less specific, there are several more *general measures* to be considered. Thus patients with Cotard's syndrome are often so distressed that suicide can be a definite risk. Although they may protest that they are already dead, they may at the same time contemplate suicide. Because of this, close observation is essential, especially if the patient is suffering from a depressive illness. Such close surveillance is even more essential when recovery begins, for at this point the patient may become more active and thus be in a better position to take steps to kill herself. Overall, psychotherapeutic support is always needed; these patients are frightened and despairing people and benefit greatly from contact with the caring professions.

Prognosis

The prognosis of Cotard's syndrome must be guarded. Complete recovery may occur as spontaneously and as suddenly as its onset, even in the most severe cases. However, in milder cases that have not yet developed the complete classical picture, recovery may be rapid or gradual. If the nihilistic delusions are related to an acute psycho-organic syndrome, the prognosis is good and the condition will tend to resolve.

If it is associated with a depressive illness, it may well persist even when the other symptoms of the depressive illness have cleared. In this situation, and where the condition becomes chronic, the delusional state of negation usually waxes and wanes in intensity, depending on the periodic fluctuations of the depressive disorder.

When the phenomenon is part of a schizophrenic illness, it usually improves when the other symptoms respond to therapy. Alternatively, it can persist for years as part of a chronic schizophrenic condition.

In a number of cases life may eventually become tolerable in spite of the symptoms, the patient exhibiting a state of double orientation. Thus she may become immersed in a fabulous pseudoreality from which she cannot detach herself and yet be able to look after herself and maintain contact with others. If the delusion becomes completely encapsulated, the subject may even be able to assume a jovial mood and to engage in a philosophical discussion about her own existence or non-existence (De Martis, 1956).

References

Ahlheid, A. (1968) *Lavoro Neuropsichiatrico*, *43*, 927.
Anderson, E.W. (1964) *Psychiatry*, *1st edn*. Ballière, Tindall and Cox, London.
Arieti, S. (1974) *American Handbook of Psychiatry*, *2nd edn*. Basic Books, New York.
Arnaud, F.L. (1892) *Annales Medico-Psychologiques*, *50*, 387.
Berrios, G.E., Luque, R. (1995a) *Comprehensive Psychiatry*, *36*, 218.
Berrios, G.E., Luque, R. (1995b) *Acta Psychiatrica Scandinavica*, *91*,185.
Bianchi, L. (1924) In *Trattu di Psichiatra*, Ed. U.T. Idelson. Naples.
Bolzani, L. (1958) *Archivio di Psicologia, Neurologia e Psichiatria*, *19*, 453.
Bourgeois, M. (1980) *Annales Medico-Psychologiques (Paris)*, *138*, 1165.
Campbell, S., Volow, M., Cavenar, J.O. (1981) *American Journal of Psychiatry*, *138*:10, 1377.
Capgras, J., Daumezon, G. (1936) *Annales Medico-Psychologiques*, *94*, 806.
Charland-Verville, V., Bruno, M.-A., Bahri, M.A., Demertzi, A., Desseilles, M., Chatelle, C., et al. (2013) *Cortex*, *49*, 1997.
Chiu, H.F. (1995) *Gen Hosp Psychiatry*, *17*, 54.
Coen-Bonifante, A. (1926) *Note Riv. Psychiatr.*, *14*, 467.
Consoli, A., Soultanian, C., Tanguy, M.L., Laurent, C., Perisse, D., Luque, R., et al. (2007) *Bipolar Disord.*, *9*, 665.
Cotard, J. (1880) *Ann Med Psychol (Paris)*, *4*, 168.

Cotard, J. (1882) *Archives of Neurology*, 4, 152–170, 282–296.

Cotard, J. (1891) *Maladies Cérebrales et Mentales*. Ballière, Paris.

Cremieux, A., Cain, J. (1948) *Annales Medico-Psychologiques*, 106, 76.

De Berardis, D., Brucchi, M., Serroni, N., Rapini, G., Campanella, D., Vellante, F., et al. (2015) *Riv Psichiatr*, 50, 95.

De Berardis, D., Serroni, N., Campanella, D., Marasco, V., Moschetta, F.S., Di Giannantonio, M. (2010) *Prog Neuropsychopharmacol Biol Psychiatry*, 34, 1347.

De Martis, D. (1956) *Riv. Sper. Freniatriá*, 80, 491.

Degiovanni, A., Faure, M., Leveque, J.P., Gaillard, P. (1987) *Annales Medico-Psychologique*, 145, 874.

Dieguez, S. (2018) *Front Neurol Neurosci*, 42, 23.

Dietrich, M. (1971) *Nervenartz*, 42, 140.

Dobzhansky, T. (1967) *The Biology of Ultimate Concern*. The New American Library, New York.

Dugas, M. (1985) *Neuropsychiatric Enfance Adolsc*, 33, 493.

Eccles, J.C. (1989) *Evolution of the Brain*. Routledge, London and New York.

Fattovich, G., Niccolani, F. (1938) *Arch. Gen. Neurol. Psichiatr. Piscol.*, 19, 200.

Fava, G.A., Kellner, R. (1993) *Acta Psychiatr Scand*, 87, 225.

Flechsig, P. (1920) *Anatomie des Menschlichen Gehirns und Rückenmarks auf Myelogenetischen Grundlage*. Leipzig: Thieme.

Förstl, H., Beats, B. (1992) *British Journal of Psychiatry*, 160, 416.

Fuster, J. (1955) *Rev. Psiquiat. v. Psic. Med*, 2, 29.

Greenberg, D., Hochberg, F.H., Murray, G.B. (1984) *American Journal of Psychiatry*, 141.12, 1587.

Grover, S., Aneja, J., Mahajan, S., Varma, S. (2014) *J Neurosci Rural Pract*, 5, S59.

Halfon, O., Mouren-Simeoni, M.C., Dugas, M. (1985) *Annales Medico-Psychologiques*, 143, 876.

Helldén, A., Odar-Cederlöf, I., Larsson, K., Fehrman-Ekholm, I., and Lindén, T. (2007) *BMJ*, 335, 1305.

Joseph, A.B. (1986) *American Journal of Psychiatry*, 47, 605.

Joseph, A.B., O'Leary, D.H. (1986) *Journal of Clinical Psychiatry*, 47, 518.

Kearns, A. (1987) *British Journal of Psychiatry*, 150, 112.

Kierkegaard, S. (1941) *Fear and Trembling and the Sickness unto Death* Trans. W. Lowrie, Princeton University Press, Princeton N.J., Oxford.

Kondo, S., Hayashi, H., Eguchi, T., Oyama, T., Wada, T., Otani, K. (2003) *Prog Neuropsychopharmacol Biol Psychiatry*, 27, 719.

Kretschmer, E. (1952) *Textbook of Medical Psychology*, Trans. E.B. Strauss. Hogarth Press, London.

Kuppili, P.P., Gupta, R., Pattanayak, R.D., Khandelwal, S.K. (2017) *Asian J Psychiatr*, 30, 26.

Lafand, A.M. (1973) *Du d·lire chronique des n·gations comme survivance asilaire* (thesis No 112). Paris, France.

Leroy, E. (1920) *Annales Medico-Psycholgiques*, 160.

Lopes, R., Costa, I., Curral, R., Esteves, M., Roma-Torres, A. (2013) *Rev Bras Psiquiatr*, 35, 212.

Machado, L., Filho, L.E., Machado, L. (2016) *Case Rep Med, 2016*, 5101357.

Majeron, F., Finavera, L. (1975) *Minerva Medica*, 66, 4269.

Mamaeva, T., Christensen, D.S., Nielsen, C.T. (2016) *Ugeskr Laeger*, *178*, V04160230

Maruo, J., Haraguchi, Y., Tateishi, H., Noguchi, T., Mizoguchi, Y., Kato, T.A., et al. (2016) *Psychogeriatrics*, *16*, 283.

Matsukura, S., Yoshimi, H., Sueoka, S., Chihara, K., Fujita, T., Tanimoto, K. (1981) *Lancet*, *1*, 162.

Mignot, H., Lacassagne, A.M. (1937) *Annales Medico-Psychologiques*, *95*, 246.

Mughal, F., Menezes, S.B. (2013) *Ment Illn*, *5*, e3.

Nardi, M.G. (1935) *Riv. M. Parol. Nerv. Ment*, *45*, 664.

Nejad, A.G. (2002) *Acta Psychiatr Scand*, *106*, 156.

Nejad, A.G., Anari, A.M.Z., Pouya, F. (2013) *Iranian Journal of Psychiatry and Behavioral Sciences*, *7*, 91.

Ozkan, N., Caliyurt, O. (2016) *Aust N Z J Psychiatry*, *50*, 600.

Parks, N.E., Rigby, H.B., Gubitz, G.J., Shankar, J.J., Purdy, R.A. (2014) *Cephalalgia*, *34*, 717.

Pearn, J., Gardner-Thorpe, C. (2002) *Neurology*, *58*, 1400.

Poli, C. (1942) *Rass. Stud. Psichiatr*, *31*, 394.

Perris, C. (1955). *Noropsychiatrica*, *11*, 175.

Régis, E. (1893) *Gazette Méd. Paris* *2*(6), 61.

Reich, M., Comet, B., Le Rhun, E., Ramirez, C. (2012) *Palliative and Supportive Care*, *10*, 135.

Saavedra, V. (1968) *Rev. Neuropsichiatrico*, *31*, 145.

Sahoo, A., Josephs, K.A. (2018) *J Neuropsychiatry Clin Neurosci*, *30*, 58.

Séglas, J. (1897) *La Délire de Negation*, Vol. 1. Masson, Paris.

Shiraishi, H., Ito, M., Hayashi, H., Otani, K. (2004) *Progress in Neuropsychopharmacology and Biological Psychiatry*, *28*, 607.

Silva, J., Leong, G., Weinstock, R., Gonzales, C. (2000) *Journal of Forensic Sciences*, *45*, 188.

Sottile, F., De Luca, R., Bonanno, L., Finzi, G., Casella, C., Calabrò, R.S. (2018) *Issues Ment Health Nurs*, *39*, 353.

Takahashi, T., Nibuya, M., Nomura, S. (2010) *J Neuropsychiatry Clin Neurosci*, *22*, E27.

Trémine, T. (1982) *Evol. Psychiatr*, *47*, 1021.

Vitetta, M. (1962) *Rass. Stud. Psichiatr*, *51*, 39.

Walloch, J.E., Klauwer, C., Lanczik, M., Brockington, I.F., Kornhuber, J. (2007) *Psychopathology*, *40*, 61.

Yarnada, K., Katsuragi, S., Fujii, I. (1999) *Acta Psychiatr Scand*, *100*, 396.

Young, A.W., Leafhead, K.M. (1996) in *Method in Madness: Case Studies in Cognitive Neuropsychiatry*. Hove, Psychology Press.

Young, A.W., Leafhead, K.M., Szulecka, T.K. (1994) *Psychopathology*, *27*, 226.

Zilboorg, G., Henry, G.W. (1941) *A History of Medical Psychology*. Allen and Unwin, London.

Chapter 9

Folie à deux
(et folie à plusiers)

I ... pray you to remember, that when two lutes or two harps, near to one
another, both set to the same tune, if you touch the strings to the one, the
other consonant harp will sound at the same time, though nobody touch it.
Sir Kenelm Digby, *A Late Discourse Made in a Solemn Assembly* (1658)

The term *folie à deux* includes several syndromes in which mental
symptoms, particularly paranoid delusions, are transmitted from one
person to one or more others with whom the apparent instigator is in
some way intimately associated, so that he, she or they also come to share
the same delusional ideas.

Historical

The term appears to have been first coined by Lasègue and Falret in a
preliminary communication followed by a fuller account (including the
description of seven cases) to the Société Médico-Psychologique in 1873
and 1877, respectively. Accounts of similar conditions had, however,
been given earlier:

1635 Primrose
1651 Harvey (described the case of pseudocyesis affecting two sisters)
1764–1838 Whytt, Haygarth, Pritchard, Millingen, Berlyn and Idelar
("infectiousness of insanity")
1846 Hofbauer ("psychic infection")
1860 Baillarger (*folie à communiquée*)

Many synonyms have been used, most reflecting the idea of the condition's transmissibility, viz. "communicated insanity," "contagious insanity," "infectious insanity," "psychosis of association" and "double
insanity." Although the condition usually involves two people, it can
extend from the original subject to three, four, five persons, viz. *folie à*

trois, folie à quatre, folie à cinq, or even a whole family, *folie à famille* (or *folie en famille*).

Many cases have been described in the English-language medical literature, some attempting to sub-classify the condition (Marandon de Montyel, 1881; Tuke, 1887); some providing a psychopathological interpretation (Brill, 1920; Gralnick, 1942); and some to demonstrate the co-existence of *folie à deux* with other uncommon psychiatric syndromes: with Munchausen's syndrome (Janofsky, 1986); with Capgras' and de Clérambault's syndromes (Signer and Isbister, 1987); with Capgras' syndrome (Hart and McClue, 1989; Christodoulou et al., 1995); with Fregoli syndrome (Wolff and McKenzie, 1994); both of the last two are forms of delusional misidentification; with Cotard's syndrome, a nihilistic and hypochondriacal delusion (Wolff and McKenzie, 1994) and other delusional syndromes such as *koro* (Westermayer, 1989).

Gralnick (1942) claimed to have reviewed all cases reported in the English-language literature from 1879 until 1942, a total of 103. Rioux (1963) reviewed the cases recorded in the English language; McNeil et al. (1972) reviewed those in which the subject was aged over 65 years; Soni and Rockley (1974) also carried out a review, as did Mentjox et al. (1993), who included all of the case reports between 1974 and 1991, a total of 76 case descriptions and a total of 107 recipients.

Kashiwase and Kato (1997) reviewed 97 cases in the Japanese literature over a period of 90 years. A total of 75% of the cases involved two individuals. Delusion was the commonest shared symptom. Sister-sister combinations were less frequent, and younger subjects influenced the older ones more often than is the case in Western society, and acute religious delusions occurred more frequently. Recognition of the global nature of *folie à deux* is illustrated by the publication of case reports from countries such as Brazil (Nunes et al., 2016), China (Tay and Li, 2017), Nepal (Chalise et al., 2015) and India (Tikka et al., 2013).

Silveira and Seeman (1995) analysed persistent cases in the English literature from 1942 to 1993 using modern nosology and biopsychological formulations including *DSM-IV*. Arnone et al. (2006) extended this review from 1993 to 2005, without any restriction on publication language, but otherwise employing similar inclusion criteria to those of Silveira and Seeman (1995). Of the 103 cases that met the inclusion criteria, significant differences were found in some of the demographic characteristics between primary and secondary cases. For instance, primary cases were on average about six years older than the secondary cases; females outnumbered males in both groups by a ratio of about 2:1. Spousal relationships accounted for almost 40% of cases, while sibling relationships made up 28% (in 8 of the 29 sibling cases, the relationship was that of twins). In only 6–7% of cases was there a non-biological or non-spousal relationship. In terms of dyad risk factors, social isolation was considered to be a major factor in over three-quarters of all cases; the duration of the association showed a wide range from less than a month to 948 months. The commonest diagnosis in the primary cases falling in the 1942–93 period was schizophrenia. In all of these 54 instances, the diagnosis for the secondary case was pure shared delusional disorder with some co-morbidities in the form of depression, dementia and mental retardation. For the 1993–2005 period, the most frequent diagnoses in primary cases was delusional disorder and schizophrenia, while pure induced delusional disorder accounted for almost three-quarters of the secondary cases. The nature of the delusions was most commonly persecutory in all groups and time periods.

The condition (and variants of it) is recognised in *ICD-10*, where it is referred to as *induced delusional disorder* (code F24); in the beta version of *ICD-11* available at the time of writing, induced delusional disorder is categorised under 6A24.7 *delusional disorder, unspecified*. It is also included in *DSM-IV*, in which it is manifested as *shared psychotic disorder* (code 297.3). In *DSM-5*, shared psychotic disorder no longer occurs, but the condition is categorised under *other specified schizophrenia spectrum and other psychotic disorder* (code 298.8 [F28]):

Delusional symptoms in partner of individual with delusional disorder: In the context of a relationship, the delusional material from the dominant partner provides content for delusional belief by the individual who may not otherwise entirely meet criteria for delusional disorder.

(American Psychiatric Association, 2013)

Folie à deux is undoubtedly an intriguing condition of very great relevance to the understanding of human psychopathology. It is perhaps the most impressive example of a pathological relationship and, therefore, an understanding of its underlying mechanisms has theoretical implications for other kinds of disturbed interpersonal relationships.

Case reports

Case I

Margaret and her husband, Michael, both aged 34 years, were discovered to be suffering from *folie à deux* when both were found to be sharing similar persecutory delusions. They believed that certain persons were entering their house, spreading dust and fluff and "wearing down their shoes." Both had, in addition, other symptoms supporting a diagnosis of paranoid psychosis, which could be made independently in either case.

Michael had first been admitted to hospital two years previously with an atypical depression accompanied by delusions of both wickedness and grandiosity which responded to ECT, following which he was discharged and prescribed chlorpromazine as an outpatient. During his hospital admission, it was recorded that Margaret had expressed similar delusional ideas when seen by the hospital social worker.

The following year Michael was admitted once again for a further month, with a delusion on this occasion that he was a multiple murderer and with marked feelings of guilt on this account. Although given ECT again, this failed to benefit his condition. This did, however, gradually respond to chlorpromazine so that his suicidal impulses gradually disappeared and his delusions faded. Six months later Margaret was seen as an outpatient at her own request, allegedly to discuss her husband's condition. It was observed, once more, that she too was markedly deluded, her delusions being focussed on her neighbours, whom she accused of deliberately annoying her and of entering her house when she was asleep or out in order to damage her furniture.

Margaret was the dominant partner who initiated the delusions which she and her husband shared. She, herself, had no insight into her condition and denied being ill in any way. Her personality was well preserved; she was of good average intelligence and worked as a clerk. While being quite uncompromising about her delusional beliefs, she nevertheless accepted that she would have to continue to tolerate her situation, stating that those who were responsible for persecuting her and her husband were persons of authority who, because the curtains were drawn, had access to the flats on either side and entered theirs through a trap door.

Michael was of lesser intelligence than his wife. His personality was inadequate; he had some sociopathic traits and was prone to bouts of heavy drinking. He had a poor work record and was described by his wife as childish and irresponsible. He believed for his part that their "persecutors" gained entry by using a skeleton key in order to gain revenge for his having killed some German prisoners of war when, he alleged, he was a child of 7 years.

Three years after his second admission to hospital, he was admitted for the third time, with a mixture of depression and schizophrenic symptoms. Again he was treated with ECT and chlorpromazine so that when discharged from hospital his condition was somewhat improved.

Case 2

Edward, aged 72 years, and his sister, Susannah, aged 79 years, were both admitted to hospital sharing delusions that their neighbours were trying to poison them, influencing them through the grates and accusing them of bestiality with dogs and of causing foul murders on the local heath. They had complained to every conceivable authority including various councils, the police, the vicar and their general practitioner. Six years previously they had tried to rid themselves of this "persecution" by moving house, but within a few months they began to develop similar delusions about their new neighbours. Their house was in fact very clean and tidy, with everything kept in its rightful place and cash set aside ready to pay bills as they fell due. They, too, were clean, well kept and well nourished. They had lived together all their lives, very much isolated even from their local community, and for most of the time had been in conflict with their neighbours.

Susannah was the dominant personality, somewhat more intelligent and garrulous than the brother, although both were of low average intelligence. However, both also possessed a certain degree of native cunning and competence, as was reflected by the fact that they managed their affairs and their house well.

Susannah, who was known to have suffered from paranoid schizophrenia for many years, had dominated her brother, who had accepted and shared her delusions for over 12 years before their first hospital admission.

These shared delusions were first noted when, seven years previously, Edward was admitted to hospital after being accused of indecently exposing himself to a young girl. He was depressed and suffered with a paranoid psychosis, some of his delusions being shared by his sister. Following their joint first admission to hospital, both were given thioridazine, which alleviated their symptoms, although they recurred when they discontinued the drug on discharge. Because of this both had to be readmitted for a few months for the second time. A year later, Susannah, now over 80 years, was again readmitted in a very feeble physical state. She died towards the end of the year, still firmly clinging to her paranoid delusions which she had shared with her brother for many years.

Case 3

A family consisting of a mother, aged 66 years, a son, Cyril, aged 41 years, and a daughter, Dorothy, aged 43 years, were diagnosed as suffering from *folie à trois*. They shared the delusion that their neighbours "up the road" and "round the corner" were persecuting them in order to get them out of their house. It was mother who appeared to be the dominant personality who had initiated these delusions which both son and daughter completely shared, adding evidence of their own in support. Their mother was diagnosed as suffering from a paranoid psychosis (paraphrenia) and both the son and daughter from paranoid schizophrenia.

The history of their shared delusions was of five years' duration before first being seen and for 12 years thereafter. While mother had never been referred to a psychiatrist, it was found that both Cyril and Dorothy had a 14-year history of psychiatric disorder, both initially having been diagnosed as suffering from neurotic illness. Cyril was the first to seek psychiatric help when he began to complain of giddiness, an inability to mix or travel on public transport, imagining also that he had various physical complaints. He had worked as a lead glazier until eight months previously. He was diagnosed as suffering from an anxiety state, but it was noted at the same time that "he does not want to work as he thinks he is not well treated there." He was seen again two years later and diagnosed as suffering from a severe obsessional neurosis together with sexual infantilism that was treated with testosterone implants from which he himself defaulted. A year after this, he was observed to have emotional flattening and affective incongruity and to be rambling in speech. He was considered, therefore, to be suffering from schizophrenia.

In Cyril's initial case record, Dorothy was recorded as having been ill for three years before Cyril, although she had not then sought psychiatric help. She was, however, first seen by a psychiatrist three years after her brother's initial consultation. She had worked as a domestic, a cinema usherette and in her mother's shop. Her periods were always regular and normal, although she too had an "infantile" appearance. When seen she complained of something prickly in her throat, pains in the back, especially on eating or drinking, being unable to lift anything because of headaches and having to wear soft shoes. Her condition was initially diagnosed as conversion hysteria, although the bizarre nature of her complaints, her inability to come to the point and her claim to come from a noble family were noted. She reiterated her numerous bizarre hypochondriacal complaints when seen again two years later.

While at the time of Dorothy's initial consultation her mother was reported as being over-protective, there was, then, no evidence of a clear paranoid psychotic illness in her case. Only 10 years later was a state of *folie à trois* found to be present, her mother admitting at this juncture to persecutory ideas of five years standing. While for a time all three remained at home, Dorothy's general condition soon began to give cause for concern. She was very distressed and preoccupied with her bizarre hypochondriacal symptoms while exhibiting thought disorder and frank delusions. Hers was the first of a series of hospital admissions, always with marked hypochondriasis. She would complain of a hole in her chest and of "lumps of flesh in my tummy coming up to my throat." This was a feature of both her first two hospital admissions during which she was also very depressed. She always improved in hospital but soon deteriorated on returning home to her mother and brother. While in hospital she was treated with phenothiazines, which she discontinued on returning home. Cyril was also admitted the same year under a compulsory order, having become very agitated, excited and hostile. In hospital a diagnosis of paranoid schizophrenia was confirmed, and he too was treated with phenothiazines, improving behaviourally, although his delusions persisted. Later he and his mother were seen by a psychiatrist who visited their home on two widely separate occasions in order to examine Dorothy. All three of them were found to be markedly deluded about their neighbours, with complete lack of insight and refusing to consider any kind of help or treatment.

Case 4

(We are grateful to Professor Andrew Sims for permission to include this case and also to the *British Journal of Psychiatry* in which it was first published.) *John*, aged 40 years, when first seen as an outpatient, was an electrician with an added interest in electronics. He complained that six months previously a very large industrial concern had put "bugging" devices in the wall of his brother George's house, that the company's agents had been following him in order to stop him interfering, and that they had also "bugged his telephone." He knew that the telephone was "bugged" because it sometimes made a crackling noise and also that his brother's walls were "bugged," not only because George told him so but because he had showed him blemishes on the walls. He agreed that blemishes in the hospital wall plaster looked similar but insisted that the house was "bugged" although the hospital was not. He also took as further evidence the fact that vertical lines sometimes appeared on George's television screen. This, he believed, proved that the devices interfered with the television "like a radar set." Then when his own television set showed vertical lines, he knew that his house had been "bugged" as well, believing that some men had put a device on his garage roof when doing some work on the house.

George lived next door to an old woman who had, at one time, also worked for the same major industrial electronic concern as he had done. Although she lived on her own, both John and his wife, Rose, believed they had heard men's voices coming from her home and that the men "operated from there," adding that George had recognised four of their voices. John said the reason for the company's interest in George was that he had worked for them but had to resign through ill health. The company, John said, was trying to find out if George was ill or not and whether he was entitled to a pension. He stated, "I can't understand why they are doing it. They know the tablets he is on."

John suffered from asthma as a child. Although he described a "nervous breakdown" when aged 18 years, not requiring admission to hospital, he was well enough three months later to be called up for National Service. Following discharge from the army, he had an excellent work record with two firms, during which time he had no history of psychiatric treatment. He remained off work for four weeks because he was upset and frightened, apparently on account of reprisals which he imagined might occur on account of his trying to help his brother. He refused admission to hospital but was prescribed phenothiazines as an outpatient. His condition was diagnosed, at this juncture, as paranoid schizophrenia.

At subsequent intervals he said that he was feeling better and had returned to work. He stated that the "bugging devices" were still there, "but I don't take any notice of them anymore. If we had the money to go to a solicitor we would do something about it." His beliefs remained unchanged for over a year. He was irritated that the men following him had not been removed and refused to take what had been prescribed, "because I don't believe in tablets."

Rose, John's wife, aged 42 years, who had been treated for anxiety for several years, was concerned about her husband's health, feeling that worry was making him ill as well. They had been married for eight years but had no children because she had been told she could develop Huntingtons' chorea, having apparently a positive family history of this disorder. Initially she corroborated John's story and said that "bugging" devices had been placed to find out what disablement category George was entitled to for compensation purposes: "You can see hammer marks from devices in the communal wall." She also said that the GPO (General Post Office) had been to the house and confirmed the findings but had done nothing about it. Clearly Rose shared John's beliefs.

Later on she said that life had become intolerable on account of all the precautions her husband had forced her to take against bugging devices being put in their house. For example, he insisted that she buy extra locks. She said that she did not know "how much electronic equipment Ruby's neighbour had" and that she should need proof "before being convinced that anything was going on." She stated that her husband now believed that their home was also bugged. However, she now no longer believed in all this apparent intrigue and had begun to feel that her husband and his relatives were mentally ill, denying at the same time that she had ever been credulous.

George, aged 43 years, John's brother, was interviewed at his home which he shared with his sister, Ruby. He looked rather vacuous, talked little and was submissive towards his sister. He had never married. Over the previous 20 years, he had frequently received drug treatment in various hospitals where he had been considered to be suffering from chronic anxiety neurosis. After working with one firm for 15 years, he was made redundant. He was then employed by the same industrial electronic concern as his brother John for over two years but was dismissed for infrequent attendance. He felt that he should have been discharged with a disability pension as he suffered from frequent migraine. After his dismissal he felt that the old lady next door had started to watch him through her window and had planted "bugging" devices in the telephone, the gramophone and also the electric lights. He believed that portions of the walls and ceilings had been removed to insert more devices and cables and that people worked at night in the space between the chimney breast and the wall and between the false ceiling of the breakfast room and the floor above. He was quite convinced that "bugging" was continuous and operated from the device in the television set. He could tell this by the crackling over the telephone, the rolling picture on the television and the needle jumping on the record player. He also believed that the firm had taken over the empty house next door. He thought that surveillance was carried out to assess the extent of his disability but did not know why it should happen to him.

Ruby, aged 57 years, John's sister, was also interviewed at home. She was obese, sociable and humorous, and clearly the most intelligent and dominant member of the household. In 1962, she had been referred for psychiatric opinion when she complained of stumbling, shaking and feeling giddy. Her condition, then, was diagnosed as "an acute–upon–chronic–anxiety reaction with hysterical features." No psychotic symptoms were elicited at that time.

When interviewed, she talked volubly of the "bugging devices." She appeared agitated and knocked the walls in various places to demonstrate that they were hollow. She passed her hands over the walls to demonstrate bumps in the plaster under which she said the devices were hidden. But although seemingly convinced of their presence, she made, nevertheless, no effort to guard her speech. It appeared that a secret dossier was being compiled by the doctor assigned to carry out the medical examinations for the assessment of disablement benefits. She sent John to the hearing over George's disablement claim because she thought that George would be upset by it. She now felt this was why John was being watched, believing that "they" might even try to kill him if he took the matter further. Following the social worker's visit, Ruby wrote her a letter saying that she had been followed around by two men in a car.

After this two of John's maternal aunts were visited, because Ruby believed that they also might be involved in the plot against her and George. But they apparently knew nothing whatsoever of the family's delusions. Next, Rose's mother, aged 70 years, was visited at her home. She confirmed the family history of Huntingtons' chorea and said that she herself had suffered from neurological symptoms 15 years before. Despite this she herself now showed no intellectual impairment, choreiform movements, tremor or other neuropsychiatric abnormality. Because there were lines going across her television set, John claimed that there were "bugging" devices in her house, claiming also that he had seen three men with ladders on her roof setting these up. Rose's mother, however, said that the whole matter was rubbish: "No firm would waste all that money on one person." She considered Ruby had started the story, that George was very dependent on her and that Ruby had stopped him working so that he could do more of her housework. She had met George's neighbour and considered her to be a "nice woman." She admitted that there were sometimes large cars outside her house, and men going in, but could not explain this. She was certain, however, that George's neighbour was not involved in any plot concerning George.

Roger, Rose's brother, aged 38 years, was considered to be ill by Rose and John and thought to be suffering from Huntingtons' chorea. In fact he had been treated for recurrent depression. There was no evidence of dementia or choreiform movements and he, apparently, knew nothing whatsoever of any "conspiracy."

Case 5

The following example involves five members of a family of six, of whom the sixth might well be included.

Stanley, aged 48 years, was the dominant personality who initiated the family's delusions. His daughter, Joan, aged 23 years, shared her father's delusions, holding them with greater firmness than any other family member. Her mother also shared the delusions but not actively, while her brother, Terence, aged 24 years, also shared the delusions but again not so firmly as in the case of his father and sister, so that they did not interfere so prominently with his day-to-day behaviour. A younger sister, Andrea, aged 15 years, expressed views which betrayed that she too shared her father's delusions, while the youngest sibling of all, an 11-year-old sister, behaved as if she believed her father's delusions but never expressed them.

The family involved were very close-knit, living in a remote rural part of England, very much isolated even from their local community. For a number of years they had been in conflict with various people and agencies, including the neighbours, the council, the Electricity Board and solicitors who had once acted on their behalf.

A climax was reached when the Electricity Board took steps to cut off their electricity as a result of persistent non-payment of bills, although the Board had recognised the correspondence relating to this matter appeared to be rather bizarre if not actually abnormal. The family, and in particular Stanley and his daughter, Joan, aggressively resisted when officials of the Board and a policeman called at the farm to cut off the electricity, becoming even more aggressive when police reinforcements arrived. The Board officials and the police did not wish to prefer any charges, believing that their behaviour was the result of mental illness. It was on this account, therefore, that Stanley and Joan were first referred for psychiatric opinion.

When they were first seen, Stanley expressed very bizarre delusions, insisting that he was "S.H. – deceased." He would brandish a piece of paper on which the words "S.H. – deceased" were written many times, shouting at the top of his voice, "Which of these is dead?" It was difficult, however, to ascertain whether he unequivocally believed that he himself was dead or that others believed that he was dead. However, he seemed to regard the piece of paper with the words "S.H. – deceased" as proof of this. He also signed his letters "S.H. – deceased." Certainly some of his bizarre behaviour arose directly from this central delusion. He refused to pay bills directly, for example to the Electricity Board, saying that it was because he was dead that he could not do so. However, he was prepared to send official letters and cheques in payment of bills to the solicitors who had formerly acted for him but who were now no longer prepared to do so. They had large amounts of correspondence from him that they kept unopened in a basket, having told him on numerous occasions to come and fetch them.

Ten years before, Stanley had leased a property that he wanted to sublet. Protracted negotiations occurred with the council during which his letters became more persecutory in tone and revealed that he believed "someone" was trying to deprive him of the property. His solicitors, at the time, received letters demanding to know who had been given permission for certain buildings to be erected on the site, although no such permission had been given by anyone. These letters were described as "confusing" and "difficult" and largely nonsensical. Seven years later, another episode caused the family much distress. Sewage from a neighbour's property did in fact flow on to their land. Stanley won a court action over this but had to pay £90 towards costs "because of his attitude." He refused to pay and got involved in a long legal action in an attempt to reverse the decision over costs. He failed and then refused to pay his own solicitor, thus adding greatly to his legal costs. Eventually the Official Receiver was called in and Stanley was made bankrupt. In order to try and preserve the family's living, the Official Receiver sequestrated rents until Stanley's debts were cleared, so that he, at one time, was indeed in credit to the amount of £1,500, but he refused to accept this money. He continued to refuse to pay his bills, which led, as described, to his difficulties with the Electricity Board, which brought the situation to a head.

Joan, who was seen at the same time as her father, completely shared his delusions about their being persecuted. She was aggressively non-cooperative. Neither father nor daughter had any insight and were therefore admitted to hospital under compulsory order. It was noted that Stanley was actively aggressive and deluded, possessed a gun and was, on his account, considered to be a danger to others.

The period in hospital under observation confirmed that Stanley had a series of bizarre delusions regarding himself and his affairs. He was diagnosed, therefore, as suffering from a paranoid psychosis. Joan was found to be solitary, lacking in initiative with poverty of ideation. She also exhibited flattening of affect and was diagnosed as suffering from a schizo-affective psychosis. Her history revealed that she had had paranoid traits for several years, on one occasion believing that she had lost her job because of a conspiracy at work.

Both patients were prescribed thioridazine and improved behaviourally. However, on discharge they did not attend for follow-up or visit their doctor for further prescriptions. Stanley began paying his bills until recently, when he again started to write bizarre letters, and the local police received a complaint about a clash with a neighbour.

His wife shared Stanley's central delusion, having no real insight into its true origin, but while she resented the fact that her husband and daughter had been admitted to hospital, she clung less firmly to their delusions and was not as aggressive as they were. Terence, a nice, pleasant and mild-mannered lad, also, at one time, believed unequivocally that his father's delusions were true. Andrea, the 15-year-old daughter fully supported her father, sharing his delusions. She was resentful and aggressive and expressed these ideas verbally. The 11-year-old daughter did not verbalise her ideas but was also resentful and supported the family's opposition to the authorities.

Epidemiology

There have been, as described, several reviews of the cases in the English medical literature. Exact figures for the incidence and prevalence of *folie à deux* are not available. Spradley (in Grover, 1937) noted a frequency of 29 persons in 1,700 consecutive admissions (1.7%) to an American state hospital, but there is no detail regarding the methodology underlying this figure. Cases have been reported beyond Western societies, including in Nigeria and India (Ilechukwu and Okyere, 1987; Pande and Gulabani, 1990). It has been emphasised that the condition does occur in people over the age of 65, but the incidence appears to be the same as in the population as a whole (McNeil et al., 1972).

Folie à deux is certainly more common than when the authors first reported. Increasing reports appear in the literature, and in addition many go unrecognised because such patients rarely seek treatment and there is a neglect of the assessment of the families of patients who are recognised as psychotic (Sacks, 1988).

As is expected, the condition becomes less common as the number of persons involved increases. Glassman et al. (1987) found only 20 cases in the literature where whole families were involved. *Folie à deux* is one of the conditions we have researched for over 50 years which remains, apparently, uncommon. It becomes less so with the interest that other authors have shown as a result of their researches. It is certainly more common in isolated communities and families where there is a great urge to defend the *status quo*.

Sex distribution

Women are found to be predominant in the reported cases (Lasègue and Falret, 1877; Gralnick, 1942), constituting 72% of principals and 54% of associates in those cases in which sex was reported (Mentjox et al., 1993). This was also found to be the case, for both principals and associates, in the reviews from 1942 to 1993 (Silveira and Seeman, 1995) and 1993 to 2005 (Arnone et al., 2006), as described earlier in this chapter. Gralnick suggested that the reason for this was the restricted social roles of women, while Mentjox et al. (1993) suggested that it was because of the frequent caring role of women within relationships. However, with the changing role of women in modern society, and yet an apparent increase in the condition, this hypothesis would not seem adequately to explain the situation.

Relationship between subjects

Usually these are relationships within families such as husband and wife, mother and child and two siblings. Gralnick (1942), for example, reported 103 cases with a total of 238 subjects involved. The following relationships were found:

- Two (or more) sisters – 34%
- Husband and wife – 22%
- Mother and child – 20%
- Two (or more) brothers – 9%
- Brothers and sisters – 5%
- Father and child – 2%
- Non-consanguineous fellow patients or friends – 8%

Some cases involving twins have been reported (Gralnick, 1942; Kendler et al., 1986; Lazarus, 1986; Shiwach and Sobin, 1998; Florez and Gomez-Reino, 2001; Francois et al., 2017; Shah et al., 2017), including a case of *folie a quatre* involving monozygotic twins (Ohnuma and Arai, 2015).

Mentjox et al. (1993) reported on 76 cases with 107 associates. The commonest relationship was mother-child with a frequency of 21%, followed by wife-husband – 19%; woman-sibling – 17%; husband-wife – 13%.

The corresponding figures in the reviews from 1942 to 1993 (Silveira and Seeman, 1995) and 1993 to 2005 (Arnone et al., 2006) were referred to earlier in this chapter.

Clinical features

The clinical features of the syndrome are:

- The primary feature is the occurrence of shared delusions in two or more persons who live in close proximity and who are usually relatively isolated from the outside world and its influences.
- The delusions are usually of a persecutory or hypochondriacal content.
- Only one of the persons involved suffers with an inherent psychotic disorder, usually schizophrenia but sometimes affective in nature. This subject is the "primary patient," "inducer" or "principal" who transfers his delusions to the secondary "partner," "acceptor" or "associate," both then supporting each other in their beliefs and thus helping to sustain the condition.
- On separation, providing that it is sufficiently complete and prolonged, the shared delusions in the second partner *may* clear.
- The majority of patients are blood relatives with certain combinations within a family being more frequent than others. Most frequently two sisters are affected. A mother-child combination is more often found than a father-child combination. In non-consanguineous groups, husband-wife combinations are most common.
- The relationship of this affected pair or of members of a family is usually, if not always, one of dominance and submission. It is the dominant member of the pair or family who usually is the first to become ill. Apart from his (or her) dominance, he is usually a more obviously forceful personality, more intelligent, better educated and the one looked up to by the submissive partner. The submissive partner usually shows evidence of a disturbed pre-morbid personality, often being over-dependent and suggestible with a history of having had neurotic traits during earlier years, often of being seclusive, suspicious, shy and sometimes irritable and depressed. He/she is thereby the secondary patient (Munro, 1986).

It should be noted that the shared psychiatric disorder could be non-psychotic in nature. Mergui et al. (2010) described a married couple in which the wife developed the same obsessive-compulsive disorder symptomology as her husband; neither spouse exhibited any evidence of psychosis. Similarly, Grover and Gupta (2006) described shared obsessive-compulsive disorder in two sisters.

Subgroups

Within a decade of its introduction, Marandon de Montyel (1894) proposed the division of *folie à deux* into three subtypes: *folie imposée*, *folie simultanée* and *folie communiquée*; a fourth variety, *folie induite*, being added by Lehmann, 1885. Although the subtypes are of limited value, they have come by common usage to be regarded as classical subdivisions of *folie à deux* and therefore are described in more detail as follows.

Folie imposée

This is said to be the commonest form of the condition in which the patient who suffers from the primary psychosis is dominant. Lasègue and Falret (1877) regarded him as the "active element; more intelligent than the other, he creates the delusion and progressively imposes it upon the second, who constitutes the passive element." The second individual, who is both submissive and suggestible, does not suffer from a true psychosis but is simply "*un malade par reflet*" who, when separated from his dominant partner, will abandon his own seemingly delusional ideas.

Folie simultanée

The term was first used by Régis, 1881 and describes a form of the condition in which delusions occur simultaneously but independently in two persons in close association for a long time who are hereditarily predisposed to psychotic illness. As there is no dominant partner, separation does not in itself improve the condition of either. We agree with Dewhurst and Todd (1956) that one person always develops the delusion first, albeit for only a short period. Therefore *folie simultanée* could be regarded as redundant.

Folie communiquée

First described by Baillarger (1860), it refers to a similar form in which two persons, also hereditarily predisposed to psychotic breakdown, are living in close association but in which the second subject develops psychotic symptoms only after a variable period of time. While initially the second patient shares the content of the delusional ideas of the first, these later assume an autonomy of their own and have a fresh delusional content not derived from initiation by the first subject. Again, separation of the two subjects does not effect improvement in the condition of either.

Folie induite

This, as Marandon de Montyel pointed out, is really no more than a variant of *folie communiquée* whereby one who is already deluded "enriches his delusions" with those of a fellow patient, when both are lodged in the same hospital. It is said to be very uncommon. Dewhurst and Todd (1956) regarded *folie induite* also as redundant because the cases can be classified under other subtypes. Munro (1986) regards only the division into *folie imposée* and *folie simultanée* as useful, because the management of cases differ, *folie communiquée* and *folie induit* being variants of *folie simultanée*. Indeed it appears that the distinction into subtypes is only useful in as much as it comments upon the diagnosis of the secondary patient and indicates if any treatment is required.

Aetiology and psychopathology

Heredity is likely to be of significance only in cases involving pairs of identical twins. Organic factors may assume greater importance where the sufferers are elderly. Both genetic and organic factors may possibly also occupy a more prominent aetiological position in the subgroup *folie simultanée*. In the majority of cases, however, it is psychological and environmental forces which play the more prominent aetiological roles.

A key aspect is the nature of the relationship between the inducer and the induced. Traditionally, this has been viewed in terms of a dominant–submissive axis. Psychodynamically, the submissive induced person unconsciously acquires the characteristics of the more dominant inducer. This relationship has also been described and explained in terms of learning theory.

A factor of supreme importance is that of the wider environment, more specifically, social isolation. Social isolation allows the domination of the weaker partner by the stronger of the pair; transmission of the delusion is mediated by the mechanism of suggestion.

The model proposed by Coleman and Last (1939) laid down the fundamental aetiological prerequisites for a case of *folie à deux* to develop. They are as follows:

> The inducer must be in the early stages of illness – that is, before he becomes completely withdrawn from reality – in order to be able positively to influence the induced.
> The inducer and induced must be in close proximity for a relatively long time, to provide the opportunity for the former to influence the latter.
> Sharing the induced delusion must be of some advantage to the induced person.
> In the eyes of the induced, the inducer must represent an authority figure. The condition most commonly develops when the persons involved are living in poverty.

Dewhurst and Todd (1956) listed the following as prerequisites for the diagnosis:

* Definite evidence that the partners had been in intimate association
* A high degree of commonality in the content of the delusion, although the formal psychosis may differ
* Unequivocal evidence that the partners share, support and accept each other's delusions

Although there have been some modifications of these views and more detailed, perhaps deeper, interpretations made, especially by the psychodynamic and psychoanalytic schools, much of Coleman and Last's contentions are clearly valid.

Contagious or not?

Early authors were intrigued by the phenomenon of *folie à deux* and the apparent wholesale transfer of delusions, without modifications, from one person to another. It implied (almost) a bizarre form of infective process – the concept of "mental contagion" discussed by Lasègue and Falret. It was clear, however, that such a mechanism only occurred under certain circumstances. After all, the transfer of delusional ideas from one unrelated patient to another detained in a psychiatric ward was extremely uncommon, despite their close proximity and the length of time spent in the shared environment (this concept of contagion will be revisited later in this chapter).

Heredity

The fact that the vast majority of cases seem to occur in family groupings suggests that either hereditary aspects, tensions within the family relationships, or both are the pathogenic factors.

Although the overwhelming representation of related individuals found in the reported examples of *folie à deux* could hint at the importance of genetic factors, heredity alone cannot explain the occurrence of the condition in husband-wife combinations or other non-consanguineous relationships. Hereditary influences could, however, possibly play a more prominent role in the cases in which the sufferers represent a pair of twins.

In the context of a case report of *folie simultanée* in monozygotic twins, White (1995) reviewed 16 twin cases from the English literature, most of which also involved monozygotic twins. Some authors have emphasised the over-representation of the subgroup *folie simultanée* in this sample. It has been suggested that in such cases the two individuals who share an identical high genetic loading for psychosis are influenced by environmental factors in the same manner. This process thereby determines the timing and presentation of the psychosis in each of the sufferers. It should not be forgotten, however, that the over-representation of monozygotic twins could simply represent a form of reporting bias. More recent reviews support a genetic component in the manifestation of *folie à deux*, with the finding that affected monozygotic twin pairs tend to be diagnosed with delusional disorder, while affected non-monozygotic pairs tend to have a diagnosis of schizophrenia in the inducer and of delusional disorder in the induced (Shiwach and Sobin, 1998; Shah et al., 2017).

Biological factors

Organic factors may play a role where the condition occurs in elderly subjects, approximately one-third of whom (according to McNeil et al., 1972) have organic brain syndromes. *Folie simultanée* is also said to be more commonly represented in this sample.

Folie à deux has been reported to be associated with a number of organic disorders in the inducer, for example, Huntingtons' disease (Huntingtons' chorea) (Roth et al., 2010). Caribé et al. (2013) described a case of *folie à trois* in which the inducer was diagnosed with systemic lupus erythematosus with psychotic features.

It is instructive to consider the case of a 32-year-old man who presented to a Texan dermatology clinic with a main complaint of "bugs flying out of my skin and swarming around my head," with resulting pruritic lesions; no dermatological lesions were found (Martin et al., 2012). Furthermore, this distraught patient reported that his 27-year-old girlfriend suffered from the same complaints and had recently been seen by a different dermatologist; again, no physical findings, apart from dermographism, were found by this doctor. Although this couple presented as a case of *folie à deux*, subsequent examination of glass slides, with the apparent "bugs" taped to them, provided by the couple revealed the presence of thrips, which are small insects of the order Thysanoptera and which are present in Texas. A diagnosis of thysanoptera dermatitis was confirmed in both cases. It should be noted, however, that Ekbom's syndrome (delusional parasitosis) may present with *folie à deux*; this is described further in the next chapter.

At this juncture it is convenient to mention the remarkable case of an organically induced *folie à deux*. Both partners, neither of whom had had previous functional psychosis, each developed a psychotic illness with shared identical paranoid delusions following the intravenous abuse of the stimulant drug, methylphenidate. When separated, the psychosis remitted and the drug abuse ceased. Although some atypical features were present, there were many psychodynamic similarities to non-drug-induced cases of *folie à deux*, such as shared paranoid delusions, the element of submission – dominance, dependency needs, hostility and the intimate relationship of the two partners. There are also reports involving the intake of cannabis (Dalby and Duncan, 1987).

Whatever the significance of work such as this, for the majority of cases of *folie à deux*, psychological and environmental factors are obviously of greater aetiological importance than overt organicity.

Psychodynamic factors

Various psychodynamic interpretations have engendered some interest. For example, Pulver and Brunt (1961) have advanced the interesting idea that the dominant partner provokes the submissive one into accepting his delusions rather than risk the deterioration of a close and gratifying relationship. *Folie à deux* thus keeps the pair united but increases their detachment from the world of reality. It has also been suggested that for the inducer, it is a final way to keep in touch with the world of reality by maintaining a meaningful relationship with at least one other human being; the alternative to this is total withdrawal and isolation.

This points directly to the need to explain the submission of the partner to the pressure and acceptance of the inducer's delusions, with eventual mutual sharing and sustaining of their unitary delusional state. This is not merely passive acquiescence or a pretence at sharing. The submissive partner may end up, as is often the case with converts, in being even more forceful in upholding the delusions than the person who originally induced them.

Although it has been suggested that the primary inducer is the more powerful, more intelligent, often older, and in a position of greater seniority and authority, this is not in itself a wholly adequate explanation of why the submissive partner eventually succumbs to pressure. His initial resistance, which ultimately collapses, calls for a deeper explanation, the more so as final and complete submission together with the sharing of the inducer's delusions implies increasing withdrawal from the world of reality, surely quite a sacrifice, even for a passive, immature personality? It must be assumed, therefore, that the latter gains something from associating, over the years, with the inducer. Probably it is because the situation fulfils his dependency needs.

The recipient, after all, is already very much identified with the dominant partner, and *identification* is a psychological mechanism of paramount importance in the production of the condition. Although it was Freud (1921) who introduced the term "identification," he nevertheless did not apply it to *folie à deux*. Freud believed that through identification the patients are able to represent not only their own experiences but the experiences of a great many persons. Brill (1920) was the first to apply this mechanism to *folie à deux*, emphasising that identification is an unconscious process. Oberndorf (1934) likewise believed that identification played a far greater role than either that of mere proximity or constitutional pre-disposition in the production of the condition. Deutsch (1938) took the matter further still, stating that:

> Close living together from the beginning is an expression of those unconscious forms which later bring both parties to similar delusional ideas; the common delusion appears to be an important part of an attempt to rescue the object through identification with it or its delusional system.

The term "identification" implies an element of adoration and love which, it may be suggested, governs the attitude of the submissive partner towards the inducer. Psychodynamic formulations suggest that the out-standing features of the recipient consist of ambivalence, a love-hate re-lationship. Thus while he is dependent on the inducer for so much, the recipient, at the same time, despises both the inducer and himself on ac-count of this dependency. Despite this, the recipient needs to maintain the relationship and to continue to keep the favour of his partner, hence his continuing submission even to the point of sharing his delusions. Yet at times he realises and will admit to his aggressive feelings towards the other. The same applies to the dominant partner; he also has a need for a passive, submissive companion, if only, as already implied, to keep as long as possible in touch with reality; yet his love easily and quickly turns to hate, especially when it can be seen that his partner threatens to desert him. Thus their relationship contains not only dependence but ambivalence on both sides.

In some cases a powerful emotional bond between the partners of the same sex, and the active-passive polarity of their personalities, combine to raise the suspicion that latent homosexuality may be a factor in the psychopathology of *folie à deux* (Heuyer, 1935; Deutsch, 1938). In this connection it may be significant that the partners often occupy the same bed. Others, such as Coleman and Last (1939), suggest that the second partner already has his own repressed fantasies, "ripe for the picking" so that he easily succumbs to the dominant partner's initiative. Such a fantasy, they suggest, will concern the oedipal situation; thus the inducer is identified in the mind of his partner with one or other parent.

This particular explanation meets the very crucial contention of Layman and Cohen (1957) that *folie à deux* "is not a distinctive psy-chopathological entity in itself, but should be considered as a 'fortuitous phenomenon.'" They add, contrary to the emphasis placed on the matter by every other author, that the delusions of *folie à deux* are not forcibly imposed on the dependent person by the dominant one, nor are they contagious, and as such communicated or transmitted. Instead they are "adopted by the dependent person." Although the background may be present for acceptance and the pressure of the dominant partner active, transmission of some sort must take place before the sharing of the delusion can become a reality. It is this which points so clearly to the uniqueness of this condition, for even if it cannot be fully explained, it cannot be explained away. Sacks (1988) argues that it is a description of a relationship and possible influence between individuals who may have very different disease processes, ranging from being "impressionable" to an autonomous delusional disorder.

Environmental and social factors

That environmental factors also play a major aetiological role is clear; those affected are often isolated from society and have a close emotional relationship (Prochwicz, 2009). The very definition of the condition denotes an intimate relationship over the years and a common sharing of delusions when these have become established. In contrast, separation, which in effect brings about an essential change in the environment of both partners, is (traditionally) regarded as the most important measure in reversing the condition. Rhein (1922) emphasised the importance of environment, in particular during the earlier period of development of the psychosis, while Postlé (1940) pointed out how emotional influences and early conditioning could be crucial even in the presence of strong hereditary predisposition. Floru (1974) has shown how close-knit communities isolated from outside influences (especially very small families living separately, even from their own community) are fertile ground for the development of *folie à deux*. He added that because World War II had led, in Europe, to there being a relatively large number of unmarried women between the ages of 40 and 60 years, this was an important factor in increasing the number at risk. He also implicated early retirement as further aggravating the situation, indicating that those who live in increasing isolation tend to become increasingly mistrustful, feeling themselves threatened by a seemingly increasingly hostile atmosphere which in turn leads to the production of a paranoid reaction and eventually a paranoid psychosis. *Folie à deux* becomes, therefore, a way of coping with such hostility and aggression. The pertinence of social factors is underlined in the case described by Salih (1981), where two women friends presented as a suicide pact. Their shared delusion was based on their life situation. Social intervention, which included obtaining employment, led to a marked attenuation of the delusion in both partners simultaneously.

Physical abuse has been reported to play an aetiological role. Tay and Li (2017) reported the case of a 42-year-old female patient who had physically abused her father until he submitted to her delusions; subsequently, they both shared persecutory delusions regarding their neighbours. Early life stress, in the form of being physically abused in childhood, can also give rise to *folie à deux*. Nunes et al. (2016) reported the case of a 9-year-old Brazilian boy who was neglected by his parents and had been abused by his mentally ill grandmother, by whom he was meant to be being cared, until he shared similar auditory and visual hallucinations and delusional beliefs to those suffered by his grandmother.

American studies, such as that of Faris and Dunham (1939), confirmed that social isolation, especially in women, is conducive to the production of psychosis of the paranoid kind, while Floru (1974) found that the rigid authoritative conservative family structure was also a potent factor. This kind of mechanism also strongly suggests another factor that has been implicated in the psychodynamics of *folie à deux* – namely, imitation and sympathy (empathy). Partenheimer (cited by Rhein, 1922),

Tuke (1887) and Brande (1888) (cited by Gralnick, 1942) have independently emphasised the role of imitation and/or sympathy in the psychopathology of *folie à deux*. Dewhurst and Todd (1956) have shown how the withdrawal from social intercourse greatly favours the domination of the weaker by the stronger and how a "leader-follower" relationship exists between the partners long before the dominant one becomes psychotic. They also believed that in the psychosis of association, the dominant partner uses the powers of suggestion, which in its essentials resembles hypnosis, to convey his delusions to the weaker partner, although emphasising that the essential dominance which is a prerequisite for this to occur arises from several and varied factors, such as superiority in age, intelligence, education and aggressive drive. Indeed, in their study of an hypnotic model of *folie à deux*, Freeman et al. (2013) were able successfully to model the transference of delusional beliefs from a "primary" to "secondary" individual using hypnosis; many highly hypnotisable individuals were found to adopt the beliefs expressed by the primary, although only when the status of the primary was portrayed as "credible" did secondaries elaborate on the suggested delusion. Brussel (1935) described a case of *folie à deux* in which a partially blind individual gained dominance over a totally blind one, thus illustrating the old adage, "in the Kingdom of the Blind, the one-eyed man is king."

The implication that a "shock," especially that which results from observing that the dominant partner has become psychotic, induces the psychosis in the second, has been suggested by Tuke but cannot be supported. However, as has been shown, *stress* within the family may well be a precipitating factor, especially if it occurs in a state of poverty, leading to material and financial deprivation, deteriorating relationships and generally declining powers from old age. Apart from such mechanisms, an interesting idea has been put forward by Schmidt (1949), who suggested that the *folie à deux* phenomenon can be explained on the basis of *learning theory*. Thus the induced learns the abnormal behaviour from the more dominant, more driving inducer and so becomes and behaves psychotically.

Some other collective mental disorders

Folie à plusiers is not the only situation in which several individuals can share the same psychopathology. There are, for example, some collective mental disorders in which large groups of people become *infected*, as it were, by irrational ideas leading them into untoward mass behaviour. Although there may be some reluctance to accept that the basic mechanisms operative in such cases (dominance –submission, identification and a need to cling together against a seemingly hostile world) may resemble those of *folie à deux*, nevertheless in some instances this certainly does appear to be the case.

As mentioned in Chapter 6, a case of *pseudologia fantastica à deux* has been described by Dimitrakopoulos et al. (2014). *Folie à deux by proxy* in a family has been described by Jolfaei et al. (2011), in which a mother who was admitted to a medical ward with hypernatraemia was found to share a persecutory delusion with her adult daughter and found not to have fed her 8-year-old son as a result of the delusion. In another case of *folie à deux by proxy*, a delusion of parasitosis shared by both parents was projected on their 18-month-old child (Daulatabad et al., 2017).

Several forms of herd behaviour, such as the sixteenth-century dancing mania of Europe, or outbreaks of giggling, sneezing and fainting among groups of adolescent schoolgirls which are periodically reported in the press, or some of the activities of the audiences during "pop" concerts, appear to be the result of sudden epidemics of hysteria. These examples might be termed *mass hysteria*, or under circumstances in which a state of religious fanaticism or primitive superstitious practices are important and relevant factors, *shared religious fanaticism*. The mass suicide in 1978 of 913 members of the Peoples Temple cult, including Jim Jones, their leader, and 276 children, was probably an example of this last phenomenon. It has been noted that as a member of a group an individual is in danger of losing his/her self-consciousness and may therefore fail to exercise self-criticism and self-restraint (Abse, 1974). Further, when a group is particularly associated with a pathological, especially histrionic and paranoid leader, hostile impulses can be directed outwards onto others.

There are recordings of other rather rarer instances, however, in which a situation by no means dissimilar to *folie à plusiers* arises. An example of this is that of Father Divine, who, together with his 18 disciples, were all admitted to the same mental hospital with similar delusions. Another earlier instance was that of Sir William Percy Honeywood Courtnay, who, in 1838, led a series of riots in Brosendon Wood, in England; many of his followers, who were yokels, sharing his belief that he was "the Son of God." In this case there appears to have been no other identifiable motive for their actions, other than an unshakeable belief in the delusional ideas of their colourful and flamboyantly dressed leader (Dewald, 1970). Of more recent occurrence has been the more sinister example in the USA of the Manson "family," in which the followers shared in the belief that their leader was "a divine" and were even prepared to kill at his command. The same mechanisms may also govern the behaviour of certain terrorist groups.

Management and treatment

Recognition

As in all rare cases, the first step to proper management and treatment is prompt recognition of the condition and situation (Suresh Kumar et al.,

2005; Delgado and Bogousslavsky, 2018). It may well be difficult to recognise the existence of a psychosis if expressed beliefs are apparently confirmed by a relative or a close friend. When assessing the condition and situation, it is always important to keep in mind the underlying clinical and social factors which, as described, are important in the production of an environment conducive to the sharing of delusion.

The importance of the "special conditions" becomes apparent when it is realised how few people in close association with deluded individuals actually do acquire the delusion. Large numbers of patients with schizophrenia live in intimate association with their relatives, yet no such sharing of delusions occurs. When it does happen, therefore, there is a need to identify the special factors which are operative in each individual's case.

On recognising the presence of *folie à deux*, it is imperative to identify the primary principal patient, i.e. the one who suffers from a true psychosis. Usually this can be done fairly easily, but if there is a difficulty then it may be necessary to hospitalise both patients together or hospitalise one and permit frequent contact. Observing two patients together will often clarify the distinction between an imposed and communicative psychosis and between the primary and secondary partners. In cases of *folie à deux*, and even more so in *folie à famille*, an interdisciplinary approach is required, involving psychiatry, psychology, social work, occupational therapy, as well as psychosocial, psycho-educational and psychopharmacological interventions (Berbara et al., 2010).

Separation

With separation of the patients the resolution of the delusions in the secondary patient is influenced by the duration of the condition, the nature of the delusions (those which are of value to the secondary in psychological terms, being given up less readily) and the suggestibility of the secondary subject. Only suggestible people and those under domination in *folie à deux* give them up more easily. Traditionally, separation of the two partners or family members has been considered to be an essential therapeutic step. Some authors, however, do doubt the value of separation. Mentjox et al. (1993) found seven cases of which only four showed a reduction in intensity of delusional beliefs on separation.

It does appear that separating elderly associates seems less successful (McNeil et al., 1972; Fishbain, 1987). Thus, separation may be contraindicated in the elderly, especially when an elderly couple have been dependent on each other in order to continue to live in the community and separation leads to irreversible institutional care (Draper and Cole, 1990). Even Lasègue and Falret (1877) themselves proposed separating the primary partner from the secondary partner but were aware that this was not invariably effective. Whereas in some cases separation may be undesirable, in others it might be crucial in order to determine the seriousness of the psychosis in each partner and for the appropriate treatment to be instituted.

Specific treatment of the principal

It has been pointed out that in almost all cases the principal and dominant partner usually suffers from a schizophrenic or allied condition. In the majority of cases, therefore, drug treatment in the form of antipsychotic medication will be necessary. However, in rarer instances the primary condition is affective in nature and an antidepressant drug, lithium therapy and even ECT may be indicated. Admission to hospital is often indicated, and sometimes it is necessary to admit under a compulsory order.

Supportive psychotherapy is also indicated. On discharge, this support should continue as well as a maintenance dose of medication and close supervision. If such follow up is not forthcoming, then a recurrence of original symptoms leading to further readmission is likely.

Specific treatment of the associate

Treatment of the associate or recipient will depend on his or her condition on separation and above all on the underlying psychiatric disorder. If there is a psychosis which is deep-rooted, then intensive antipsychotic treatment will be necessary including antipsychotic drugs. If, however, the condition is one of learning disability or dementia or other mental or physical disability which contributes to the dependence of the recipient on the inducer, then specific steps must be taken to deal with these.

In cases of *folie imposée*, recovery often accompanies a recovery of the principal. However, the conditions, including the social factors, must be dealt with to avoid recurrence. In fact, it may be difficult to treat *folie à deux* because of the refusal of co-operation and the insistence of both patients to remain together. Hence sometimes the need for compulsory admission and treatment even though only one may be truly psychotic (Munro, 1986).

It is significant that one review (McNeil et al., 1972) revealed that in about 25% of cases the recipients suffered from physical disabilities, including partial deafness, strokes and those caused by alcohol abuse. It was therefore essential to treat the underlying physical disorder to avoid continual dependence.

Treatment of the relationship and social conditions

The principal and recipient having been treated specifically, whether by pharmacotherapy or psychotherapy and/or other treatments including separation, attention should be directed towards the relationship and the social conditions of the two. The primary aim will be to maintain their mental health. It will be done by continuing each individual's specific treatment and by providing close follow-up. In addition interventions aimed at separation in psychological terms, as well as physical separation, must be considered (Rioux, 1963; Mentjox et al., 1993).

Total isolation must be avoided. Both should be given more support to become more active and have other interests, with the aim of reducing their pathological enmeshment (Sacks, 1988). This will mean, in addition to the involvement of the wider psychiatric team, the specific input of a social worker.

Deeper psychotherapy

This may be possible for one, if not both, patients with the aim of dealing with the issues of dependence, separation and aggression (Sacks, 1988). At this point psychotherapy may be of use in exploring issues of dependence and hostility (Bankier, 1988), facilitating the expression of feelings, exploring poor parental relationships and encouraging modelling of the relationship with a therapist (Potash and Brunel, 1974). The difficulty is to get one or both patients to commit themselves to a long period of therapy.

In communicated psychosis, Porter et al. (1993) considered that deliberate shifting of dependence could be beneficial, for example from a deluded dominant figure to a sane one, although for the great majority of patients the aim should be independence. Porter et al. (1993) cite various reports of separation where there is a shift of dependence which results with the resolution of psychosis in the dependent partner. Their own case was treated by a multiplicity of treatments including separation, a neuroleptic and individual and group psychotherapy. This in itself indicated the difficulties of attributing recovery to a single agent. However, *family therapy* may be an obvious indication and is of importance not only because of the fact that over 90% of cases occur within families but because, as has already been stressed, *folie à deux* is a defence mechanism, although a pathological one, which mitigates against the effects of social isolation with the threat emanating from a seemingly hostile environment. Thus the family unit is maintained in a *status quo*, even by having to resort to psychotic symptoms. If lasting improvement is to be brought about, this aspect of the matter must be fully considered and dealt with thoroughly.

Social intervention and support

This is highly relevant in the management and can be the most significant factor as illustrated by the case already mentioned of the two women friends presenting as a suicide pact, who improved markedly with social support which included gaining employment.

The review of Arnone et al. (2006) referred to earlier in this chapter also looked at management outcomes and treatment settings. Essentially, a half of the cases responded to medication only and a further quarter to a combination of medication and physical separation. Only 7% of the cases responded to physical separation alone. The majority (over a half) of both primary and secondary cases were treated in an inpatient setting.

Prognosis

There are not enough available data to give a definitive prognosis. It might be supposed that the prognosis for the associate not suffering from any underlying mental illness is good and that with separation there is complete recovery. The prognosis, however, for the principal and for the associate suffering from an underlying mental illness is probably somewhat worse. Mentjox et al. (1993) suggest that in recipients a degree of differentiation, the personality and the amount of stress to which they are exposed are determining factors for prognosis. Unfortunately, there is no specific evidence to support this view. A relapse is said to be a danger in the recipient if the inducer relapses (Fernandoh and Frieze, 1985). Certainly the prognosis will depend on the effectiveness of the initial treatment and the thoroughness of the follow-up.

As this condition is still uncommon, a single-case methodology may be the only useful approach in assessing prognosis. This methodology includes establishing a baseline value for the dependent variables, changing one independent variable at a time and repeated measures of dependent variables. Detailed accounts of this may be found elsewhere (Barlow and Herson, 1984). As we suggested in earlier editions of our book, standardised diagnostic instruments and rating scales should be used in case reporting.

Forensic aspects

Antisocial behaviour including theft, violence, murder and suicide pacts associated with *folie à deux* has been reported (Greenberg, 1956; Bourguis et al., 1992; Kraya and Patrick, 1997; Nielssen et al., 2013); *folie à deux* has been used as a legal defence in criminal and civil cases (Newman and Harbit, 2010). The potential dangerousness of some of these cases is illustrated by a 58-year-old woman suffering from delusional parasitosis trying to kill her general practitioner. Her husband shared and supported her delusional beliefs, though he lost all delusional conviction when she was compulsorily admitted to a High Secure Hospital (Bourguis et al., 1992). Kraya and Patrick (1997) also emphasised the potential risk in describing five cases of *folie à deux*, including three cases of husband-wife, one case of mother-daughter and one case of twin brothers in which the victim suffered a fatal or near-fatal outcome. Rahman et al. (2013) described a case of infanticide of a 4-month-old boy whose parents, retrospectively assessed forensically as suffering from *folie à deux*, allowed him to die of starvation and dehydration. These cases all shared religious delusions, the presence of which appears to heighten the risk.

Talamo et al. (2011) described a case of *folie à deux* in which separation, following antipsychotic and supportive treatment, of two highly interdependent and chronically psychotic sisters was associated with increasing anxiety and a fatal outcome in the primary: "She impulsively ingested an overdose of the non-dominant sister's medicines and died of cardiac arrest, despite her sister's efforts to seek medical assistance."

Catanesi et al. (2014) described a case of *folie à famille*, which developed within the context of extreme religiosity and seclusion, in which some family members met with particularly unpleasant deaths and the last surviving family member lived for over a year and a half with their mummified remains.

In the case mentioned above of *folie à trois* in which the inducer, a 50-year-old married mother of six, was diagnosed with systemic lupus erythematosus with psychotic features (Caribé et al., 2013), "the father returned home to see his oldest son killed, strangled with wire. He found his wife bloodied and angry, and she told him a goat-faced demon had invaded the house, which she had to kill to defend the family." Another forensic case involving *folie à trois* was described by Joshi et al. (2006) and involved three sisters, all in their early twenties at the time of the index offence:

> For three days before their arrest, the sisters prayed continuously without sleeping. Sister 1 became convinced that God had special plans for her and her sisters and would provide for them. She also concluded that the Bible had been tampered with and was now incorrect due to the alternate spellings of Immanuel and Emmanuel. She had become convinced that God was trying to tell her something, and she convinced her sisters of the same. On the day of the incident, the sisters disrobed in their home to "free themselves from the confines of clothing." Upon reading a Bible verse, Sister 1 believed that God wanted her to have the house that she and her sisters were accused of burglarizing. Sister 1 later told the court-appointed forensic psychiatrist that she had seen this house several months before the alleged offense and had always wanted to live in a "house like that." She had become convinced over several days that God was going to provide for all her needs in that house. She believed that her situation was similar to that of Moses when God told Moses to claim the Promised Land. The three sisters drove to the victims' house wearing only pajamas.

Mela (2005) described a case of *folie à trois* which occurred in three unrelated inpatients in the Regional Psychiatric Center in Saskatoon, Canada, a multi-level security forensic treatment centre:

The three patients incorrectly believed, despite contrary evidence, that their convictions would be overturned. They further asserted, despite incontrovertible and obvious proof, that their subsequent release from jail would occur early and not in accordance with the normal processes of the National Parole Board. They, therefore, wrote "affidavits" (legal letters) to guarantee this method of release. When they did not get the expected replies to their affidavits, they believed that their letters were being tampered with as a plan to keep them from achieving early release. They believed that their letters were opened and the contents tampered with, because the institutional logo was stamped on the envelope (stamping all letters coming through the treatment center's mailing system is a usual practice).

Suicide pacts associated with *folie à deux* are rare, and the majority of suicide pacts are not associated with the disorder. However, often one of the persons in each pact does usually suffer from a formal psychiatric disorder, most often from a depressive illness. The fact that there is evidence of dependency and social isolation suggests the presence of *folie à deux* in some suicide pacts (Rosen, 1981; Brown et al., 1995).

Postscript

Folie à deux is not only a colourful and intriguing condition; it also serves to emphasise how rarely psychotic symptoms are actually contagious: almost never, in fact, except under those rather specific conditions which have been enumerated, especially social isolation.

References

Abse, D.W. (1974) In *American Handbook of Psychiatry, Vol. 3*. Basic Books, New York.
Arnone, D., Patel, A., Tan, G.M. (2006) *Annals of General Psychiatry*, 5, 11.
American Psychiatric Association (2013). *Diagnostic and Statistical Manual of Mental Disorders, Fifth Edition (DSM-5)*. American Psychiatric Association, Washington, D.C.
Baillarger, J.G.F. (1860) *Gaz. Hôp. Paris*, 33, 149.
Bankier, R.G. (1988) *Canadian Journal of Psychiatry*, 33, 251.
Barlow, D.H., Herson, M. (1984) *Single Case Experimental Designs: Strategies for Studying Behaviour Change*, 2nd edn. Pergamon Press, New York.
Berbara, C., Almeida, S., Cermelli Reber, M., Cortez, S., Gonzales, M. (2010) *Vertex*, 21, 105.
Berlyn, C. (1819) *Z. Psychiatr. Aerzte Leipzig*, 2, 530.
Bourgeois, M.L., Duhamel, P., Verdoux, H. (1992) *Br J Psychiatry*, 161, 709.
Brill, A. (1920) *Medical Records (New York)*, 97, 131.
Brown, M., King, E., Barraclough, B. (1995) *British Journal of Psychiatry*, 167, 448.
Brussel, J.A. (1935) *American Journal of Psychiatry*, 92, 215.

Caribe, A.C., Daltro-Oliveira, R., Araujo, R.H., Cardoso, A.P., Guimaraes, P.B., Miranda-Scippa, A., et al. (2013) *Compr Psychiatry*, *54*, 1032.

Catanesi, R., Punzi, G., Rodriguez, W.C., 3rd, Solarino, B., Di Vella, G. (2014) *J Forensic Sci*, *59*, 274.

Chalise, P., Subedi, S., Sharma, P. (2015) *JNMA J Nepal Med Assoc*, *53*, 295.

Christodoulou, G.N., Margariti, M.M., Malliaras, D.E., Alevizou, S. (1995) *Journal of Neurology, Neurosurgery and Psychiatry*, *58*, 499.

Coleman, S., Last, S. (1939) *Journal of Mental Science*, *85*, 1212.

Dalby, J.T., Duncan, B.J. (1987) *Canadian Journal of Psychiatry*, *32*, 64.

Daulatabad, D., Sonthalia, S., Srivastava, A., Bhattacharya, S.N., Kaul, S., Moyal, D. (2017) *Australas J Dermatol*, *58*, e113.

Delgado, M.G., Bogousslavsky, J. (2018) *Front Neurol Neurosci*, *42*, 44.

Deutsch, M. (1938) *Psychoanalytic Quarterly*, *7*, 307.

Dewald, P.A. (1970) *Psychiatry*, *30*, 390.

Dewhurst, K., Todd, J. (1956) *Journal of Nervous and Mental Disease*, *124*, 451.

Dimitrakopoulos, S., Sakadaki, E., Ploumpidis, D. (2014) *Psychiatriki*, *25*, 192.

Draper, B., Cole, A. (1990) *Australian and New Zealand Journal of Psychiatry*, *24*, 280.

Faris, E., Dunham, H.W. (1939) *Mental Disorders and Urban Areas*. University Press, Chicago.

Fernando, F.P., Frieze, M. (1985) *British Journal of Psychiatry*, *146*, 315.

Fishbain, D.A. (1987) *Canadian Journal of Psychiatry*, *32*, 498.

Florez, G., Gomez-Reino, I. (2001) *Eur Psychiatry*, *16*, 501.

Floru, L. (1974) *Forschitte Neurologie Psychiatrie*, *42*, 76.

Francois, D., Bander, E., D'Agostino, M., Swinburne, A., Broderick, L., Grody, M.B., et al. (2017) *Clin Schizophr Relat Psychoses*, *11*, 61.

Freeman, L.P., Cox, R.E., Barnier, A.J. (2013) *Conscious Cogn*, *22*, 1285.

Freud, S. (1921) *Group Psychology and the Analysis of the Ego*. Hogarth, London.

Glassman, J.N., Magulac, M., Darko, D.F. (1987) *American Journal of Psychiatry*, *144*, 658.

Gralnick, A. (1942) *Part I. Psychiatric Quarterly*, *16*, 230; *Part II. Psychiatric Quarterly*, *16*, 491.

Grover, M.M. (1937) *American Journal of Psychiatry*, *93*, 1045.

Greenberg (1956). *Journal of mental Science Oct:*, *102*, 722–9.

Grover, S., Gupta, N. (2006) *Psychopathology*, *39*, 99.

Hart, J., McClue, G.M. (1989) *British Journal of Psychiatry*, *54*, 552.

Haygarth, J. (1800) *Of the Imagination as a Cause and a Cure of Disorders of the Body*. R.Crutwell, Bath.

Heuyer, G.R. (1935) *Annales Medico-Psychologiques*, *93*, 254.

Hofbauer, J.L. (1846) *Oest. Med. Uschr*, *118*.

Idelar, K.W. (1838) *Grundriss der Seelenmeilkunde (Berlin)*, *2*, 530.

Ilechukwu, S.T., Okyere, E. (1987) *Canadian Journal of Psychiatry*, *32*, 216.

Janofsky, J.S. (1986) *Journal of Nervous and Mental Disease*, *174*, 368.

Jolfaei, A.G., Isfahani, M.N., Bidaki, R. (2011) *J Res Med Sci*, *16* (Suppl. 1), S453.

Joshi, K.G., Frierson, R.L., Gunter, T.D. (2006) *J Am Acad Psychiatry Law*, *34*, 511.

Kashiwase, H., Kato, M. (1997) *Acta Psychiatrica Scandinavica*, *96*:4, 231.

Kendler, K.S., Robinson, G., McGuire, M., Spellman, M.P. (1986) *British Journal of Psychiatry*, *148*, 463.

Kraya, N.A., Patrick, C. (1997) *Aust N Z J Psychiatry*, *31*, 883.

Lasègue, C., Falret, J. (1877) *Annales Medico-Psychologiques*, *18*, 321.

Layman, W.A., Cohen, L. (1957) *Journal of Nervous and Mental Disease*, *125*, 412.

Lazarus, A. (1986) *British Journal of Psychiatry*, *148*, 324.

Lehmann, G. (1885) *Arch. Psychiatr. Nervenkr*, *14*, 145.

Marandon de Montyel, E. (1881) *Annales Medico-Psychologiques*, *5*, 28.

Marandon de Montyel, E. (1894) *Annales Medico-Psychologiques*, *19*, 266.

Martin, J.T., Richmond, A., Davis, B.M., Krejci-Manwaring, J. (2012) *Arch Dermatol*, *148*, 864.

McNeil, J.N., Verwoerdt, A., Peak, D. (1972) *Journal of the American Geriatrics Society*, *20*, 316.

Mela, M. (2005) *J Am Acad Psychiatry Law*, *33*, 310.

Mentjox, R., Van Houten, C.A., Kooiman, C.G. (1993) *Comprehensive Psychiatry*, *34*, 120.

Mergui, J., Jaworowski, S., Greenberg, D., Lerner, V. (2010) *Aust N Z J Psychiatry*, *44*, 859.

Millingen, J.G. (1839) *Curiosities of Medical Experience*. Richard Bentley, London.

Munro, A. (1986) *Canadian Journal of Psychiatry*, *31*, 233.

Newman, W.J., Harbit, M.A. (2010) *J Am Acad Psychiatry Law*, *38*, 369.

Nielssen, O., Langdon, R., Large, M. (2013) *Cognitive Neuropsychiatry*, *18*, 390.

Oberndorf, C. (1934) *International Journal of Psychoanalysis*, *15*, 14.

Ohnuma, T., Arai, H. (2015) *Case Rep Psychiatry*, *2015*, 983212.

Pande, N.R., Gulabani, D.M. (1990) *British Journal of Psychiatry*, *156*, 440.

Porter, T.L., Levine, J., Dinneen, M. (1993) *British Journal of Psychiatry*, *162*, 704.

Postlé, B. (1940) *Archives of Neurology and Psychiatry*, *43*, 372.

Potash, H., Brunell, L. (1974) *Psychotherapy: Theory, Research and Practice*, *11*, 270.

Primrose, J. (1651) *De Vulgi in Medicina Erronbus*, Trans. R. Willie. Archives of General Psychiatry, London.

Pritchard, J.C. (1835) *A Treatise on Insanity and Other Disorders Affecting the Mind*. Sherwood, Gilbert & Piper, London.

Prochwicz, K. (2009) *Psychiatr Pol*, *43*, 19.

Pulver, A., Brunt, M. (1961) *Archives of General Psychiatry*, *5*, 257.

Rahman, T., Grellner, K.A., Harry, B., Beck, N., Lauriello, J. (2013) *American Journal of Psychiatry*, *170*, 1110.

Régis, E. (1881) *Encephahle (Paris)*, *1*, 43.

Rhein, J. (1922) *New York Medical Journal*, *116*, 269.

Rioux, B. (1963) *Psychiatric Quarterly*, *37*, 405.

Rosen, B.K. (1981) *Psychological Medicine*, *11*, 525.

Roth, C., Stuwe, R., Boger, A., Serafin, S., Franz, M. (2010) *Psychiatr Prax*, *37*, 43.

Sacks, M.H. (1988) *Comprehensive Psychiatry*, *29*, 270.

Salih, M.A. (1981) *British Journal of Psychiatry*, *139*, 62.

Schmidt, A.O. (1949) *Journal of Abnormal and Social Psychology*, *44*, 402.

Shah, K., Breitinger, S., Avari, J., Francois, D. (2017) *Schizophr Res*, *182*, 142.

Shiwach, R., Sobin, P. (1998) *Med Hypotheses*, *50*, 369.

Signer, S.F., Isbister, S.R. (1987) *British Journal of Psychiatry*, *151*, 402.

Sims, A., Salmons, P., Humphreys, P. (1977) *British Journal of Psychiatry*, *130*, 134.

Soni, S.D., Rockley, G.J. (1974) *British Journal of Psychiatry*, *125*, 230.

Silveira Jose, M., and Seeman Mary, V. (1995). Department of Psychiatry, University of Toronto, *40*(7), 389–395.

Suresh Kumar, P.N., Subramanyam, N., Thomas, B., Abraham, A., Kumar, K. (2005) *Indian J Psychiatry*, *47*, 164.

Talamo, A., Vento, A., Savoja, V., Di Cosimo, D., Lazanio, S., Kotzalidis, G.D., et al. (2011) *Clin Ter*, *162*, 45.

Tay, J.L., Li, Z. (2017) *East Asian Arch Psychiatry*, *27*, 121.

Tikka, S.K., Goyal, N., Tikka, D.L., Sinha, V.K., Mathew, K.J., Rai, S. (2013) *Asian J Psychiatr*, *6*, 629.

Tuke, D. (1887) *British Medical Journal*, *2*, 505.

Vargas Alves Nunes, A., Odebrecht Vargas Nunes, S., Strano, T., Pascolat, G., Schier Doria, G.M. and Nasser Ehlke, M. (2016) *J Med Case Rep*, *10*, 339.

Westermayer, J. (1989) *Journal of Clinical Psychiatry*, *50*, 181.

White, T.G. (1995) *Canadian Journal of Psychiatry*, *40*, 418.

Whytt, R. (1764) *The Words of Robert Whytt*. Royal College of Physicians, Edinburgh.

Wolff, G., McKenzie, K. (1994) *British Journal of Psychiatry*, *165*, 842.

Ekbom's syndrome (delusional infestation) and body dysmorphic disorder

So, naturalists observe, a flea
Hath smaller fleas that on him prey;
And these have smaller fleas to bite'em,
And so proceed *ad infinitum*.

Jonathan Swift (1667–1745)

This is a condition in which patients suffer from delusions of infestation. The sufferer believes with absolute certainty that insects, lice, maggots or other small vermin are living or otherwise thriving in the skin and sometimes the body.

Historical

The condition is named after Karl-Axel Ekbom, a Swedish neurologist who described its principal manifestations (1937; 1938). However, it was probably first described in 1894 in France by Thieberge, and again in 1896 by Perrin, both of whom were dermatologists. The condition gave rise to misnomers such as zoophobia, parasitophobia (Eller, 1929) and acarophobia (Myerson, 1921). Later, Annika Skott (1978) published a monograph on the subject referring to Ekbom's use of the term *Dermatozoenwahn*, which literally translated means "skin-animal-delusion."

The condition may occur in association with other psychiatric symptoms, or the delusion may exist as an isolated phenomenon. In modern classificatory systems, the latter condition finds its expression as an example of *delusional disorder* in *ICD-11* and its precursor *ICD-10*, and *delusional disorder – somatic type* in *DSM-5* and its precursor *DSM-IV-TR*. The *DSM-5* criteria for *delusional disorder* (297.1 [F22]) include (American Psychiatric Association, 2013; slightly modified):

A The presence of one (or more) delusions with duration of at least one month.

B   Criterion A for schizophrenia (see below) has never been met. Hallucinations, if present, are not prominent and are related to the delusional theme; for example, the sensation of being infested with insects is associated with delusions of infestation.
C   Apart from the impact of the delusion(s) or its (their) ramifications, functioning is not markedly impaired, and behaviour is not obviously bizarre or odd.
D   If manic or depressive episodes have occurred, these have been brief relative to the duration of the delusional periods.
E   The disturbance is not attributable to the physiological effects of a substance or another medical condition and is not better explained by another mental disorder, such as body dysmorphic disorder (see later in this chapter) or obsessive-compulsive disorder.

In *DSM-5*, "somatic type" should be specified: "This subtype applies when the central theme of the delusion involves bodily functions or sensations." Criterion A for schizophrenia (295.90 [F20.9]) is as follows (American Psychiatric Association, 2013; slightly modified):

Two (or more) of the following, each present for a significant portion of time during a one-month period (or less if successfully treated). At least one of these must be (1), (2) or (3):

1   Delusions
2   Hallucinations
3   Disorganised speech (e.g. frequent derailment or incoherence)
4   Grossly disorganised or catatonic behaviour
5   Negative symptoms (i.e. diminished emotional expression or avolition)

Nomenclature

The use of the term "delusions of parasitosis," or "delusional parasitosis," for the disorder known as Ekbom's syndrome, was introduced by Wilson and Miller (1946) as a replacement of the name "acarophobia," on the basis that this last name was etymologically inappropriate, both in respect of the cause ("acaro-") and the fact that the condition is a delusion rather than a phobia.

More recently, Freudenmann and Lepping (2009) have argued for a further change in nomenclature to "delusional infestation":

The name "delusion of parasitosis" was introduced in 1946 … and it became the most common name in the literature. An alternative was "delusional parasitosis." However, in recent years, patients have reported the presence of specific parasites less commonly, and the name thus has the disadvantage of covering only one sort of pathogens. We therefore recommend the use of the broader term "delusional infestation" in the future. This name highlights the core psychopathological feature (a thought disorder) and covers all kinds of (even "newly emerging") imaginary pathogens by referring to the delusional theme "infestation" and not to a single species.

Case reports

Case 1

This patient was a single woman aged 43 years who was referred by a dermatologist. Her problem first presented itself as a case of disseminated pruritis, the origin of which, the patient believed, was the invasion of her house, some two years previously, by various arthropod ectoparasites emanating from house martins' nests (these being swallow-like birds which commonly nest under the eaves of buildings). The infestation paradoxically seemed to her to be worse during the winter months. She stated that she had been bitten on many occasions but had failed to find a cause for this. She admitted that her mother, who lived with her, did not experience any similar bites. Upon admission to hospital, the only physical abnormality discovered was extensive excoriation which underwent considerable improvement during the short period of time she was an inpatient.

Interestingly enough, it came to light that she was employed as a veterinary officer in the Ministry of Agriculture and Fisheries and had, during the course of her career, suffered an attack of ringworm from contact with cattle. She had also suffered from an attack of scabies while a student at college, although it is not known from whom or how she acquired this, as not only was she a single woman but she tended to avoid contact with the opposite sex. She also mentioned that her skin reacted adversely to flea bites so at one time it seemed reasonable to assume that her physical contact with others may have been closer than she cared later to admit. Likewise, perhaps, these other skin conditions may have been significant in "sensitising" her psychologically for what was to come. Apart from these misfortunes, she appeared to be physically healthy. There was also no history of mental illness to be elicited, either from the patient herself or in her family.

Case 2

This patient, also female, was aged 68 years, and the features of her case were much more in line with many of those described by others. While she initially made no direct complaint of infestation, there was an unequivocal past history of this. Nine years previously she had presented elsewhere complaining of "something crawling up my private," asking also whether it was possible to catch worms from the cat. She did not seem to be depressed, but on admission to hospital her zoopathic symptoms were more marked than they had originally appeared to be or, in addition, she began to insist that the worms had also invaded her rectum and affected her spine. She also claimed to have suffered from paraesthesiae in various parts of her body including her head. She was reported to have spent days searching for worms and to have seen these in her faeces. On this occasion she was treated with ECT, to which her condition responded fairly rapidly. However, following discharge from hospital, her condition soon underwent relapse. The diagnosis made at the time was of masked depression with hypochondriacal features. When seen a year later, her condition was found to be much as it originally had been, in view of which she was again admitted and treated on this occasion with anti-depressive drugs. Once more her mood improved, but her zoopathic occupations did not entirely disappear.

When she came under our care in 1981, her presenting complaints, although not altogether dissimilar to those made previously, had nevertheless undergone some change. While she no longer claimed to be infested, she still complained of peculiar crawling sensations in her vagina, rectum and buttocks which she insisted went through to her spine.

She presented as a well-dressed woman, somewhat frail in appearance, although not overtly agitated or depressed. She spoke rapidly and coherently, but it was difficult to get her to talk of anything but her bowels. On examination of her sensorium there was evidence of some degree of arteriopathy. Her blood pressure was 180/100 mmHg, and a chest radiograph showed left ventricular hypertrophy. Given nine further electroconvulsive treatments and the prescription of phenothiazines, which served to control some paraphrenic-type hallucinations (i.e. voices addressing her in the third person and commenting on her actions) which she developed shortly after her readmission to hospital, her condition on discharge was found to be greatly improved, although her prognosis was considered to be guarded.

Case 3

This patient was also a single woman, a 23-year-old of Jamaican origin and a Jehovah's Witness. She too was referred by a dermatologist to whom she had presented with the fixed belief that there were insects crawling through her hair and over her body, a belief she appeared to have held for eight years and since she had been an adolescent. It is perhaps significant that during this period of her life and shortly before her ideas of infestation emerged, she had, whilst still living in Jamaica, fallen accidentally into an open latrine.

She stated that she had seen "little white streaks in her hair" but never any insects. The itching sensation spread from her head to her axillae and pubis, which led her to shave her hair from these secondary areas. Although she had seen nothing in her scalp, she nonetheless felt "creepy crawlies" there, and they bit her scalp and crawled about making "a cracking noise." She was unable to relieve these discomforts by combing or washing her hair or by treating herself with various lotions. At the time she was first seen she felt her symptoms were worsening and that the itching sensations were spreading over her entire body. She then began to believe that those with whom she was associated, her illegitimate daughter and her sister, were similarly infested and that she knew this was so because she had seen her sister scratching. On talking to the latter, it became clear that she knew nothing about this or indeed very little about the patient's complaints.

On mental state examination, the patient appeared to be an alert, outgoing, reasonably intelligent and well kept young woman. There was no evidence of her being depressed. She seemed clear in her mind and seemingly not unduly obsessional about cleanliness etc She stated that she slept well, and her appetite was good and her weight steady. There was no evidence of any suicidal intent.

Apart from clearly expressed ideas of parasitic infestation, there seemed to be no evidence of thought disorder or other symptoms suggestive of schizophrenia or any other major psychotic condition. She was treated with pimozide, which, while it has been said by a number of investigators to be particularly effective in this condition, brought about no improvement in her case by the time she came to be discharged from hospital. She has not been seen since.

While the first patient described above seems to be a case of delusional disorder occurring in the pure form, the second developed her delusions of infestation and later that of her bowels, etc. being interfered with, in a setting of depression possibly associated with some degree of cerebral arteriosclerosis. In contrast, the third patient's disorder, although clearly bordering on psychosis, could nevertheless possibly be regarded as obsessional in nature. The following illustrative composite case is interesting because the patient, also a female, presented in a forensic fashion and demonstrates the lengths to which some sufferers will go when acting under the influence of their beliefs.

Case 4

This patient, a 50-year-old woman, was referred for a psychiatric opinion after she had been charged with obtaining a number of prescribed drugs by means of forged prescriptions. A variety of drugs were obtained, usually antibiotics, antifungals or anti-helminths, although sometimes she also acquired warfarin and nifedipine. She bought the drugs from reputable pharmacy outlets and spent all of her savings (several thousands of pounds) in the process.

There was no history of any previous criminality or illicit drug abuse.

She gave a history of being infested with a parasite for seven years. She said that around that time she had passed some sort of intestinal worm that was small but thick and motile. This fell on to her leg and quickly disintegrated. She had then shown the remains to a doctor and had been told that "it was a larval type creature."

During the ensuing years she had attended numerous medical practitioners – generalists and specialists – in the NHS and on a private basis but had never been satisfied with the responses received. She began to think that each doctor she saw was covering up for a medical mistake or a misdiagnosis made at an earlier stage in the process. On one occasion she even sought help from a veterinary surgeon. She explained that although she knew she was breaking the law, she felt that because of the failure of the medical profession she had no choice but to act as she did, otherwise her condition would become life-threatening.

She was otherwise in good physical and mental health.

Epidemiology

The incidence and the prevalence of the syndrome are unknown. In our experience the condition is uncommon; in a search through hospital records of 1,690 patients admitted to a small general hospital psychiatric unit over a period of 18½ years where it could have been expected that such patients might present themselves only three cases were discovered. The following research has been published.

Maneros 1988 estimated the incidence to be about 7 per 10,000 psychiatric admissions.

Skott (1978) listed 354 cases in 82 separate publications between 1954 and 1961. However, 40 of these reports were confined to single instances; in only six of the remainder did the number of case reports reach double figures. (Ekbom himself only reported seven of his own cases.) Dohring (1960), a German psychiatrist, identified 66 cases.

It has been suggested that the disorder is more likely to present to dermatologists (Musalek and Kutzer, 1989), and therefore a more accurate reflection of the true incidence can be obtained by reference to dermatological populations. Indeed, in their cross-sectional study of 200 patients with primary psychiatric disorders compared with 200 controls, Moftah et al. (2013) found a significantly higher prevalence of skin diseases in general in the psychiatric patients (72% versus 22% in the controls), with a higher prevalence in the psychiatric patients of infectious skin diseases (48% versus 11%); in the psychiatric patient group, the proportion of infectious versus non-infectious skin diseases varied according to the primary psychiatric diagnosis. Infectious skin diseases by far outnumbered non-infectious (by a ratio of about 8.5:1.5) in cases of schizophrenia whereas in obsessive-compulsive disorder this pattern was reversed. The ratio was closer to 1:1 in mood and mood-related disorders.

Bourgeois et al. (1986) reported 150 cases presenting to French dermatologists; Reilly and Batchelor (1986) in a postal survey identified 365 patients with a presumptive diagnosis of delusional parasitosis (now known as delusional infestation), seen by 144 dermatologists over a five-year period; Schrut and Waldron (1963) described three cases and referred to 100 others having been seen in a dermatological clinic over a period of five years.

A number of epidemiological studies were published between 1991 and 2014, including a relatively large population-based study by Bailey et al. (2014) of residents in Olmsted County, Minnesota. This study produced an estimated incidence of 1.9 cases per 100,000 person years. Other studies, typically based on surveys of medical practitioners and health facilities, provide a range of estimated prevalence rates from 0.1–4.5 cases per 100,000 population (Trabert, 1991; 1993; Lepping et al., 2010; Pearson et al., 2012). The Bailey et al. (2014) study reported the incidence of delusional infestation by age at diagnosis with increasing age, in a step-wise fashion from a low of 0.2 per 100,000 person years in the 0–19 year age group. Incidence was higher in females than males between the ages of 20 years and 79 years. Thereafter, a steep rise in incidence in males was observed (16.2 per 100,000 person years compared with 7.2 per 100,000 person years in females). These authors also studied the age-adjusted incidence by year of diagnosis and showed a significant increase in recorded incidence in both sexes between the years 1986 and 2010. Finally, in a more recent on-line questionnaire study of Scottish dermatologists, Wong et al. (2018) found that, of 55 members of the Scottish Dermatology Society who responded, 98% reported that they had encountered patients suffering from delusional infestation.

Clinical features

The clinical features of the disorder are:

- A delusion of infestation. The description "worms of the mind" by Prakash et al. (2012) seems particularly apposite.
- Other psychiatric features may also be present: tactile and visual hallucinations, delusional memories.

- Sometimes occurs as a symptom of another psychotic illness such as schizophrenia or depressive psychosis.
- Sufferers typically give a detailed account of the parasite's behaviour, frequently producing "evidence" in the form of skin fragments, keratin or other kinds of debris.
- A physical examination of the skin shows this to be normal or sometimes provides evidence of picking, scratching or dermatitis caused by antiseptics.
- The development of *folie à deux* occurs with a high frequency. It has been estimated that such an outcome arises in up to one in four or five cases (Skott, 1978; Mester, 1975). Several such cases have recently been described (Kim et al., 2003; Colombo et al., 2004; Sawant and Vispute, 2015; Giam et al., 2017). Friedmann et al. (2006) described delusional infestation (parasitosis) presenting as *folie à trois*, treated successfully with risperidone. Sometimes several members of the same family become involved, so-called *folie en famille* or *folie partagée*, as in the case reported by Evans and Merskey (1972) in which both parents and their two daughters all shared the belief of dermal infestation. As mentioned in the previous chapter, Daulatabad et al. (2017) described a case of *folie à deux* and delusional infestation by proxy; further details are given in that chapter.
- Morris et al. (1988) and Morris and Jolly (1987) have made a particular study of elderly sufferers and have also reported a novel variant of the condition in which the patient believes his environment is infested and not his own person.

Hylwa et al. (2012) studied psychiatric comorbidity in delusional infestation. Of 109 delusional infestation patients seen at the Mayo Clinic over a seven-year period who were referred to a Mayo Clinic psychiatrist, 54 (50%) underwent a psychiatric consultation. Of these, 14 (26%) were diagnosed as suffering from delusional infestation alone, while the remaining 40 (74%) were diagnosed with a co-morbid psychiatric condition, as follows: 44% (24 of 54) depression; 19% anxiety; 19% drug dependence/abuse; 9% pain disorder; 9% somatisation disorder; 7% schizoaffective disorder; 7% posttraumatic stress disorder; 6% mood disorder, not otherwise specified; 6% hypochondriasis; 6% bipolar disorder; 6% obsessive-compulsive disorder; 4% schizophrenia; 4% psychosis, not otherwise specified; 4% panic disorder with agoraphobia; 4% panic disorder, not otherwise specified; 4% cognitive disorder; 4% seasonal affective disorder; 4% dependent personality disorder; and 31% other psychiatric diagnoses.

In the above-mentioned recent on-line questionnaire study of Scottish dermatologists, Wong et al. (2018) reported on both physical and psychiatric co-morbidities in 47 patients with delusional infestation. These authors found that in 81% of the sample there was no material dermatological history or co-morbidity. However, a range of psychiatric co-morbidities occurred in over two-thirds of the cases, with depression being the most common diagnosis, found in 36% of the sample.

Related conditions include those in which patients suffer with a delusion that they emit a foul odour and where the delusion concerns some perceived bodily defect, a dysmorphic delusion. The clinical presentations of these conditions are now described.

Delusions of emitting a foul odour

These patients may have a delusion that they emit a bad odour either from the mouth (halitosis) or from the anus as an alimentary stench. This belief is reinforced by the patient misinterpreting the attitudes of people around him, accusing them of showing disgust or avoidance behaviour. Patients will insist that a foul smell emanates from leakage of flatus from the bowel, which results in demands to be referred to a gastroenterologist, or to abnormalities in the sweat with an insistence on being referred to a dermatologist.

A significant subgroup of patients complain of halitosis and are often referred to dentists or ENT specialists. A small percentage of these cases appear to have an olfactory hallucination, for they are able to describe the odour in detail. This has been described as "hallucinatory halitosis" and an "olfactory reference syndrome" (Iwu and Akpata, 1990). Iwu and Akpata (1990) reviewed 32 cases of delusional halitosis, none of whom had a prior history of psychiatric care or drug abuse, and all but one had continued with their occupations.

There is no doubt that sufferers of this condition do experience great distress. They do not respond to normal dental management and at times, although rarely, will suffer depression and even attempt suicide (Davidson and Mukherjee, 1982). Malasi et al. (1990) emphasise the difficulty of sometimes distinguishing overvalued ideas, delusions and hallucinations in the clinical setting.

Case 5

A married woman of 52 years with two children sought dental help for apparent periodontal disease, but her main complaint was of a bad taste and smell in her mouth which had persisted for about 10 years. Initially, she claimed that the bad taste and smell related to certain teeth. However, when these were dealt with, she would then point to other teeth as being the cause. She also complained that because of the emission of a bad odour she had had "a lot of reaction from other people." She described how they checked whether the bad odour came from her or them. As a result she became very inhibited, whereas previously she had been a gregarious person, easy-going and outward-looking.

She did have familial stress in that her mother had had a recent stroke, there was some marital disharmony and some tensions at her place of work. However, she was not overtly depressed, and there was no other form of psychiatric disorder. She was preoccupied with the bad smell and taste in her mouth, and this reached delusional intensity so that she could not be convinced otherwise. She was treated successfully with a combination of pimozide and supportive psychotherapy. After about 18 months, she discontinued the pimozide and experienced a recrudescence of her symptoms. The symptoms resolved when the pimozide was restarted.

Dysmorphic delusions

The term "dysmorphophobia" was coined in 1886 by Morselli, who described it as "a subjective feeling of illness or physical defect which a patient feels is noticeable to others, although his appearance is within normal limits." The concept has been confined to those complaints arising out of psychological mechanisms; the symptoms are usually regarded as being manifestations of a disturbed body image.

The sufferer's preoccupation is most often with the nose but sometimes with the chin, penis, falling hair, the breasts, acne or wrinkles. The disorder is not a phobia but is nearer to an obsession or overvalued idea. The diagnosis, which was once recognised, also depended on the presence of certain personality features – sensitivity, introversion and a hypochondriacal bent. The condition has now come to be known as *body dysmorphic disorder* (BDD) and the term "dysmorphophobia" is obsolete (Munro and Stewart, 1991).

BDD, which has an estimated prevalence of 1–2% in the general population (Mackley, 2005) and around 13% in those seeking cosmetic surgery (Dey et al., 2015), is classed under "obsessive-compulsive or related disorders" in *ICD-11*, with the code 6B21 (WHO 2018). The *DSM-5* diagnostic criteria for BDD (code 300.7 [F45.22]) (American Psychiatric Association, 2013) are as follows:

A   Preoccupation with one or more perceived defects or flaws in physical appearance that are not observable or appear slight to others.

B   At some point during the course of the disorder, the individual has performed repetitive behaviours (e.g. mirror checking, excessive grooming, skin picking, reassurance seeking) or mental acts (e.g. comparing his or her appearance with that of others) in response to the appearance concerns.

C   The preoccupation causes clinically significant distress or impairment in social, occupational, or other important areas of functioning.

D   The appearance preoccupation is not better explained by concerns with body fat or weight in an individual whose symptoms meet diagnostic criteria for an eating disorder.

Specify if:

With muscle dysmorphia: The individual is preoccupied with the idea that his or her body build is too small or insufficiently muscular. This specifier is used even if the individual is preoccupied with other body areas, which is often the case.

Specify if:

Indicate degree or insight regarding body dysmorphic disorder beliefs (e.g. "I look ugly" or "I look deformed").
With good or fair insight: The individual recognizes that the body dysmorphic disorder beliefs are definitely or probably not true or that they may or may not be true.
With poor insight: The individual thinks that the body dysmorphic disorder beliefs are probably true.
With absent insight/delusional beliefs: The individual is completely convinced that the body dysmorphic disorder beliefs are true.

BDD is a chronic non-psychotic somatoform disorder in which there is a persistent subjective belief of bodily abnormality. The patient is convinced the abnormality is obvious to others: in some cases a relatively minor physical abnormality does exist but is totally insufficient in degree to warrant the concern shown by the sufferer and his/her persistence. Veale and Bewley (2015) have provided a checklist, based on the history and observations, to make the diagnosis. The checklist has two components: questions to the patient (e.g. Do you currently think a lot about the feature you dislike?) and observations of the patient made by the physician (e.g. Does your patient have long hair to hide his or her face?).

The appearance, therefore, is very much like that of the once-called *monosymptomatic hypochondriacal psychosis* now termed *delusional disorder – somatic type* except that the complaint does not reach delusional intensity. It has, rather, the form of an overvalued idea. It has been suggested that BDD has features similar to obsessive-compulsive disorder, as was stated about dysmorphophobia initially. This similarity is perhaps enhanced by the response of both conditions to serotonergic antidepressants such as clomipramine.

It has been claimed that a minority of BDD cases become transiently psychotic, as in the case of other disorders such as morbid jealousy (McElory et al., 1993; Phillips and McElroy, 1993). This state may be indistinguishable from delusional disorder. However, the descriptions are more suggestive of brief psychotic episodes, and the patients may respond to serotonergic antidepressants, whereas cases of delusional disorder appear to improve only with neuroleptic drugs.

Whatever the nature of their relationship, both conditions (BDD and delusional disorder) can present to plastic and cosmetic surgeons, with sufferers demanding surgical intervention. In the UK, a scandal relating to a relatively high risk of bursting of Poly Implant Prothèse breast implants led to a major review of cosmetic surgery, starting in 2012, led by the then medical director of the National Health Service, Sir Bruce Keogh (Latham, 2014). Subsequently, the General Medical Council (2016) issued guidance for doctors who offer cosmetic interventions, the main aims of which were to ensure that such doctors:

- Are appropriately trained and experienced to practise safely
- Work with each individual patient to make sure their expectations about the outcomes that can be achieved for them are realistic
- Follow current guidelines or protocols for safe, effective provision of cosmetic interventions
- Consider the psychological needs of their patients
- Do not allow any financial or commercial interests in a particular intervention, or an organisation providing cosmetic interventions, to adversely affect standards of good patient care

Similarly, the Royal College of Surgeons (2013) have advised surgeons who offer cosmetic surgery to:

- Make attempts to identify the psychologically vulnerable patient and, where they have concerns, be prepared to avoid or defer operation pending psychological assessment.
- Refer a patient to a mental health expert when they consider that the psychological state of the patient may affect the patient's satisfaction with the outcome of surgery.

    Examples of situations that might trigger a referral to a psychologist include:

    - When surgeons consider that the expectations of the outcome of surgery are unrealistic, and this discrepancy is not resolved as part of the consultation.
    - When the patient has a history of repeated cosmetic procedures, particularly where those are in one anatomical area and there is evidence of dissatisfaction.
    - When the patient's mental health history reveals co-existing psychological disturbances.

Piras et al. (2016) have recently reviewed forensic and medicolegal aspects of cosmetic surgery. In failing to receive such treatment, BDD patients will turn to other surgeons and if again thwarted may revert to litigation.

In the case of dysmorphic delusional disorder, it appears to be the case that surgery should certainly be avoided, since it rarely satisfies the patient and often results in demands for further treatment (Greenberg et al., 2019). Connolly and Gipson (1978) reported that out of 86 patients who underwent rhinoplasties for largely cosmetic reasons, after a period of 15 years 32 exhibited a severe neurosis and six were suffering from schizophrenia. However, of 101 patients who received similar surgery for disease or injury, only 9 were severely neurotically disabled and 1 had schizophrenia.

This is an area where focussed research is very much necessary and should be undertaken by psychiatrists and cosmetic surgeons together. The problem has become even greater because of the nature of the society in which we live, where bodily perfection, of a type frequently portrayed in the media, has become of paramount importance as far as many individuals are concerned.

Case 6

A divorced man of 40 years, who looked much younger than his years, presented with a demand for surgery to correct his "misaligned jaw which gives me a lot of pain." He was totally preoccupied with the fact that his jaw was misaligned and that as a consequence his teeth collided and overlapped.

He had a three-year history of a change in behaviour; he had become isolated. He readily agreed that he was "a perfectionist in all I do in life." He hated looking into the mirror, something that he stated had begun with a difficult extraction when he was young – when his jaw was "pulled out of place and became more prominent."

He had a happy childhood, although even then he showed some obsessional personality traits. He, himself, stated, "I was always very confident and capable of doing anything that I put my mind to." He then added, referring to his present problem: "I wish this was totally in my hands, but I depend on other people to put it right; either they won't or can't and so I cannot put it out of my mind – cannot put it to rest at all." He had been happy at school but did not achieve the academic standards he knew he could have. He married at the age of 20, but there was a clash over children, and he was divorced by the age of 26. He had had other long-term relationships, but he thought that his current partner suffered as a result of their isolation.

There was a history of depressive episodes and suicidal thoughts. Paradoxically, he stated that it was when he realised that suicide was one avenue of escape that his tensions lessened. Apart from the one unshakeable hypochondriacal belief regarding his jaw, the patient's mental state appeared normal, although he had obvious obsessional personality traits.

He was initially treated with clomipramine, which had no effect. He was then successfully managed with a prescription of pimozide while remaining under the care of the dental practitioners as well as the mental health team.

Case 7

A young man of 18 years presented with complaints about the size of his ears. He stated that he had been mocked and bullied at school, and he recalled when he was aged 11 being teased about the way his ears stuck out. He was particularly conscious of his ears when he went swimming and, increasingly, he gave up this and other sporting activities so that he became isolated.

As his preoccupation grew, he became increasingly incapacitated. He was not able to go out and seek a job and became depressed. He superficially cut his forearm as a suicidal gesture.

He originated from a close-knit family. His grandmother was a dominating figure in the family where there were eight children and 25 grandchildren. His father was an authoritarian, and his mother suffered from "nerves." His early development was slower than that of the other children. He had a markedly obsessional personality, being preoccupied with hygiene and his general appearance.

On examination he was tense and depressed and preoccupied with the size and shape of his ears. He could discuss the possibility that his re-actions were exaggerated, but he believed that plastic surgery was the answer, even though the outcome might be unsatisfactory. There was no evidence of any formal depressive illness or psychosis. His IQ fell on the dull side of the average range.

The diagnosis was BDD, and he was treated with a course of cognitive behaviour therapy.

Psychopathology and aetiology

The syndrome is almost certainly non-specific and exists either in isolation, when it is an example of a paranoid disorder, or as a symptom of other conditions, both functional and organic. The pure form of the disorder almost certainly bears a relationship with the wide range of other hypochondriacal conditions. These extend from neurotic anxiety about health at one end of the scale – which varies from a constant obsessional preoccupation of being afflicted by various diseases – to, at the other, a delusional certainty at having some dire disease or deformity. This range may include dysmorphophobia, venerophobia and cancerophobia, for example. Furthermore, as Laupland and Valiquette (2016) have pointed out, "Delusional infestation challenges the infectious diseases specialist who must diligently rule out the presence of a true infection."

Heredity

A family history of mental disorder is frequent in that about 40–45% of siblings are said to suffer other forms of psychiatric disturbance.

Skott (1978) identified a number of cases where organic brain disease appeared to be present. Other physical conditions which seemed to her to be contributory include hypertension, heart failure and cerebral arteriopathic degenerative changes, although she concluded that the physical conditions, while prominent in some patients, neither constituted a single cause nor the most important factor underlying their delusions.

More recently other investigators have also reported an apparent association between delusional parasitosis and other physical disorders. These include hypoparathyroidism (Trabert, 1985), Huntington's chorea (Morris, Moss and Jolly, 1988), Alzheimer's disease and complex visual hallucinations (Renvoize et al., 1987; Kanazawa and Hata,1992; Johnson et al., 2017), multi-infarct dementia (Bhatia et al., 2015), HIV infection (Yang et al., 2016) and HIV dementia (Musso et al., 2013), CADASIL (cerebral autosomal dominant arteriopathy with subcortical infarcts and leukoencephalopathy) (Berhili et al., 2016), pontine lesions at the root of the trigeminal nerve (Frazier et al., 2010); peripheral neuropathy (Sales et al., 2013) and in haemodialysis patients (Trigka et al., 2012; Herbert et al., 2015; Omri et al , 2015). The majority of cases, however, are not associated with overt organic brain disorder.

There is a relatively strong association with drug use. In order to assess the aetiological role of recreational psychoactive substance use in patients with delusional infestation, Marshall et al. (2017) studied the following two groups of delusional infestation patients attending their London clinic: a retrospective review of 86 consecutive patient records (mean age 56 years; female:male 1.4:1) to determine current or previous recreational drug use; and 24 consecutive patients (mean age 54 years; female:male 3:1) prospectively offered a urine test for recreational drugs. Around a fifth of the first group had used or were still using such drugs, particularly cannabis, cocaine and amphetamines. In the second group, of the 18 patients who actually provided a urine sample, one-third were positive for recreational drugs, namely cannabinoids and amphetamines. Thus in the assessment of delusional infestation it is important not only to ask about psychoactive substance misuse but also to consider testing urine samples for undeclared use (Marshall et al., 2017).

The question arises as to whether or not patients with delusional infestation may actually suffer from skin infestation. Hylwa et al. (2011) studied the results of skin biopsies and patient-provided specimens in delusional infestation. Of 108 delusional infestation patients seen at the Mayo Clinic over a seven-year period, 80 underwent skin biopsies, 80 brought their own specimens and 52 belonged to both groups. Not a single biopsy showed evidence of infestation. One patient-provided specimen contained a true parasite, namely a pubic louse. These results indicate that there is no need to carry out formal skin biopsies in such patients; Hylwa et al. (2011) concluded that "in patients with suspected delusional infestation, neither skin biopsies nor examination of patient-provided specimens provided objective evidence of skin infestation."

The first published study of delusional infestation using voxel-based morphometry of structural MRI brain scans of patients and controls was that of Wolf et al. (2013). They scanned 16 patients: six met the *DSM-IV-TR* criteria for delusional disorder, somatic type; three had delusional infestation secondary to psychotic depression; seven had delusional infestation secondary to an organic disorder (five with subcortical vascular encephalopathy, one with hearing loss and blindness, and one with hyperthyroidism); all met the delusional infestation criteria of Freudenmann and Lepping (2009). Their control group consisted of 16 healthy subjects who were matched with the patients in respect of sex, age and handedness. Compared with the controls, the delusional infestation patients showed reduced grey matter volume in left medial, lateral and right superior frontal cortices, left anterior cingulate cortex, bilateral insula, left thalamus, right striatal regions and in lateral and medial temporal cortical regions; and increased white matter volume in right middle cingulate, left frontal opercular and bilateral striatal regions. Wolf et al. (2013) suggested that their findings pointed to disruption of prefrontal control over somatosensory representations in delusional infestation.

The last study, by Wolf et al. (2013), included different types of delusional infestation patients, who were dichotomised by the authors into patients with "psychiatric delusional infestation" (meeting the *DSM-IV-TR* criteria for delusional disorder, somatic type or secondary to psychotic depression) and those with "organic delusional infestation" (secondary to an organic disorder). A further, source-based morphometry analysis of the data using this dichotomisation showed that the grey matter volume changes in the delusional infestation patients were independent of aetiology, while the aberrant white matter volume appeared to be restricted to cases of delusional infestation of organic aetiology (Wolf et al., 2014).

Case reports of delusional infestation have also been reported to be associated with pharmacotherapy for Parkinson's disease (Swick and Walling, 2005; Flann et al., 2010; Kölle et al., 2010; Ojeda-Lopez et al., 2015). This finding is consistent with decreased striatal dopamine transporter function in delusional infestation, leading to increased synaptic dopamine levels, particularly when dopaminergic reuptake is blocked by drugs such as methylphenidate and cocaine (Ojeda-Lopez et al., 2015; Wolf et al., 2013). Furthermore, Ojeda-Lopez et al. (2015) have gone on to suggest that:

> The striato-thalamo-parietal network has been presumed to play a key role in the explanation of somatic symptoms, supporting the sensorialistic approach of delusional parasitosis in which an impaired perception leads to the fixed false belief of infestation. Dysfunction in

this "somatic loop" has been supported by a case series of secondary organic delusional parasitosis with lesions in the putamen [Huber et al., 2008].

In [Parkinson's disease], central processing of sensory stimulation has been shown to be decreased in functional Imaging studies. When compared with controls, patients with [Parkinson's disease] show reduced activation of contralateral basal ganglia and primary and secondary sensory cortical areas, along with motor, premotor, and cingulate cortices [Ceballos-Baumann et al., 1999]. Then, dopamine supplementation combined with structural susceptibility may lead to the onset of delusional parasitosis in [Parkinson's disease].

More recently, Wolf's group have carried out a detailed structural MRI study of the cerebral cortex in 18 patients with delusional infestation, comparing them with 20 healthy controls matched for age, sex and handedness (Hirjak et al., 2017); 16 of the patients were the same as those in the previous two studies by the same group mentioned above (Wolf et al., 2013; 2014). Compared with the control group, the delusional infestation group showed:

* Increased cortical thickness of the right orbitofrontal gyrus
* Decreased cortical areas of the right lingual and right orbitofrontal gyri
* Decreased cortical folding of the left precentral, right inferior parietal, right middle temporal and right precentral gyri

Hirjak et al. (2017) suggested that their findings were noteworthy for several reasons:

First, the precentral gyrus is specialized in the control of response inhibition (Li et al., 2006). Therefore, it might be suggested that [local gyrification index] alterations in precentral cortices result in impaired inhibition of motor response ... [which] implicate a potential neurobiological mechanism underlying impulsive and self-destructive behavior such as skin picking and excoriation when attempting to remove the pathogens. Second, the postcentral gyrus is the location of the primary somatosensory cortex that is involved mainly in proprioception, thermoreception, and nociception. Alterations of the somatosensory cortex might explain disturbed body perception and proprioception, which can result in the experience of intolerable pruritus misattributed as being caused by pathogens scrabbling under the skin (Wolf et al., 2013). This is also in line with previous study conducted by Eccles [et al. (2015)] who found that [delusional infestation] patients exhibited exaggerated responses to infestation-relevant stimuli in the posterior insula/ secondary somatosensory cortex, which is the primary interoceptive area. Further, ... patients exhibited heightened activity in the amygdala, which plays a crucial role in states of fear and anxiety. According to these findings, the authors concluded that the aberrant connectivity between posterior insula and amygdala might cause altered interpretation of skin sensations, which are reinforced by failed amygdala habituation (e.g. negative emotional stimuli) (Eccles et al., 2015). This neuronal failure might initiate a process leading to the development of [delusional infestation]. Third, aberrant cortical folding might represent the shared neurodevelopmental marker of different psychotic syndromes ... Fourth ... we observed alterations of cortical folding in parietal regions. The inferior parietal lobule is involved in a general attention role ... , inhibitory control ... , reorienting attention ... , self reflection, self perception ... and interpreting of sensory input ... Together with previous studies supporting the notion of the dorsal "somatic" loop (putamen/dorsal striatum – thalamus – parietal cortex) being involved in [delusional infestation] ... this evidence allows us, cautiously, to assume that structural alterations within the [inferior parietal lobule] might substantially contribute to abnormal bodily perception and poor insight in patients with [delusional infestation]. Taken together, the present data support previous studies and support the hypothesis that [delusional infestation]-associated symptoms are associated with aberrant frontostriatal and parietothalamic pathways which are considered to be intricately linked to delusion formation, especially in somatic delusions (Corlett et al., 2010; Freudenmann and Lepping, 2009).

Psychodynamic factors

Whatever the underlying psychiatric disorder which causes the emergence of delusions of infestation, whether this be affective, schizophrenic, paranoid or organic, psychodynamic formulations are important. The two most important aspects in this regard are *guilt* and *projection*.

One odd feature is that delusions of infestation occur more commonly in females (with a higher incidence in females up to the age of 79 years), whereas dysmorphophobic conditions (*anorexia nervosa apart*) are much more frequent in men and younger men at that. It is probable that the form which hypochondriasis actually takes is influenced by sexual role and activity. Thus it may be postulated that in the case of a woman who is made pregnant, possibly unwillingly, or who is ashamed at her loss of virginity or who has been venereally affected (not necessarily by syphilis but even by scabies) may well come to feel that she has been contaminated or even infested. Males with BDD, on the other hand, may believe themselves to have a misshapen nose or other deformities leading, they are convinced, to lack of social or sexual prowess.

Traditionally, paranoid psychoses of a persecutory or even of a grandiose type have been conceptualised as representing a projection of a patient's feelings into the environment so that these, being reflected back to him, lead him to believe that others torment or persecute him or, in the case of manic paranoid states, that he is in some way exulted and beyond such persecution. In Cotard's syndrome, when nihilistic delusions of death and decay occur, the patient may be seen as his own accuser and inquisitor. Likewise she who complains of being infested with fleas, lice or whatever else may be giving vent to a psychotic self-accusation of being unclean, an idea which, as has already been suggested, may have a guilt-ridden sexual connotation.

Nosology of the delusional disorders

Ekbom's syndrome is one striking example of delusional disorders, a category recognised in *ICD-11* and *DSM-5*. Prior to this, delusional disorders were known as paranoia, which up until the end of the nineteenth century was a well-recognised illness. However, by 1977 Gregory and Smelzer were advocating the demise of the diagnosis and, in a 1980 *British Medical Journal* editorial stated that "paranoia is no longer a fashionable term." But as Bernard Shaw said, "fashions are already out of date," and it was no surprise that the concept was reintroduced in 1987 in *DSM-III-R* albeit in the guise of "delusional disorders."

Paranoia/delusional disorder is an important concept because it is an illness characterised by a constant and persistent delusional system, to which the patient adheres with fanatical intensity, although it is quite encapsulated and leaves the rest of the personality and psychosocial functioning intact. Hallucinations very rarely occur, and if they do, are not prominent and are typically related closely to the delusional belief. The illness is chronic and often lifelong, but the principal characteristics of schizophrenia are crucially absent.

There is a specific spectrum in these conditions which is more pronounced than in many other psychotic conditions. On the one hand, there appears to be more contact with reality. The severity of the delusions can fluctuate markedly at different times. At certain times insight appears to be preserved. However, on the other hand, insight can be completely lost, and the delusional belief is then impervious to any reasoning to the contrary.

Treatment and management

The treatment approach to Ekbom's syndrome is based on the following principles:

- If the disorder occurs as a symptom of another condition, then the treatment must be directed at the latter. For example, if a strong affective element is present, ECT or other antidepressant treatment may be reasonably successful in bringing about a degree of relief (Gupta et al., 1986; Dowson, 1987).
- In those cases where the disorder exists in isolation, antipsychotic medication is the treatment of choice. Pimozide may be worth a trial, but despite its advocates (Munro, 1978; Avnstorp et al., 1980; Lindskov and Baadsgaard, 1985; Mitchell, 1989), any claim for superiority over other neuroleptics is uncertain and issues of drug safety must be borne in mind (Freudenmann and Lepping, 2009). Other antipsychotics which have been advocated include aripiprazole (Carpiniello et al., 2011; Yeh et al., 2014), blonanserin (Bhatia et al., 2013), clozapine (in combination with citalopram) (Cupina and Boulton, 2012), olanzapine (Kansal et al., 2012), paliperidone (Albayrak et al., 2011; Altinoz et al., 2014) and ziprasidone (Contreras-Ferrer et al., 2012; De Berardis et al., 2013). In a study of 17 consecutive delusional infestation patients attending an Italian psychiatric outpatient clinic, Huber et al. (2011) reported that the vast majority (88%) benefitted from antipsychotic treatment, with an average duration of treatment of 3.8 years. However, in a cross-sectional study of 69 patients with delusional infestation receiving treatment at a London psychodermatology clinic, Ahmed and Bewley (2013) found that the compliance with psychotropic medication, which included second-generation antipsychotic drugs and antidepressant drugs, was around only 59%.
- A psychotherapeutic approach, especially when combined with appropriate medication, may be helpful. A symptom-free remission in an "infested" patient who was the dominant partner in a *folie imposée* following weeks of supportive psychotherapy alone has been described (Macaskill, 1987).

Prognosis

In most cases of delusional parasitosis, the symptom, once established, often appears to be intractable. Cases in which the symptom either exists in isolation or is organically determined may carry a worse prognosis with a greater tendency to become chronic. In their 10-year dermatology case series of delusional infestation patients, Wong et al. (2018) found that an associated psychiatric disorder and chronic pain were both associated with a poor outcome.

Suicide as an outcome has been reported (Bebbington, 1976), while Hunt and Blacker (1980) have described the case of a male patient who set fire to several dwellings in an apparent attempt to fumigate them and pointed out that such a patient could constitute a danger to others.

References

Ahmed, A., Bewley, A., (2013) British Journal of Dermatology, 169, 607.

Albayrak, Y., Ekinci, O., Ozbay, S.Y. (2011) The Israel Journal of Psychiatry and Related Sciences, 48, 291.

Altinoz, A.E., Tosun Altinoz, S., Kucukkarapinar, M. and Cosar, B. (2014) Australasian Psychiatry, 22, 576.

Avnstorp, C., Hamaan, K., Jepsen, P.W. (1980) Ugeskrift for Laeger, 142, 2191.

American Psychiatric Association (2013) Diagnostic and Statistical Manual of Mental Disorders, Fifth Edition (DSM-5). American Psychiatric Association: Washington, DC.

American Psychiatric Association (2013) Diagnostic and Statistical Manual of Mental Disorders, Fifth Edition (DSM-5) Washington, D.C.: American Psychiatric Association.

Bailey, C.H., Andersen, L.K., Lowe, G.C., Pittelkow, M.R., Bostwick, J.M., Davis, M.D. (2014) The British Journal of Dermatology, 170, 1130.

Bebbington, P. (1976) British Journal of Psychiatry, 128, 475.

Berhili, N., Bout, A., Hlal, H., Aarab, C., Aalouane, R., Ramniouz, I. (2016) The Pan African Medical Journal, 24, 130.

Bharia, M.S., Gautam, P., Kaur, J. (2015) Journal of Clinical and Diagnostic Research , 9, VD03.

Bhatla, M.S., Rathi, A., Jhanjee, A. (2013) The Journal of Neuropsychiatry and Clinical Neurosciences, 25, E54.

Bourgeois, M., Rager, P., Peyrie, F. Nguyen-Lan, A., Etchepare, J.J. (1986) Annales Medico-Psychologiques, 144, 659.

Carpiniello, B., Pinna, F., Tuveri, R. (2011) Case Reports in Medicine, 2011, 103652.

Ceballos-Baumann, A., Weindl, A., Conrad, B., Munz, F., Boecker, H., Siebner, H. R., et al. (1999) Brain, 122, 1651.

Colombo, G., Caimi, M., Dona, G.P. (2004) European Psychiatry,, 19, 115.

Contreras-Ferrer, P., de Paz, N.M., Cejas-Mendez, M.R., Rodriguez-Martin, M., Souto, R., Bustinduy, M.G. (2012) Case Reports in Dermatology, 4, 150.

Connolly, F. and Gipson, M. (1978) British Journal of Psychiatry, 132, 458.

Corlett, P.R., Taylor, J.R., Wang, X.J., Fletcher, P.C., Krystal, J.H. (2010) Progress in Neurobiology, 92, 345.

Cupina, D., Boulton, M. (2012) Psychosomatics, 53, 301.

Daulatabad, D., Sonthalia, S., Srivastava, A., Bhattacharya, S.N., Kaul, S., Moyal, D. (2017) Australasian Journal of Dermatology, 58, e113.

Davidson, M., Mukherjee, S. (1982) The American Journal of Psychiatry, 139, 1623.

De Berardis, D., Serroni, N., Marini, S., Rapini, G., Valchera, A., Fornaro, M. et al. (2013). Case Reports in Psychiatry, 2013, 913248.

Dey, J.K., Ishii, M., Phillis, M., Byrne, P.J., Boahene, K.D., Ishii, L.E. (2015) Facial Plastic Surgery, 17, 137.

Dohring, E. (1960) Munchener medizinische Wochenschrift, 102, 2158.

Dowson, J.H. (1987) Journal of Neural Transmission, 23, 121.

Eccles, J.A., Garfinkel, S.N., Harrison, N.A., Ward, J., Taylor, R.E., Bewley, A.P., et al. (2015) Neuropsychologia, 77, 90.

Ekbom, K.A. (1937) Om. de. s. k. parasitofobierna. Svenska Psykiatriska Foreningens Fordandlingar, Stockholm. Cited in Skott (1978). Reports from the Psychiatric Research Centre, St Jorgen Hospital, University of Goteborg, No 13 (Goteborg University Press).

Ekbom, K.A. (1938) Acta Psychiatrica Scandinavica, 13, 227.

Eller, J.J. (1929) *New York Medical Journal*, 129, 481.

Evans, P., Merskey, H. (1972) *British Journal of Medical Psychology*, 45, 19.

Flann, S., Shotbolt, J., Kessel, B., Vekaria, D., Taylor, R., Bewley, A. *et al.* (2010) *Clinical and Experimental Dermatology*, 35, 740.

Frazier, L.G., Azad, A., Scholma, R.S., Joshi, K.G. (2010) *Psychiatry (Edgmont)*, 7, 33.

Freudenmann, R.W., Lepping, P. (2009) *Clinical Microbiology Reviews* , 22, 690.

Friedmann, A.C., Ekeowa-Anderson, A., Taylor, R., Bewley, A. (2006) *The British Journal of Dermatology*, 155, 841.

General Medical Council (2016) https://www.gmc-uk.org/ethical-guidance/ethical-guidance-for-doctors/cosmetic-interventions/about-this-guidance. Accessed February 2019.

Giam, A., Tung, Y.L., Tibrewal, P., Dhillon, R., Bastiampillai, T. (2017) *Asian Journal of Psychiatry*, 28, 152.

Greenberg, J.L., Weingarden, H., Wilhelm, S. (2019) *Journal of American Medical Association Facial Plastic Surgery*.

Gregory, I., Smelzer, D.J. (1977) *Essentials of Clinical Practice with Examination Questions, Answers and Comments*. Little Brown, Boston.

Gupta, M.A., Gupta, K.A., Haberman, H.F. (1986) *Journal of the American Academy of Dermatology*, 14, 633.

Herbert, J., Cameron, K., Battistella, M. (2015) *CANNT J*, 25, 40.

Hirjak, D., Huber, M., Kirchler, E., Kubera, K.M., Karner, M., Sambataro, F. *et al.* (2017) *Progress in Neuro-Psychopharmacology & Biological Psychiatry*, 76, 72.

Huber, M., Karner, M., Kirchler, E., Lepping, P., Freudenmann, R.W. (2008) *Progress in Neuro-Psychopharmacology and Biological Psychiatry*, 32, 1967.

Huber, M., Lepping, P., Pycha, R., Karner, M., Schwitzer, J., Freudenmann, R.W. (2011) *General Hospital Psychiatry*, 33, 604.

Hunt, N.J., Blacker, V.R. (1980) *British Journal of Psychiatry*, 150, 713.

Iwu, C. O., Akpata, O. (1990) *The British Dental Journal*, 168, 294.

Hylwa, S.A., Bury, J.E., Davis, M.D., Pittelkow, M., Bostwick, J.M. (2011) *Archives of Dermatology* , 147, 1041.

Hylwa, S.A., Foster, A.A., Bury, J.E., Davis, M.D., Pittelkow, M.R., Bostwick, J.M. (2012) *Psychosomatics*, 53, 258.

Johnson, K., Nasol, E., Wood, S., Chien, J. (2017) *Psychogeriatrics*, 17, 493.

Kansal, N.K., Chawla, O., Singh, G.P. (2012) *The Indian Journal of Psychological Medicine*, 34, 297.

Kanazawa, A. and Hata, T. (1992) *Psychopathology*, 25, 209.

Kim, C., Kim, J., Lee, M., Kang, M. (2003) *Journal of Korean Medical Science*, 18, 462.

Kölle, M., Lepping, P., Kassubek, J., Schönfeldt-Lecuona, C., Freudenmann, R.W. (2010). *Pharmacopsychiatry*, 43, 240.

Laupland, K.B., Valiquette, L. (2016) *The Canadian Journal of Infectious Diseases and Medical Microbiology'*, 2016, 9091838.

Latham, M. (2014) *Medical Law Review*, 22, 384.

Lepping, P., Baker, C., Freudenmann, R.W. (2010) *The Journal of Clinical and Experimental Dermatology*, 35, 841.

Li, C.S., Huang, C., Constable, R.T., Sinha, R. (2006) *The Journal of Neuroscience*, 26, 186.

Lindskov, R., Baadsgaard, O. (1985) *Acta Dermato-Venereologica*, 65, 267.

Macaskill, N.D. (1987) *British Journal of Psychiatry*, 155, 261.

Mackley, C.L. (2005) *Dermatologic Surgery*, *31*, 553.

Malasi, T.H., el-Hilu, S.M., Mirza, I.A., el-Islam, M.F. (1990) *The British Journal of Psychiatry*, *156*, 256.

Maneros, M., Deister, A., Rohde, O. (1988) *Psychopathology*, *21*, 267.

Marshall, C.L., Williams, V., Ellis, C., Taylor, R.E., Bewley, A.P. (2017) *Journal Clinical and Experimental Dermatology*, *42*, 41.

McElory, S.L., Phillips, K.A., Keck, P.E. Jr, Hudson, J.I., Pope, H.G. Jr (1993) *The Journal of Clinical Psychiatry*, *54*, 389.

Mitchell, C. (1989) *British Journal of Psychiatry*, *155*, 556.

Mester, H. (1975) *Psychiatric Clinics of North America*, *8*, 339.

Moftah, N.H., Kamel, A.M., Attia, H.M., El-Baz, M.Z., Abd El-Moty, H.M. (2013) *Journal of Epidemiology and Global Health*, *3*, 131.

Moro, A., Munhoz, R.P., Moscovich, M., Arruda, W.O., Teive, H.A.G. (2013) *Parkinsonism & Related Disorders*, *19*, 751.

Munro, A. and Stewart, M. (1991) Body Dysmorphic Disorder and the DSM-IV: The Demise of Dysmorphophobia. *Canadian Journal of Psychiatry*, *36*, 9110.1177/070674379103600203.

Morris, M., Jolly, D.J. (1987) *British Journal of Psychiatry*, *151*, 272

Morris, M,, Moss, G.M., Jolly, D.J. (1988) *Geriatric Medicine*, *18*, 57.

Morselli, E. (1886) *Boll Accad Sci Med Genova*, *6*, 100.

Munro, A. (1978) *Archives of Dermatology*, *114*, 940.

Musalek, M., Kutzer, F. (1989) *Wiener Klinische Wochenschrift*, *101*, 153.

Munro, A. and Stewart, M. (1991) *Canadian Journal of Psychiatry*, *36*, 91.

Musso, M.W., Jones, G.N., Heck, M.C., Gouvier, D. (2013) *Applied Neuropsychology: Adult,*, *20*, 66.

Myerson, A. (1921) *Boston University School of Medicine*, *184*, 635.

Ojeda-Lopez, C., Aguilar-Venegas, L.C., Tapia-Orozco, M., Cervantes-Arriaga, A., Rodriguez-Violante, M. (2015) *Psychosomatics*, *56*, 696.

Omri, S., Damak, R., Ben Brahim, H., Mechri, A. (2015) *La Tunisie médicale*, *93*, 484.

Pearson, M.L., Selby, J.V., Katz, K.A., Cantrell, V., Braden, C.R., Parise, M.E. *et al.* (2012). *PLoS One*, *7*, e29908.

Perrin, L. (1896). *Annals of Dermatology Syphilgraph*, *7*, 129.

Phillips, K.A., McElroy, S.L. (1993) *The Journal of Nervous and Mental Disease*, *181*, 699.

Piras, M., Delbon, P., Conti, A., Graziano, V., Capasso, E., Niola, M., *et al.* (2016) *Open Medicine (Wars)*, *11*, 327.

Prakash, J., Shashikumar, R., Bhat, P.S., Srivastava, K., Nath, S., Rajendran, A. (2012) *The Indian Journal of Psychiatry*, *21*, 72.

Reilly, T.M., Batchelor, D.H. (1986) *International Clinical Psychopharmacology*, *1*, 340.

Renvoize, E.B., Kent, J., Klar, H.M. (1987) *British Journal of Psychiatry*, *150*, 403.

Royal College of Surgeons (2013) *Professional Standards for Cosmetic Surgery*. Royal College of Surgeons, London.

Sales, P.M., Thomas, F.P., Gondim Fde, A. (2013) *Arquivos de Neuro-Psiquiatria*, *71*, 131.

Sawant, N.S., Vispute, C.D. (2015) *Indian Journal of Psychiatry*, *24*, 97.

Schrut, A.H., Waldron, W.G. (1963) *Journal of the American Medical Association*, *186*, 429.

Skott, A. (1978) *Delusions of Infestation, Ekbom's Syndrome*. Goteburg University Press, Goteburg, Sweden.

Swick, B.L., Walling, H.W. (2005) *Journal of the American Academy of Dermatology*, 53, 1086.

Thieberge, G. (1894) *Annales Psychiatrie Neurologie*, 5, 730.

Trabert, W. (1985) *Psychiatrie, Neurologie and Medizinische Psycholoie (Leipzig)*, 37, 648.

Trabert, W. (1991) *Nervenarzt*, 62, 165.

Trabert, W. (1993) *Delusional Parasitosis. Studies on Frequency, Classification and Prognosis (Dissertation)*. Homburg/Saar: Universitat des Saarlandes.

Trigka, K., Dousdampanis, P., Fourtounas, C. (2012) *The International Journal of Artificial Organs*, 35, 400.

Veale, D., Bewley, A. (2015) *BMJ*, 350, h2278.

Wilson, J.W., Miller, H.E. (1946) *Archives of Dermatology and Syphilology*, 54, 39.

WHO (2018). *International Classification of Diseases, 11th Revision (ICD-11)* Geneva: World Health Organization.

Wolf, R.C., Huber, M., Depping, M.S., Thomann, P.A., Karner, M., Lepping, P. *et al.* (2013) *Prog Progress in Neuro-Psychopharmacology & Biological Psychiatry*, 46, 19.

Wolf, R., Huber, M., Lepping, P., Sambataro, F., Depping, M.S., Karner, M. *et al.* (2014) *Progress in Neuro-Psychopharmacology & Biological Psychiatry*, 48, 112.

Wong, Y.L., Affleck, A., Stewart, A.M. (2018) *Acta Dermato-Venereologica*, 98, 441.

Yang, C., Brandenburg, J., Mozingo, E.B. (2016) *Primary Care Companion for CNS Disorders*, 18, 10.4088.

Yeh, T.C., Lin, Y.C., Chen, L.F., Chiang, C.P., Mao, W.C., Chang, H.A. *et al.* (2014) *Australian and New Zealand Journal of Psychiatry*, 48, 681.

Possession states and allied syndromes

The mind is its own place, and in itself
Can make a Heaven of Hell, a Hell of Heaven

John Milton (1667)

In this chapter, so-called possession states and a number of other related disorders and phenomena will be considered. A possession state can be defined as the presence of a belief, delusional or otherwise, held by an individual (and sometimes by others) that their symptoms, experiences and behaviour are under the influence or control of supernatural forces, often of diabolical origin. We make no judgement concerning the absolute reality or not of demonic possession. What is acknowledged, however, is that despite centuries of so-called enlightened thinking, such beliefs still retain a powerful hold upon some individuals within our society and culture. Indeed, there is some evidence to suggest that such beliefs may be more frequently held today than in recent former times (see below).

Furthermore, it is also accepted that there is (whatever its nature) a spiritual dimension to the human condition, and all human beings, to varying extents, have spiritual needs. It is not surprising, therefore, that the anguish and distress associated with severe mental illness on occasions is manifested in pathological thoughts, perceptions and other abnormal experiences which contain a diabolical content. It follows, therefore, that it is incumbent upon all practising psychiatrists to maintain some awareness of these aspects so as to ensure that the practitioner is always in a position to offer appropriate help to his/her patients.

Historical

So much has been written on demonic possession and related subjects that a fully comprehensive review is clearly impossible within the confines of a single chapter in a book such as this. Spirit possession beliefs can be found in the majority of human communities across the globe (Bourguignon, 1970). For a review of the subject from a transcultural perspective, the reader is referred to Littlewood (2004). We have confined ourselves to those writings of major historical importance or which are relevant to the psychopathological understanding of possession syndromes. What follows is inevitably heavily euro-centric in its nature.

The early Church

There is no doubt, according to all four Gospels found within the New Testament, that the casting out of demons played a major part in the ministry of the man later known as Jesus Christ; for example,

> Just then a man with an evil spirit in him came into the synagogue and screamed "what do you want with us, Jesus of Nazareth? Are you here to destroy us? I know who you are – you are God's holy messenger!" Jesus ordered the spirit "Be quiet, and come out of the man!" The evil spirit shook the man hard, gave a loud scream, and came out of him.
>
> Mark 1:23–26

It is also clear that, although allied to the healing of diseases, exorcisms such as that recorded above were nevertheless regarded as being in some way distinct:

> The news about him spread through the whole country of Syria, so that people brought to him all those who were sick, suffering from all kinds of diseases or disorders: people with demons, and epileptics, and paralytics – and Jesus healed them all.
>
> Matthew 4:24

The exorcism of demons had become an established practice during the early years and centuries of the church as is clear from the account of St Paul's ministry (Acts, 16:18; Acts, 29:12) and the writings of some of the early Church Fathers, for example Tertullian (Apologet., 23, P.L., I, 410) and Origen (C.Celsum, VII, 4 P.G. 1425). These traditions have persisted in the church down to the present day.

Mediaeval times/early Modern Age

In 1484, there appeared the *Papal Bull of Innocent VIII,* followed three years later by the publication of Sprenger and Kraemer's (1489)*Malleus Maleficarum.* This latter work provided a detailed account of the signs of witchcraft along with the procedures to be adopted when arresting and examining (often with the aid of torture) suspected witches. Witchcraft was often considered to be the basis of possession, and witches were thought to be agents of the devil or to participate in intimate relationships with him. This publication lay at the heart of the witch hunts of the late Middle Ages.

Many striking examples of mediaeval possession can be found in both the historical and fictional literature. Indeed, according to Levack (2013), in a comprehensive historical review of this topic, the phenomenon of demonic possession probably reached epidemic proportions in the late Middle Ages/early modern era. This development is thought to have been associated with the profound religious anxiety that characterised that particular era, and also coincided with the start of witch hunting in the early fifteenth century. One such is the case of Soeur Jeanne des Anges, the mother superior of the Ursuline Convent in Loudun, who, in 1632, together with her nuns, claimed to have become possessed as a result of the machinations of the Jesuit priest Urbain Grandier. A psychopathological interpretation of this affair was provided by Legué and Gilles de la Tourette's in 1886. The same subject was later treated by Aldous Huxley (1951) and the playwright John Whiting (1961).

The convulsions demonstrated by Soeur Jeanne and her companions were similar to those of Abigail and her associates in the case of the Witches of Salem so vividly characterised by Arthur Miller (1956) in his play *The Crucible*.

The modern era

In 1921, Traugott Konstantin Oesterreich distinguished *true* possession from instances where the features of possession were clearly manifestations of mental disorder:

> These are cases of mere delusion ... which may have a very different origin. The mildest cases concern uneducated people who, in order to explain maladies, particularly of a psychic nature, adopt the vulgar notion of possession. The more serious ones concern paranoiacs, paralytics, and other persons suffering from diseases of the mind which produce hallucinatory ideas and in whom the delusion of possession arises. Such affections defy exorcism, or if not, a new illusory idea will immediately take the place of the former one.

It should be noted that by *true* possession, Oesterreich did not necessarily intend it to be thought that possession as such could actually occur. He was of the opinion that so-called *true possession* occurs in two main forms: A "somnambulistic" or *hysterical* form and a "lucid" or *obsessional* form. What distinguishes the obsessional from the hysterical form is a lack of ego participation, which seems to prevent the supposed devil from taking over completely, although the sufferer cannot by any power of will be free of the compulsion to behave in a grossly distorted and unwanted manner as the devil inside seemingly dictates.

In contrast, that variety of possession described as somnambulistic or of hysterical origin is more striking. Just as the somnambulist or sleep-walker is able to perform a whole series of complicated actions without any apparent awareness of so doing, so apparently is the hysterically possessed subject, who, doing likewise, seems to be at the complete mercy of his or her personal demon.

Sigmund Freud (1946) also wrote on possession, including an analysis of the diary and paintings of the painter Christoph Haizmann, a celebrated case of possession – *a Neurosis of Demonical Possession in the Seventeenth Century*. Freud regarded *true* possession to be a manifestation of gross neurotic illness. Thus he wrote:

> Cases of demonical possession correspond to the neurosis of the present day; in order to understand the latter we have once more to have recourse to the conception of psychic forces. What in days gone by was thought to be evil spirits to us are base and evil wishes, the derivatives of impulses which have been rejected and repressed. In one respect only do we not subscribe to the explanation of these phenomena current in mediaeval times; we have abandoned the projection of them into the outer world, attributing their origin instead to the inner life of the patient in whom they manifest themselves.

In 1975, Jan Ehrenwald, a Czech-American psychoanalyst, distinguished four different forms of the possession syndrome:

a   Those who *act out* their "possession" by projecting inner mental conflicts onto external reality – struggling with repressed instinctual desires (Oersterreich's *obsessional* form) or by dramatisation giving rise to a trance state based on dissociation (*hysterical* form).
b   Where personal or culture-bound factors act upon an organic or functional pathology leading to a pathoplastic colouring to the content of a psychosis.
c   Where ideas of possession are based on "initiation and contagion," i.e. mass suggestion.
d   *Paranormal* forms, "such as the ability of the gifted trance medium to detect subtle telepathic cues" and weave them into the fabric of a seemingly autonomous personality.

Other recent writers have further advocated that not all cases of demonic possession can be attributed to recognisable mental disorder. The former is said to include features not characteristic of mental illness and the sufferers – unlike those with psychosis – do not lose their object reality (Cooper, 1975; Sall, 1970). Sall in particular, although agreeing that most deviant behaviour may be explained in terms of natural causes, does not preclude the possibility of possession in the current day and age. Prins (1990) seemed to agree with this, stating, "It would appear to be a tenable view that theological (Divine) explanations are necessary, because in some cases, when all of the facts are examined, other explanations seem insufficient." This of course is something about which the reader must form his/her own view.

Even in the late twentieth century, periodically cases arose where death occurred in the setting of beliefs of possession or attempts at exorcism. A good example is that which occurred in Ossett in South Yorkshire in March 1975, when, following an all-night exorcism ceremony to rid him of demons, a 31-year-old man returned home and, it was alleged, brutally killed his wife to rid her also of an evil spirit (Times, April 24, 1975).

During the very week this chapter was first written for the second edition of this book, there were two such reports in a single day. One was of two Roman Catholic priests in the former West Germany charged with causing the death of a woman with epilepsy who had starved to death while they were trying to drive out the devils whom she believed possessed her. The other was that of a 24-year-old French woman known to her neighbours as "The Sorceress" who had a farm worker aged 46 years strapped to his bed and given nothing except salt and water, which she had blessed, in order to "exorcise" him of demons. Fortunately, the matter was brought to the attention of the police so that after a week the victim was released, weakened but otherwise unharmed.

More recently, in Norwich, a 42-year-old Chinese man killed his mentally ill sister by stamping on her during a bizarre attempt to exorcise the demonic forces he believed possessed her (Eastern Daily Press, September 13, 1994).

According to Levack (2013), in the latter part of the twentieth century the number of reported cases of demonic possession rose. This rising trend is also reported to be continuing in the first two decades of the twenty-first century (Rowan and Dwyer, 2015). This phenomenon is possibly related to the changing cultural profile of actively religious communities in the UK.

Case reports

Case I

S.W., a 22-year-old West Indian woman who came originally from St Kitt's, was first admitted to hospital complaining of "terrible feelings" especially in her pelvic region, of "pains all over," of "feeling hollow as if something were eating her out," together with loss of appetite, weight and sleep and a foreboding of imminent death.

She insisted that all the symptoms were the result of having been bewitched, stating that when she was a child an aunt, with malign intent, had given her some noxious substance to eat and had tampered with her panties. Three years earlier, at the age of 19 years, she married; she became pregnant but shortly afterwards miscarried, which misfortune she explained as being caused by her bewitchment. This led her to return from England to the West Indies, whereupon she visited a witch doctor in Guadeloupe, who gave her some tablets which, she insisted, saved her life. Following this she recounted how she had vomited a piece of fresh fat covered with hairs, shortly afterwards voiding other similar pieces per rectum. At about the same time she claimed to have had a "visitation" by night of the Holy Spirit.

After returning to England, her condition again deteriorated so that when first admitted to hospital she was vomiting again and was found to have a swinging pyrexia from an intercurrent urinary infection which was soon brought under control. The only other discoverable physical abnormality was ankylostomiasis, which also responded satisfactorily to treatment.

Although she had been strictly brought up and her childhood marred by nightmares and nocturnal enuresis, she described herself, nonetheless, as having grown up to be a cheerful person but prone to mood swings. She said also that she was shy and somewhat easily embarrassed seemingly about sexual matters. It was also noteworthy that religion played a very important part in her life and that her main interest lay in reading the Bible. Her grandfather had been a Methodist preacher.

She was given 11 applications of ECT, to which treatment her condition slowly responded. At one time her prognosis seemed to be impeded by unusual distress on account of a delayed menstrual period. (Pregnancy apart, there is apparently a West Indian belief, which the patient shared, that if a woman's menstrual period is overdue then her husband is having and extramarital affair. However, she was able to accept that there might well be an alternative explanation in her case.) Finally, after several more psychotherapeutic sessions and after claiming another "nocturnal visitation" of the Holy Spirit, her condition greatly improved and she was discharged.

For a time she remained perfectly well, became pregnant again and successfully gave birth to a son. A few weeks after this happy event, she was seen, together with her infant, in the course of a routine follow-up appointment and discovered to be free from symptoms. Asked on this occasion about her illness and her ideas about its origin, she smiled and with slight embarrassment said she had forgotten all about it.

Three years later she was readmitted in a state of severely retarded depression with marked hypochondriacal delusions. She complained of multiple somatic symptoms including a terrible rumbling in her abdomen "like the pots of hell boiling," abdominal pain, "feeling dead inside" and of delusional ideas of bewitchment precisely similar to those she had held during her initial illness. She was convinced that others could hear her stomach rumbling and that this was a subject of discussion. Once again she was treated with ECT and made a moderate improvement after seven treatments, following which she discharged herself. She was admitted later the same year with some increase in her depressive state. On this occasion she refused ECT so was treated instead with Amitriptyline. Her main complaints were, as before, of abdominal rumbling and frigidity since the birth of her son, which she again attributed to her bewitchment. With treatment her depression lifted so that her somatic symptoms and her ideas of reference concerning these disappeared and her frigidity improved. She still maintained, however, that she had been bewitched.

Two years later she was admitted once more with much the same symptoms as on previous occasions. At first she improved spontaneously but relapsed to some extent following a deep vein thrombosis in her right calf. Given three ECT treatments, together with antidepressant drugs, there was some waning of the strength of her delusional ideas of bewitchment. She stated on discharge that she now felt better than she had done for several years. Following this she remained relatively well although was admitted for a three-day period during which her behaviour was observed to be more overtly attention seeking than on previous occasions. At times she lay on the floor staring into space, at others she danced around the ward, often laughed and made half-hearted attempts to hurt people. However, as none of her previous depressive symptoms were evident and her disturbed behaviour settled within 24 hours, and because she decided to discharge herself, there was thought to be no good reason for detaining her further.

In most respects this patient's illness can be seen as one of a fairly straightforward recurrent depressive illness. The features of possession/bewitchment are examples of pathoplastic colouring and can be understood in the context of the patient's cultural background. The particularly interesting feature, however, is the history of vomiting and voiding pieces of fat covered with hairs. This particular aspect was described in mediaeval demonological writings. Thus, Guazzo (1608) in his *Compendium Malificarum,* quotes Cornelias Gemma's account of a 15-year-old girl who, in 1571, both vomited and voided a remarkable variety of objects including "hairs ... like those which fall from old dogs."

Cases 2 (an illustrative composite case) and 3 represent patients who displayed what were considered to be dissociative symptomatology, a phenomenon sometimes referred to as an hysterical possession state. The cases share common features: pseudohallucinatory experiences of a stereotypical nature and a belief of being under the control of an external being. In keeping with the practice followed in the fourth edition of this book, only core features are reported so as to ensure patient anonymity.

Case 2

A young adult male who was seen in prison where he was serving a sentence following a conviction for several burglaries.

He behaved violently in prison and would spend much of his time talking and writing about the Devil and vampires. No features that could be attributed to psychosis were present other than a persistently held belief that his actions (including his offences) arose because he had been under the direct control of an external personage since the age of 8 years. This being – whom he had named – would talk to him, often giving instructions in a "deep, husky" voice and had a strange habit of omitting words from sentences. He also described being repeatedly woken up at night by a "big thing" which he saw and felt, sitting on his chest, jumping up and down and preventing him from breathing.

As an aside, his experience of waking to the presence of something sitting on his chest is interesting but readily explicable. It is a phenomenon called *incubus*, which occurs during slow wave sleep and was described in the Middle Ages when the Devil was thought to be responsible for its occurrence. The word "nightmare" is derived from such an experience. In this case it is essentially a normal phenomenon that has been elaborated by the patient's abnormal personality.

Case 3

A mature adult male who was serving an indeterminate sentence for a number of extremely serious offences. He had a long history of relatively minor offending, an inability to maintain interpersonal relationships, long-term institutionalisation and deliberate self-harm at times of stress. These features indicated a severe personality disorder with prominent antisocial and histrionic traits.

He gave an account (provided to a psychiatrist before the last series of serious offences) of how he was controlled by an external being, somebody he had known but who had died during his childhood. This being would appear before him and give him verbal instructions and commands which he felt impelled to carry out.

Clinical features

There are no clinical manifestations of possession which are in themselves of specific diagnostic significance. The core feature is the belief (whatever its nature) that the sufferer is possessed by an external being such as an evil spirit, demon, ghost or the Devil. If the supposed malign force falls short of a personified form, then the term "bewitchment" may be more appropriate to use.

Clearly such a vaguely defined symptomatology can be found in many conditions throughout the spectrum of psychiatric disorder:

- Organic psychosis – acute confusional states and delirium can be associated with vivid visual hallucinations the content of which may be heavily influenced by the background belief systems of the sufferer. The intake of certain illicit drugs may produce similar features.
- Schizophrenia – the bizarre passivity experiences of this condition may be interpreted by patients as the work of a malign external force such as a demon or devil.
- Depressive psychosis – the characteristic guilt and sense of worthlessness which forms part of this condition can readily lead to a pathoplastic state in which the patient believes that he or she is being punished or tormented by a demon.
- Dissociative conditions/dissociative identity disorder – in which trance-like states and apparently multiple identities may occur.
- Neurosis – particularly in obsessive-compulsive disorder where the intrusive impulses and images may briefly be attributed by the patient to external diabolical forces.
- Personality disorders – where there is a gross disturbance of identity and where many aspects of the individual's life are chaotic, leading to dabbling in drug abuse, sexual deviancy, Satanism and other occult activities. The development of a hysterical possession state in a disturbed personality with prominent histrionic traits has already been described. This condition is characterised by repetitive and stereotypical visual and auditory pseudohallucinations.
- Bereavement reactions – recently bereaved people may see the apparition of the loved one just lost and also hear and feel their presence. It is not uncommon for the recently bereaved to seek solace by resorting to spiritualism.

Some authors (albeit mostly non-medical) distinguish what may be referred to, for the sake of argument, as *true* or *genuine* possession on the one hand and a *possession syndrome* arising during the course of formal medical or psychiatric illnesses or disorders on the other (Cooper, 1975; Richards, 1984; Robbins, 1984; Perry, 1987). Quite apart from what this distinction implies for aetiology and causation, this latter condition is said to often exhibit peculiar features of its own. Such writings also date back into the Middle Ages: for example, in his *Compendium Maleficarum*,

Guazzo (1608) lists 47 indications of demonical possession and another 20 of simple bewitchment:

> Those afflicted are subject to sudden frights, their heads seem to swell to an enormous size, their brains seem as if tightly bound or pierced or stricken by a sword. Some suffer from constriction of the throat, feeling as if they are being strangled. Others have an acute pain in the guts, feeling a forcible inflation of the stomach, a constriction of the heart as though it had been unmercifully beaten or eaten away.

The various features recorded by these authors are not described as being invariably present in every case. They can be categorised in the following manner:

- History – involvement in the occult; a lifetime of wicked or immoral behaviour.
- Physical features – psychosomatic pains; the vomiting of unusual objects; a bilious complexion; physical wasting; an habitual frightening facial expression; great physical strength.
- Voice changes – compulsive utterances, usually obscenities; glossolalia (speaking in tongues); speaking in a voice that is not that of the sufferer, often a deep and uncouth voice; an ability to understand and converse in a language unknown to the sufferer; making the noises of an animal.
- Behavioural changes – forced movements including convulsions; resistance to participation in prayer; a tendency to curse and blaspheme; marked fear when in the presence of religious symbols or ritual.
- Mental phenomena – a trance-like state; amnesia on recovery.
- Other "paranormal" activities – powers of clairvoyance; poltergeist phenomena.

In addition, Prins (1992) refers to the "saneness" of the thought processes of a sufferer apart from those connected with possession, and how, unlike the mentally ill who have a demonic content to their symptomatology, avoid discussing the subject of demons or possessions unless directly approached upon the subject.

Aetiology and psychopathology

Where aspects of possession occur within a wider clinical picture of obvious and established mental disorder, then the syndrome can be understood as arising in a *pathoplastic* fashion. That is, the patient's belief structure and cultural background influences and is represented in the content of the symptoms exhibited. This concept is as equally applicable to states of gross personality disorder as it is to psychotic conditions.

The question of whether or not *true* possession exists – i.e. the actual reality of demons occupying a person's body and mind – as suggested by some authors, cannot be answered and is largely a matter of faith or lack of it. The existence of demons has neither been proved nor disproved by scientific enquiry. It is, however, possible to consider some of the factors which may underpin the development of possession syndromes or possession states in our culture without attempting to answer the fundamental question.

Psychological factors

It has been postulated that the concept found in the writings of mediaeval demonology can be readily replaced with those of psychodynamic psycho pathology. Trethowan (1963) put this to the test in a comparative study of the putative causes of Impotence as advanced by Guazzo in 1608, under the heading *Of Tying the Points*, with those put forward by Strauss in 1950. While Strauss formulated his ideas in psychoanalytical terms and Guazzo in those of the Devil's work, what emerged so clearly was how close was the resemblance between the various types of impotence described quite independently by each author. Trethowan considered it easy to draw an analogy between these two formulations despite their separation by over three centuries. In order to translate the demonopathological view of impotence into an understanding of its psychodynamics, he recast the original notion of the Devil in terms of the Freudian concept of the "id."

The principle of psychological *causality* seems to lie at the heart of the phenomenon of bewitchment. Psychological causality refers to the belief that events take place because some person or something which has become personified has willed their occurrence. This provides a basis for magical beliefs, together with a wide range of ritual behaviour.

Another factor to consider is the sheer power of human belief. Shakespeare was fully aware of this particular principle. So, in *Henry IV* part one, we find Owen Glendower boasting to Hotspur that he could "call sprits from the vasty deep." This earns him Hotsput's rebuke:

> And I can teach thee, coz to shame the Devil
> By telling the truth: tell truth and shame the Devil
> If thou have power to raise him, bring him hither
> And I will be sworn, I have power to shame him hence.

(III, i)

What the description and dismissal of so-called primitive or unsophisticated attitudes does not do, however, is fully explain why beliefs such as demonic possession continue to exert such a powerful hold upon a range of individuals of varying degrees of intelligence and cultural sophistication in such a modern, complex and scientifically dependent society as our own.

Sociological factors

Prins (1992) in his review of possession and possession states remarked that historical evidence suggests that possession and other so-called paranormal phenomena tend to occur during periods of great social upheaval. He also stressed that media interest in occult practices has increased considerably in this country from the 1970s onwards. Allegations concerning the sexual abuse of children during the practice of occult rituals was certainly regularly discussed in contemporary radio and television news programmes.

Arthur Miller's play about the witches of Salem, *The Crucible*, is fundamentally a story about a witch hunt and was written against the background of a very modern witch hunt, hearings in the United States chaired by Senator McCarthy. It is certainly the case that humans obtain much vicarious enjoyment from this particular process, hence the perpetuation of the term "witch hunting" in current parlance.

Management and treatment

The treatment of possession syndromes is that of the underlying condition. In all cases, even in that of a psychotic disorder with a pathoplastically determined content, it is essential that a very careful and detailed medical and social history be obtained. Psychodynamic as well as the phenomenological aspects of the symptoms have to be understood. It is also important not to show disrespect for the belief systems of the patient.

Once appropriate treatment has been instigated, some patients may still feel the need to discuss their troubles with a priest or member of the clergy. At such time it is essential that effective liaison takes place between the psychiatrist and the priest so that each patient can receive the best and safest care appropriate for their individual needs.

Exorcism – this can be defined simply as the act of driving out demons or evil spirits from persons, places or things which are believed to be possessed by them. The role of exorcism in psychiatry is, at the very least, extremely controversial. Many patients seek and demand to be exorcised. This is a topic where it is not possible to give any absolute recommendations, and the best advice that can be given is simply to judge each individual case on its merits and follow the Hippocratic dictum of avoiding harm.

Exorcism is permitted by both the Roman Catholic and Anglican denominations, and the position adopted by both churches is essentially unchanged from that reported in the fourth edition of this text. With respect to the former denomination, Canon 1172 of the Code of Canon Law states that "no one is able to legitimately undertake exorcisms of the possessed unless express and individual permission has been obtained from the Ordinary of the place (the Bishop)." Further, "this permission is to be granted by the local Ordinary only to a priest who is endowed with piety, knowledge, prudence and integrity of life."

The Anglican Communion refers to a ministry of "deliverance," which, following the Osset tragedy of 1975, is only carried out by experienced persons so authorised by the diocesan bishop. In many dioceses there is an advisory team of individuals which includes clerical and lay members. It is usual practice for this team to seek professional psychiatric advice on a case-by-case basis.

It is reported that in Italy, where according to Levack (2013) the number of exorcisms has increased, there is increasing collaboration between the Catholic church and psychiatrists in order to distinguish "real possession" from "mere psychopathology" (Innamorati et al., 2019). Interestingly, a study of beliefs held by clergy in the UK found that among mainstream clergy beliefs about the reality of demonic possession are "equivocal," whereas in the case of Pentecostal churches and evangelical clergy, such beliefs are "integral" (Leavey, 2010).

Glossolalia

Glossolalia (speaking in tongues) was regarded by Oesterreich (1966) as automatic speech in which the mouth speaks without the subject willing or even knowing what he or she says. It is a phenomenon linked with automatic writing and doubling of the personality. It can occur in a variety of states; in hypnosis, in mediumistic trances, in certain pathological mental states, such as hysterical dissociation and in schizophrenia, and also in religious ecstasy. It has aroused the interest of a number of investigators, particularly in the USA.

Vivier (1968) reached the conclusion that there were two types of glossolalic experience: one which occurred in association with a kind of mass hysterical reaction which forms part of the high emotional state accompanying Pentecostal religious ceremonies; the other, in contrast, occurring in circumstances of quiet meditation, contemplation and dedication. He observed furthermore that although glossolalia occurred among the early Christians and indeed is mentioned in the Bible (Corinthians), the phenomenon is not confined to Christianity but may also occur outside the ambit of a strictly religious setting, e.g. in spiritualistic séance etc. Having examined a number of subjects, he concluded that glossolalia was not necessarily associated with neuroticism, although he wondered nevertheless whether the accompanying emotional catharsis served some psychotherapeutic function. Again, in a religious context, he observed that glossolalics were those who had acquired the habit of renunciation and who, possibly because of superego pressures, were prepared to accept moral restrictions and goals of higher achievement.

According to Cutten (1927), the words spoken during glossolalia are for the most part pseudolanguage which may, however, be mistaken for a foreign tongue. When a real foreign language is spoken, this may be what Jung (1917) called *hypermnesia*, a state of heightened memory of things long consciously forgotten but brought back into mind in a dissociated or trance state. In line with this, Sargent (1973) has pointed out that it has never been satisfactorily proved that anyone in a trance has spoken a foreign language with which they have no previous acquaintance but that people in hypnoid states can sometimes remember foreign words and phrases heard in the past but since forgotten. However, if in a suggestible state, they may believe they are speaking in tongues and convey the same conviction to others equally uncritical.

Pattison and Carey (1969) saw glossolalia as part of a range of behaviour which, in the more remote regions of the southern USA, included snake-handling and a full range of "convulsionary" (sic) and hysterical behaviour, this being in line with Sargent's view that glossolalia, in addition to these other types of behaviour, is a form of aggressive and dissociative abreaction. However, they also observe that more recently glossolalia is practised by more staid denominations such as Episcopalians, Lutherans and Presbyterians, and by those attending urban middle- and upper-class churches among whom it could not necessarily be interpreted as deviant or pathological. Where not occurring as part of gross hysterical behaviour, they suggested that the practice seems to aid in the reduction of emotional tension, allowing a discharge of affect which in itself is not necessarily of a regressive nature.

We have received a very remarkable and detailed account of the condition from the husband of a lady in whom it occurred over the period of the 23 years of their marriage until she deserted him and died shortly afterwards of a subarachnoid haemorrhage.

Case 4

Her "other voice," which was usually childish and different from her normal voice, most often appeared at about the time she seemed to drop off to sleep when in bed at night and also occasionally if she had a nap by day. The "other voice" was at times strangely dictatorial, and as her husband put it "controlled much of our daily doings." Thus once it asked him to buy some fish for supper when he went to town the following day.

He did so, apparently to the considerable astonishment of his wife, who said that she had gone to the same fish shop but "something told me not to bother." He related a number of other such incidents governing, for example, the buying of her birthday present on one occasion.

According to her husband, his wife in her glossolalic state also revealed clairvoyant and precognitive abilities. She could, he said, on being given the page numbers, identify pictures on the pages of a closed book. She also foretold the occurrence of a number of events, such as the death of a friend in an air crash, the winner of a horse race and certain events appertaining to her husband's business. She also professed an aptitude to psychokinesis, being able, it was said, to switch on the lights in a darkened room when her hands were full, and on another occasion being able to alter the speed of the idling engine of her car, when it was left running but unattended in the driveway.

Later on she would, in her sleep, recount incidents which took place in her childhood in India, sometimes speaking in a strange tongue which her husband was able to identify as Hindustani. Although the language was unfamiliar to him, he was able to take down phonetically a number of words and phrases which she uttered, some of which his wife was able to recognise and translate when in her waking state. Towards the close of all these experiences, she spoke on at least one occasion in a male-sounding voice, saying, "My name is Khotawalla," the voice apparently of a little Indian boy whom she said she had known in childhood.

In fairness to her husband, who went to considerable lengths to supply this information, together with many other interesting details, it has to be said that he believed, and still does, in an authentic explanation of his late wife's unusual behaviour. While respecting this belief, we would be inclined to regard her condition as yet another example of alternating personality, emerging when in a hypnagogic state. Once again an element of attention-seeking appeared to be apparent. This interpretation does not, however, entirely explain the occurrence of *psy*-phenomena in her case.

Reeves et al. (2014) described the case of a 44-year-old woman who reported jerking of her arm during praying/speaking in tongues. EEG recording carried out while she engaged in glossolalia silently (so as not to show "disrespect") showed that speaking (silently) in tongues was associated with right temporal lobe spikes. In contrast, when she was thinking of nothing in particular, the EEG was normal. Unrecorded episodes of glossolalia appeared to be associated with classic jerking clonic movements of the arm.

The Poltergeist phenomenon

This phenomenon appears to be worthy of inclusion, if for no other reason than completeness. So far the phenomenon seems hardly to have found a place in the psychiatric literature, which is surprising in view of the fact that it is so often associated with a disturbance of behaviour in childhood or adolescence. Although the poltergeist seems rarely to have aroused psychiatric interest and although it is relatively uncommon, it has nevertheless a very long history, extending over several centuries, during which a steady stream of cases have been reported both in the UK and many other places (Artley and Roll, 1968,;Owen, 1964; Sitwell, 1940; Thurston, 1978).

In its simplest and most usual form, the poltergeist phenomenon consist of the mysterious occurrence of noises, usually raps, bangs and other knockings, sometimes groans and other wordless utterances. A second feature is the movement of objects, even furniture, as if by unseen hands. Objects such as stones may apparently materialise, and vases or other ornaments may be cast upon the floor or thrown through the air. As indicated, these strange happenings appear to be associated with the presence of a child in the house, most often female, and do not occur while the child is outdoors or asleep. As a general rule, the poltergeist phenomenon is not associated with apparitions, ectoplasm or other supposedly spiritualistic manifestations. Most subjects of the ministrations of a poltergeist are seldom injured by flying objects, although some family members may record feeling as if touched or pushed. The other main characteristic of the phenomenon is that although it is not apparently amenable to exorcism, it tends to cease spontaneously after a period of a few weeks or months. The following case which is described was investigated by Professor Trethowan and reported in the second and third editions of this book.

Case 5

Diana F., around whom the case revolved, was first seen when a schoolgirl 14 years of age. She was very much the youngest of a family of five, being eight years younger than her next sibling, a married daughter aged 22 years. Her father was a fitter and her mother an unskilled helper at a nearby learning disability hospital.

Although somewhat physically mature for her years, Diana was educationally backward, being in the lowest stream of the bottom form of her year and having a reading level of about 9½.

Trouble first began in April 1977, when Diana refused to go to school because she said she was being bullied. During this period her grandfather, of whom she was very fond and who used to make something of a fuss of her, died. Two days after his funeral, Diana paid a visit to his grave accompanied by a friend, Carole, of about her own age. While there they visited the grave of another girl, again of about the same age, who had been run over and killed. On the grave was a photograph which Carole picked up and handed to Diana for her to look at following which it was put back. According to Diana the first "manifestation," a falling stone, occurred as they left the cemetery. Later that evening when she was at Carole's home, Carole's parents having gone out, more stones came. Diana stated that they couldn't see the stones coming but saw them land. A few days later, Carole came to Diana's house and the stones started appearing again. As a result of this, the police were called but took no action other than saying they had heard of other similar cases.

Following this there were a number of other happenings in Diana's home, these occurring after Carole had left. The doorbell would ring on a number of occasions, seemingly without any good cause. Ashtrays and other ornaments would clatter and bang on the table, glass marbles and stones bounced down the stairs as if from nowhere and on one occasion an ornament was thrown across the room, breaking a glass panel in a door separating the lounge from the kitchen. At night, bangings and knockings occurred chiefly in Diana's bedroom, and once footsteps were heard on the stairs. On another occasion her mother's dentures mysteriously disappeared from the beaker in the kitchen in which they had been placed and were later discovered under the gas fire in the lounge.

Diana's father was able to produce the stones for inspection, having collected no less than 33 which he had systematically numbered with green ink. They proved to be largish brown pebbles, each weighing about half a pound or so and of the type which father stated were not found in the garden or the vicinity of the house.

Diana herself appeared not to be unduly disturbed by these manifestations which fluctuated in frequency and intensity and did not occur at all when she was asleep or out of the house. Her family, although quite clearly believing in the authenticity of these phenomena and although somewhat bewildered, did not appear to be particularly frightened. Furthermore, it was clear that while they associated the phenomena in some way with Diana herself, not for one moment did they appear to suspect that she might be producing them herself. At one juncture they asked the local vicar to bless the house without, however, any amelioration of the situation.

No member of the family including Diana had seen any apparition. Once or twice some had felt as if a cold wind was blowing round the house. On one occasion father felt as if pushed, and on another mother discovered a piece of chewing gum in her hair. Most of the phenomena were of this essentially trivial nature, and no one seemed to have been harmed in any way. Further investigation of the matter proved difficult as it was extremely hard to disentangle what the various family members who were present had actually observed from what they imagined to have happened. None of these happenings occurred when strangers were in the house.

Finally, Diana was taken by her mother to see a medium. After one or two sessions the phenomena began to die down but did not entirely disappear until a place had been found in a new school in January 1978. Although Diana remained somewhat disturbed, there does not appear to have been a recurrence of poltergeist phenomena since the end of 1977.

This case closely resembles other fairly simple examples which have been recorded several times before. As stated, adolescent girls are often involved, outnumbering boys by more than two to one. As is also true of some other cases, no complete explanation is forthcoming, first because the phenomena never occurred when strangers were present and second because the whole family appeared unquestioningly to accept that although connected with Diana the phenomena were of supernatural origin. In this sense the situation bore some resemblance to *folie à famille*. Short of invoking an actual supernatural explanation or regarding the phenomena as caused by psychokinesis emanating in some unexplained way from Diana herself, it must be assumed that she herself was producing them in such a way as to deceive her credulous family, and possibly deceiving herself also. In any event, she was unable to offer any explanation.

References

Artley, J.L., Roll, W.G. (1968) Mathematical models and the attenuation effect in two RSPK (Poltergeist) cases. *Eleventh Annual Conference of the Parapsychological Association*, Freiburg.

Bourguignon, E. (1970) Cited by Bhavsar, V. and Bhugra, D. (2016). *Psychiatry and Clinical Neurosciences, 70*, 551.

Cooper, A. (1975) *The Scottish Baptist Magazine*, November.

Cutten, G.B. (1927) *Speaking with Tongues*. Oxford University Press, New York.

Eastern Daily Press (1994) *13 September*.

Ehrenwald, J. (1975) *Journal of the American Academy of Psychoanalysis, 3*, 105.

Freud, S. (1946) *Collected Papers*, Vol. 4. Hogarth Press, London.

Gemma, C. (1575) *De Natura Divinis Characterismus*. Plantin, Antwerp, Vol. 2, Quoted by Guazzo, F.

Guazzo, F.M. (1608) *Compendium Maleficarum (1929)*, Trans. E.A. Ashwin. John Rodker, London.

Huxley, A. (1951) *The Devils of Loudun*. Chatto and Windus, London.

Innamorati, M., Taradel, R., Foschi, R. (2019) *History of Psychology, 22*(1), 1.

Jung, C. (1917) *Collected Papers on Analytical Psychology*, Ed. C.E. Long. Baillière, London.

Leavey, G. (2010) *Transcultural Psychiatry, 47*(4), 571.

Legué, G., de la Tourette, G. (1886) *Soeur Jeanne des Anges, Autobiographie d'une hystérique possédée*. Charpentier, Paris.

Levack, B.P. (2013) *The Devil Within: Possession & Exorcism in the Christian West*. Yale University Press, New Haven, London.

Littlewood, R. (2004) *Psychiatry, 3*, 8.

Miller, A. (1956) *The Crucible*. Cresset Press, London.

Oesterreich, T.K. (1966) *Possession, Demoniacal and Other, among Primitive Races in Antiquity, the Middle Ages, and Modern Times*. University Books, New York.

Owen, A.R.G. (1964) *Can We Explain the Poltergeist?* Garrett, New York.

Pattison, E.M., Carey, R.L. (1969) *International Psychiatry Clinics*, 5, 133.

Perry, M. (1987) Ed. *Deliverance*. SPCK, London.

Prins, H. (1990) *Bizarre Behaviours*. Tavistock / Routledge, London and New York.

Prins, H. (1992) *Medicine Science and the Law*, 32(3), 237.

Reeves, R.R., Kose, S., Abubakr, A. (2014) *Neurocase*, 20, 236.

Richards, J. (1984) *But Deliver Us from Evil: An Introduction to the Demonic Dimension in Pastoral Care*. Darton, Longman and Todd, London.

Robbins, R.H. (1984) *The Encyclopaedia of Witchcraft and Demonology*. Newnes Books, London.

Rowan, K., Dwyer, K. (2015) *Mental Health, Religion & Culture*, 18(6), 440.

Sargent, W. (1973) *The Mind Possessed*. Heinemann, London.

Sall, M.J. (1970) *Journal of Psychol. Technol.*, 4, 286.

Sitwell, S. (1940) *Poltergeists*. Faber, London.

Sprenger, G., Kraemer, H. (1489) *Malleus Maleficarum (1928)*, Trans. M. Summers. John Rodker, London.

Strauss, E.B. (1950). Psychiatric Aspects of Impotence. *British Medical Journal*, 1, 697, http://dx.doi.org/10.1136/bmj.1.4655.697.

Thurston, H.S.J. (1978) *Ghosts and Poltergeists*. Folcroft, Pennsylvania.

Times (1975) *24 April*.

Trethowan, W.H. (1963) *British Journal of Psychiatry*, 109, 341.

Vivier, L.M. (1968) *Bibliotheca Psychiatrica et Neurologica*, 134, 153.

Whiting, J. (1961) *The Devils*. Heineman, London.

Other uncommon psychiatric syndromes

> [The righteous] cry, and the LORD heareth,
> and delivereth them out of all their troubles.
> The LORD [is] nigh unto them that are of a broken heart;
> and saveth such as be of a contrite spirit.
>
> *Psalm* 34:17–18 (King James Version)

This final chapter is devoted to a brief description of some further uncommon psychiatric syndromes. None of these is classified in either *ICD-11* or *DSM-5*.

Diogenes syndrome

In 1966, Duncan Macmillan and Patricia Shaw published "a study of a small group of individuals who cease to maintain the standards of cleanliness and hygiene which are accepted by their local community." As all the subjects bar one, a psychiatric patient, were over the age of 60 years, Macmillan and Shaw (1966) chose to name the condition "senile breakdown." They painted the following graphic image of a typical case:

> The usual picture is that of an old woman living alone, though men and married couples suffering from the condition are also found. She, her garments, her possessions, and her house are filthy. She may be verminous and there may be faeces and pools of urine on the floor.

Just over half the original cohort of 72 patients were "psychotic," suffering variously from senile psychosis, paranoid psychosis, chronic alcoholism, manic-depression and reactive depression. Females outnumbered males in a ratio of 5:1. Most (around 80%) were single or widowed.

Clark et al. (1975) described a similar case series of 30 patients aged between 66 and 92 years who "all had dirty, untidy homes and a filthy personal appearance about which they showed no shame. Hoarding of rubbish (syllogomania) was sometimes seen. All except two lived alone, but poverty and poor housing standards were not a serious problem." They named the syndrome after the fourth-century BCE Greek philosopher Diogenes and pointed out that, in their cohort, multiple deficiency states were found, including of vitamins, iron, water, potassium, serum albumin and proteins. It is now also known as squalor syndrome. Since 1975, it has become clear that Diogenes syndrome can occur in patients much younger than 60 years of age; it has even been described in a 28-year-old woman (Sheridan and Jamieson, 2015). A Texan study of 538 patients with self-neglect aged 65 years or over by Dyer et al. (2007) showed that a majority suffered from physical and/or psychiatric diagnoses, most commonly hypertension, diabetes mellitus, dementia and depression.

Systematic epidemiological studies of this syndrome have yet to be published. Although early cases were described in Western countries, it is now known to occur in other countries, with cases having been described in India (Nath et al., 2018) and China (Chan et al., 2007), for example.

Of the originally described aetiological factors, it has been found particularly to be associated with frontotemporal dementia (Cipriani et al., 2012), and recently an association has also been reported with autistic spectrum disorder (Sadlier et al., 2011) and Asperger syndrome (Padovan et al., 2018). In their large study (*vide supra*), Dyer et al. (2007) found strong evidence of impaired neuropsychological and physical performance and of low mood amongst sufferers with substantial overlap in impairments in physical performance, executive function and cognitive functions; based on these findings they put forward a model attempting to explain the self-neglect. Underlying medical/psychiatric conditions result in impaired executive functioning with consequent impairment in basic everyday activities and a reduced capacity for decision-making. The added presence of adverse extrinsic social factors along with inadequate support services then lead to the end result of extreme self-neglect.

Diogenes syndrome by proxy may occur (O'Mahony and Evans, 1994). It may also occur in married couples and sibling pairs, with both individuals being affected; here, by analogy with *folie à deux*, it has been named *Diogenes à deux* (Cole et al., 1992; Esposito et al., 2003).

As reported above, Diogenes syndrome is associated with many medical problems (Dyer et al., 2007; Assal, 2018; Klosterkotter and Peters, 1985). Cases have been described in which some co-morbid conditions have been life-threatening, such as folic acid deficiency (Sheridan and Jamieson, 2015) and Paget disease (Sami et al., 2014). Freeman and Byard (2014) described a case of fatal haemorrhage from an undiagnosed rectal carcinoma.

Jerusalem syndrome

In the years leading up to 2000 CE, Israel's mental health services noted an increase in "Jerusalem syndrome" (Siegel-Itzkovich, 1999):

> The temporary psychiatric condition – characterised by patients believing that they have become biblical figures such as Jesus, John the Baptist, or Moses – has been known to Israeli psychiatrists for decades. It affects mainly Christian pilgrims but is occasionally diagnosed in Jews who tour holy sites. Those affected begin to act strangely, sometimes proclaiming that they are ancient religious figures sent on a holy mission. Apocalyptic Christians expect the next millennium to herald the second coming of Jesus on the Mount of Olives in Jerusalem, so experts have warned that the number of patients may increase sharply.... Professor Richard Landes, director of the Center for Millennial Studies at Boston University, Massachusetts, explained that the problem has occurred before. In the year 1033 – the 1000th anniversary of the crucifixion – crowds of people visited Jerusalem to mark the event, and many refused to leave.

Bar-El et al. (2000), based at the Kfer Shaul Mental Health Centre in Jerusalem, Israel, classified Jerusalem syndrome into three types based on the underlying motivation for visiting Jerusalem, the mode of travel to the city and the presence or absence of pre-existing psychiatric illness. Type I is characterised by a need to accomplish a mission owing to psychiatric religious ideation, travelling alone and a documented history of psychiatric disorder. Type II cases are motivated by curiosity associated with unusual (although not psychotic) thoughts or a sense of mission, usually travelling in groups and have a previous history of non-psychotic mental disorder such as personality disorder. Finally, Type III forms (referred to as Jerusalem syndrome discrete type) tend to be regular tourists with a religious home background who travel with family or friends, often as part of an organised tour, with no previous psychiatric history. The Type I and II syndromes could be further broken down into subtypes. They gave the following example of a patient suffering from subtype I(ii), that is, psychotic identification with an idea:

> A Protestant from South America conceived a plan to destroy Islamic holy places in order to replace them with Jewish holy places. The second stage of his plan was then to destroy them in order to start the war of Gog and Magog so that the Anti-Christ would reveal himself, after which Christ would reappear. The patient succeeded in gutting one of the most holy mosques in Jerusalem. Psychiatric examination was ordered by the court, and he was diagnosed as being unable to

differentiate between right and wrong, not responsible for his deeds and therefore not fit to stand trial. He was admitted to a local psychiatric institution and later transferred to a mental health institution in his own country.

The seven clinical stages of type III are as follows (Bar-El et al., 2000):

a   Anxiety, agitation, nervousness and tension, plus other unspecified reactions.
b   Declaration of the desire to split away from the group or the family and to tour Jerusalem alone. Tourist guides aware of the Jerusalem syndrome and of the significance of such declarations may at this point refer the tourist to our institution for psychiatric evaluation in an attempt to pre-empt the subsequent stages of the syndrome. If unattended, these stages are usually unavoidable.
c   A need to be clean and pure: obsession with taking baths and showers; compulsive fingernail and toenail cutting.
d   Preparation, often with the aid of hotel bed-linen, of a long, ankle-length, togalike gown, which is always white.
e   The need to scream, shout, or sing out loud psalms, verses from the Bible, religious hymns or spirituals. Manifestations of this type serve as a warning to hotel personnel and tourist guides, who should then attempt to have the tourist taken for professional treatment. Failing this, the two last stages will develop.
f   A procession or march to one of Jerusalem's holy places.
g   Delivery of a "sermon" in a holy place. The sermon is usually very confused and based on an unrealistic plea to humankind to adopt a more wholesome, moral, simple way of life.

Witztum and Kalian (1999) have suggested that the religious atmosphere of Jerusalem should not be considered to be the primary cause of Jerusalem syndrome; rather, they argue that before journeying to Jerusalem the individuals concerned have chosen this destination because of a delusional system within the context of a pre-existing psychotic illness.

Stendhal syndrome

The Italian psychiatrist Graziella Magherini (1989) introduced this syndrome in her book of the same name, *La Sindrome di Stendhal*, which was based on over a hundred emergency admissions to the Santa Maria Nuova Hospital in Florence between 1977 and 1986. Typically, in this psychosomatic illness, "the presence of a beautiful piece of work or architecture causes dysautonomic symptoms such as tachycardia, diaphoresis, chest pains and loss of consciousness" (Palacios-Sanchez et al., 2018).

Stendhal was the pen name of the French author Marie-Henri Beyle (1783–1842), who described being overwhelmed by the cultural beauty of Florence (Stendhal, 1817):

> As I emerged from the porch of Santa Croce, I was seized with a fierce palpitation of the heart … the well-spring of life was dried up within me, and I walked in constant fear of falling to the ground.

Stendhal syndrome is also known as Florence syndrome, tourist syndrome and hyperkulturaemia (Fried, 1988; Palacios-Sanchez et al., 2018). It is the subject of the film *The Stendhal Syndrome* by the Italian director Dario Argento, which was released in 1996.

Nicholson et al. (2009) described a recent case:

> A 72-year-old fine-arts graduate and creative artist presented with insomnia and concerns about being followed and monitored. This started eight years previously after travelling from southern France to Florence (Italy), the city known as the "cradle of the Renaissance," to fulfil a lifelong wish to see the art and culture that so inspired him. He described visiting some works of art as "like seeing old friends." While standing on the Ponte Vecchio bridge, the part of Florence he was most eager to visit, he experienced a panic attack and was also observed to have become disorientated in time. This lasted several minutes and was followed by florid persecutory ideation, involving him being monitored by international airlines, the bugging of his hotel room and multiple ideas of reference. These symptoms resolved gradually over the following three weeks.
>
> Four years later, he revisited southern France, this time with no intention of returning to Florence. However, visiting this area reminded him of his trip to Florence and triggered another panic attack followed by persecutory beliefs, again involving monitoring by the airlines and which settled within a few days. There have been no anxiety or psychotic episodes since.

Paris syndrome

Described by Hiroaki Ota (1988), Paris syndrome refers to psychosomatic (e.g. anxiety, dysautonomia) and/or psychotic symptomology suffered by those visiting Paris who find that the city is not as impressive as they were expecting. It has been noted particularly in Japanese tourists, having originally been described as "voyages et déplacements pathologiques des Japonais vers la France" (Ota, 1988; Tamami, 1998).

Stockholm syndrome

Stockholm syndrome refers to the occurrence of a positive emotional bond or psychological alliance from a victim of a crime, such as being taken hostage or being abused, towards the perpetrator(s) of that crime; it is also known as "traumatic bonding," "terror bonding" and *Norrmalmstorgssyndromet* (the "Norrmalmstorg syndrome") (Eitinger and Weisaeth, 1980; Harnischmacher and Muther, 1987; Skurnik, 1988). It takes the name Stockholm syndrome after the following events that took place at the Sveriges Kreditbank, Norrmalmstorg Square, Stockholm in August 1973 (Strentz, 1980):

> During ... 131 hours ... four employees ... were held hostage.... This particular hostage situation gained notoriety primarily because the electronic media exploited the fears of the victims as well as the sequence of events. Contrary to what had been expected, it was found that the victims feared the police more than they feared the robbers. In a telephone call to Prime Minister Olaf Palme, one of the hostages expressed these typical feelings of the group when she said, "The robbers are protecting us from the police." Upon release, other hostages puzzled over their feelings: "Why don't we hate the robbers?" ... For weeks after this incident, and while under the care of psychiatrists, some of the hostages experienced the paradox of nightmares over the possible escape of the jailed subjects and yet felt no hatred for these abductors. In fact, they felt the subjects had given them their lives back and were emotionally indebted to them for their generosity.

Norrmalmstorgssyndromet (referred to as Stockholm syndrome in the English-speaking world) was described by Nils Bejerot, professor of social medicine at the Karolinska Institute, who acted as a consultant psychiatrist to the police during the above six-day attempted bank robbery (Bejerot, 1974). The dangerousness of the situation is emphasised by Bejerot (1974): "Right at the beginning the robber very nearly killed a policeman with shots from his submachine gun.... A few days afterwards another policeman was shot, and here again it was only by chance that this did not end in the murder of a policeman."

In psychodynamic terms, Stockholm syndrome may be considered to be a defence mechanism of the ego under stress; from a practical viewpoint, it reduces the likelihood that the hostage-takers may act violently towards the victims (Harnischmacher and Muther, 1987). Alexander and Klein (2009) have suggested that conditions which increase the likelihood of the occurrence of Stockholm syndrome include:

- An extended and emotionally charged environment
- An adverse environment shared by hostages and hostage-takers (e.g. poor diet and physical discomfort)
- When threats to life are not carried out (e.g. "mock executions")
- When there has to be a marked dependence by the hostages on the hostage-takers for even the most basic needs
- When there are opportunities for bonding between captives and their captors in circumstances in which the former have not been "dehumanised" (Some hostage-takers aim to dehumanise hostages by hooding them, depriving them of their names, any identifying details and possessions, treating them as "animals" and changing regularly their guards – as did Saddam Hussein with his "human shields" in Kuwait.)

There have been several famous cases in which Stockholm syndrome has been diagnosed. One potential well-known case is that of Patricia Campbell Hearst, commonly known as Patty Hearst, granddaughter of the American publisher William Randolph Hearst (1863–1951), who was kidnapped in 1974 by members of the Symbionese Liberation Army while a 19-year-old student at the University of California, Berkeley. She was subsequently raped by two members of the group. Two months after the kidnapping, she recorded a message to the effect that she had joined this group. Indeed, soon after, she appeared voluntarily to participate in violent criminal acts perpetrated by the group and became a fugitive from justice. She was arrested in 1975, and a plea of having suffered from Stockholm syndrome was not accepted. "The Patty Hearst trial undoubtedly will be one of the most memorable courtroom dramas of the century, not only because of its human interest aspects but also because of the legal and psychological questions it aired regarding terrorism, the 'crime of the 70s'" (Montgomery, 1979). She was sentenced to 35 years' in gaol, which was subsequently commuted by President Carter; she was pardoned by President Clinton. Another well-known case was that of the 10-year-old Natascha Kampusch, "who was held captive for eight years [and] bonded with her abductor to such an extent that, on his suicide immediately after her escape, she blamed the police for his death and clearly grieved his death" (Alexander and Klein, 2009; see also Hall and Leidig, 2006).

In popular culture, Stockholm syndrome has been mentioned in a number of films and television series, including the James Bond films *Never Say Never Again* (1983) and *The World Is Not Enough* (1999). It was mistakenly referred to as the "Helsinki syndrome" in the film *Die Hard* (1988), an error which was repeated in an episode of the series *Babylon 5*. It is sometimes invoked in political and sociological studies; for example, Schulman (2009) alludes to the response of indigenous Western Europeans to radical Islam in terms of the Stockholm syndrome. It has also been suggested that Stockholm syndrome may occur in children who are being commercially sexually exploited (Egu, 2018) as well as being a possible explanation of abuse occurring, and continuing, within intimate relationships (Stevens, 2014). Indeed, Graham et al. (1995) have identified the following three "Stockholm syndrome reaction" factors in abusive dating relationships of young American heterosexual college women:

- Core Stockholm syndrome, characterised by cognitive distortions and other strategies for coping with abuse
- Psychological damage, marked by depression, low self-esteem and loss of sense of self
- Love-dependence, typified by the feeling that one cannot survive without one's partner's love

Finally, it should be noted that the apparent occurrence of Stockholm syndrome may be a manifestation of Munchausen's syndrome, as demonstrated in the following case described by Spuijbroek et al. (2012):

A young female of indeterminate age called a crisis hotline several times in the course of a month, giving accounts of severe sexual abuse, kidnapping by her father, and membership in a sect in the recent past. She spoke by preference to male staff members, was difficult to understand, and used a high-pitched, childlike voice. She provided different names and addresses that proved to be wrong. "God," "men and women," and "good and evil" were regular topics. Quotations that she claimed were from the biblical New Testament book Ephesians 6 turned out to be incorrect, containing too many statements about punishment.

After a few weeks, she expressed suicidal feelings, saying she wished to go to God, and she agreed to be admitted to a local psychiatric hospital. She left, however, after one day. One month later, she was hospitalized again, using a different family name. She stated that she was 19 years of age and claimed to have been severely abused by her father and other sect members. She said her father intended to move abroad and had demanded that she go with him. Her request for help at the moment of readmission was "How to give more love to my father." Within a day, the patient again expressed a wish to be discharged, but this time her stay on the psychiatric department was continued following an involuntary commitment, based on her level of suicidal ideation and claims of unrestrained punishment by the father in case of her return to him. Her isolation from the outside world, the power imbalance, her sympathy for her abusing father, and her unwillingness to escape the life-threatening situation were consistent with the clinical picture of Stockholm syndrome.

... It became clear that she had used a false identity and had invented the story, leading to diagnoses of both Munchausen's syndrome and dissociative identity disorder. Despite a long period of treatment, she eventually suicided.

Lima syndrome

This is essentially the reverse of the Stockholm syndrome; in the Lima syndrome, there is the occurrence of a positive emotional bond or psychological alliance from the perpetrator of a crime towards the victim(s). It is named after the attack on the Japanese embassy in Lima, Peru, between December 1996 and April 1997, by members of the Túpac Amaru Revolutionary Movement. It has been said that one of the reasons the terrorists set some of the hostages free within the first few days was because of the development of a positive emotional bond from the terrorists towards (some of) their hostages.

References

Alexander, D.A., Klein, S. (2009) *Journal of the Royal Society of Medicine, 102*, 16.

Assal, F. (2018) *Frontiers of Neurology and Neuroscience, 41*, 90.

Bar-el, Y., Durst, R., Katz, G., Zislin, J., Strauss, Z., Knobler, H.Y. (2000) *British Journal of Psychiatry, 176*, 86.

Bejerot, N. (1974) *New Scientist, 61*, 486.

Chan, S.M., Leung, P.Y., Chiu, F.K. (2007) *Neuropsychiatric Disease and Treatment, 3*, 589.

Cipriani, G., Lucetti, C., Vedovello, M., Nuti, A. (2012) *Dialogues in Clinical Neuroscience, 14*, 455.

Clark, A.N., Mankikar, G.D., Gray, I. (1975) *Lancet, 1*, 366.

Cole, A.J., Gillett, T.P., Fairbairn, A.D. (1992) *International Journal of Geriatric Psychiatry, 7*, 839.

Dyer, C.B., Goodwin, J.S., Pickens-Pace, S., Burnett, J., Kelly, P.A. (2007) *American Journal of Public Health, 97*, 1671.

Egu, K. (2018) *Stockholm Syndrome in Commercial Sexual Exploitation of Young Women: An Exploration of the Impact of Trauma Bonding in the Transition out of Sexual Exploitation*, Ann Arbor, MI: ProQuest.

Eitinger, L., Weisaeth, L. (1980) *Tidsskrift for den Norske Laegeforening, 100*, 307.

Esposito, D., Rouillon, F., Limosin, F. (2003) *Canadian Journal of Psychiatry, 48*, 571.

Freeman, A., Byard, R.W. (2014) *Forensic Science, Medicine, and Pathology, 10*, 116.

Fried, R.I. (1988) *Ohio Medicine, 84*, 519.

Graham, D.L., Rawlings, E.I., Ihms, K., Latimer, D., Foliano, J., Thompson, A., et al. (1995) *Violence and Victims, 10*, 3.

Hall, A., Leidig, M. (2006) *Girl in the Cellar: The Natascha Kampusch Story*, London: Hodder & Stoughton.

Harnischmacher, R., Muther, J. (1987) *Archiv für Kriminologie, 180*, 1.

Klosterkotter, J., Peters, U.H. (1985) *Fortschritte der Neurologie-Psychiatrie, 53*, 427.

Macmillan, D., Shaw, P. (1966) *British Medical Journal, 2*, 1032.

Montgomery, B.J. (1979) *JAMA, 242*, 126.

Magherini, G. (1989). *La Sindrome di Stendhal. Firenze: Ponte Alle Grazie.*

Nath, S., Saraf, A., Pattnaik, J.I. (2018) *Asian Journal of Psychiatry, 43*, 216.

Nicholson, T.R., Pariante, C., McLoughlin, D. (2009) *BMJ Case Reports, 2009*, bcr06.2008.0317.

O'Mahony, D., Evans, J.G. (1994) *British Journal of Psychiatry, 164*, 705.

Ota, H. (1988) *Nervure, 6, 12.*

Padovan, C., Bonze, M., Rouch, I., Herrmann, M., Dorey, J.M. (2018) *International Journal of Geriatric Psychiatry, 33*, 555.

Palacios-Sanchez, L., Botero-Meneses, J.S., Pachon, R.P., Hernandez, L.B.P., Triana-Melo, J.D.P., Ramirez-Rodriguez, S. (2018) *Arquivos de Neuro-psiquiatria, 76*, 120.

Sadlier, M., Cooney, C., Philbin-Bowman, E., Lewis, A. (2011) *Irish Journal of Psychological Medicine, 28*, 224.

Sami, M., Tucker, J., Norris, K., Townsend, G., Odemuyiwa, O. (2014) *British Journal of Hospital Medicine (London), 75*, 470.

Schulman, A. (2009) *Human Rights Review, 10*, 469.

Sheridan, M., Jamieson, A. (2015) *American Journal of Medicine, 128*, e7.

Siegel-Itzkovich, J. (1999) *BMJ, 318*, 484.

Skurnik, N. (1988) *Annales Médico-Psychologiques (Paris), 146*, 174.

Spuijbroek, E.J., Blom, N., Braam, A.W., Kahn, D.A. (2012) *Journal of Psychiatric Practice, 18*, 296.

Stevens, P. (2014) *Journal of Criminal Law, 78*, 184.

Stendahl (1817) Rome, Naples et Florence en 1817 Paris: Julliard.

Strentz, T. (1980) *Annals of the New York Academy of Sciences, 347*, 137.

Tamami, K. (1998) *Nissei Byoin igaku zasshi, 26*, 127.

Witztum, E., Kalian, M. (1999) *Israel Journal of Psychiatry and Related Sciences, 36*, 260.

Index

Printed in the United States
by Baker & Taylor Publisher Services